MEDICATING RACE

EXPERIMENTAL FUTURES

Technological Lives, Scientific Arts, Anthropological Voices

A series edited by Michael M. J. Fischer and Joseph Dumit

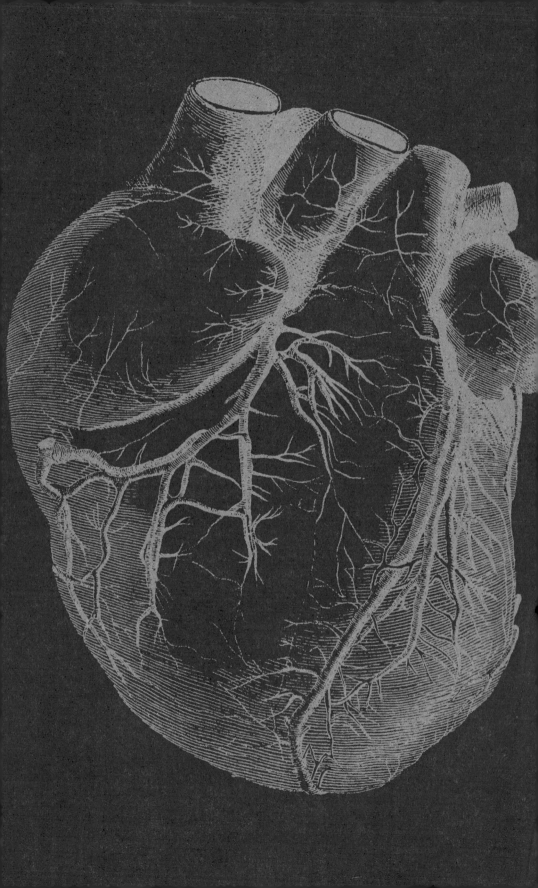

MEDICATING RACE

Heart Disease and
Durable Preoccupations
with Difference

ANNE POLLOCK

Duke University Press

Durham and London 2012

© 2012 Duke University Press
All rights reserved
Printed in the United States
of America on acid-free paper ⊛
Designed by Amy Ruth Buchanan
Typeset in Quadraat and Trade Gothic
by Keystone Typesetting, Inc.
Library of Congress Cataloging-
in-Publication Data appear on the
last printed page of this book.

CONTENTS

ACKNOWLEDGMENTS

I am grateful to the physicians and others who let me tag along in the worlds of heart disease research and race, welcoming me to their conferences, sharing insights in countless conversations, and giving comments on written work in progress. Among the many to recognize and thank are Drs. Michelle Albert, Charles Curry, Janice Douglas, Keith Ferdinand, John Flack, Clarence Grim, Kenneth Jamerson, Shawna Nesbitt, Elijah Saunders, Neil Shulman, Herman Taylor, Sean Wharton, Richard Allen Williams, and Jackson Wright. Drs. Paul Sorlie at the National Heart, Lung, and Blood Institute, Frances Henderson at the Jackson Heart Study, and Daniel Levy at the Framingham Heart Study were gracious hosts to my questions there.

This project began at the Massachusetts Institute of Technology under the guidance of Joe Dumit, David Jones, and Sherry Turkle, and I owe them a debt of gratitude. Joe Dumit has been a diligent mentor, kindred intellectual spirit, and academic inspiration. His scholarship has been deeply influential, and his generosity with his time both while at MIT and beyond has been extraordinary. David Jones's arrival at MIT was fortuitous for me both intellectually and logistically: he was a generous and exacting reader, and he organized crucial financial support and intellectual community through the MIT Center for the Study of Diversity in Science, Technology and Medicine, which was founded by Evelynn Hammonds with funding from the Mellon Foundation. Sherry Turkle has provided invaluable support for my scholarship by fostering intellectual community through her Initiative on Technology and Self, by engaging me in formative conversations about social theory, and by having faith in the importance of my story and point of view. She has both provided a superlative example of an incisively relevant intellectual voice and encouraged me to develop my own.

Many other MIT faculty also provided crucial early guidance. Elazer Edelman gave remarkably insightful lectures on cardiovascular pathophysiology; Evelynn Hammonds introduced me to the topics of race and medicine at the beginning of my graduate career; Kenneth Manning challenged me to write complicated stories that remain human stories; and Susan Silbey pushed me to present those stories more clearly. Evelyn Fox Keller, Hugh Gusterson, and Abha Sur helped me both hone my STS analysis and learn how to combine scholarship and activism. Other activist faculty were also both cherished allies and role models, including Noam Chomsky, Nancy Kanwisher, Jonathan King, and Nergis Mavalvala.

I have been fortunate to find excellent homes for developing this work and new projects since, first as a visitor at Rice University in the Department of Anthropology, and then as assistant professor of science, technology and culture at Georgia Tech in the School of Literature, Communication, and Culture. I have found rich interdisciplinary academic community at each of these institutions and beyond. My intellectual inquiry has been incomparably enriched by on-topic and off-topic conversations with colleagues including Amy Agigian, Robert Aronowitz, Wenda Bauchspies, Katherine Behar, Ian Bogost, Nichole Payne Carelock, Carol Colatrella, Carl DiSalvo, Elizabeth Freudenthal, Nate Greenslit, Narin Hassan, Anthony Hatch, Chihyung Jeon, Wen Hua Kuo, Hannah Landecker, Aryn Martin, Mara Mills, Janet Murray, Natasha Myers, Alondra Nelson, Gerald Oppenheimer, Esra Ozkan, Rachel Prentice, Kane Race, Michael Rossi, Aslihan Sanal, Janet Shim, Jenny Smith, Kaushik Sunder Rajan, Will Taggart, and Livia Wick. I owe a special debt to Ruha Benjamin, Nihad Farooq, Sara Giordano, Jeremy Greene, Jennifer Hamilton, John Krige, Melissa Littlefield, Robert Rosenberger, Miriam Shakow, Kate Weiner, and especially Candis Callison and Lindsay Smith, treasured colleagues who read and commented on draft chapters in various iterations.

I have also had the privilege of presenting material from this project and receiving invaluable comments from audiences, including at several Society for Social Studies of Science conferences; Vital Politics II and later a BIOS Roundtable at the London School of Economics; the Biopolitics of Science Seminar Series at Sydney University; the Centre for the Study of Innovation as Social Process at Goldsmiths College; the Institute for Science and Society Seminar Series at the University of Nottingham; the Science in Human Culture Lecture Series at Northwestern University; and the Science and Technology Studies Colloquium at the University of California, Davis.

Some of the material that straddles chapters 4 and 5 has been published in the *Journal of Law, Medicine and Ethics* (in 2008). Some of the material that straddles chapters 5 and 6 was published in the volume *The Value of Transnational Medical Research* (2012).

I am grateful to Ken Wissoker and Duke University Press for having faith in this project and shepherding the manuscript through revisions and into publication, and to Mark Mastromarino, Liz Smith, Jade Brooks, Maura High, and Amy Ruth Buchanan for their help through that process. The insightful reader reports from Steven Epstein, Alondra Nelson, and an anonymous reviewer helped me to sharpen the manuscript immensely.

Most of all I thank Maital Dar, whose editing acuity is a treasure and without whose love, support, and sense of humor all life's projects would be less worthwhile.

INTRODUCTION

In 2005, BiDil became the first drug ever approved by the U.S. Food and Drug Administration (FDA) for use in a specific race: it was indicated for heart failure in "self-identified black patients." As such, it became fodder for both popular and academic debate about the role of race in medicine, and the nature of racial difference more broadly. As novel as its FDA indication was, this drug represents just one moment in a long-standing and dynamic interplay of race, pharmaceuticals, and heart disease in America. *Medicating Race* examines these. In the wake of BiDil's commercial failure, this analytical contextualization helps to account for its allure and its unpalatability, as well as to open larger questions of medicine and American identities.

My analysis of race in medicine focuses on heart disease categories and their treatment. It highlights the complicated roles that physicians have long taken, advocating for the urgent needs of black patients on both scientific and social justice grounds. Whereas most scholars have situated BiDil within discussions of race and genetics and pharmaceutical marketing, I see the drug as part of narratives that precede and exceed any of these things. Enlarging the framework to pay attention to the intertwined trajectories of medical research and advocacy situates BiDil within a wider set of medical and racial ideas and practices.

The intersecting and mutually constituting trajectories of race, heart disease, and pharmaceuticals provide an excellent site to analyze what I conceptualize as the durability of preoccupations with race in medicine. Race in heart disease research and practice is *durable*: it cannot easily be gotten rid of. It is also a *preoccupation*: it cannot easily be let go. *Durable preoccupation* thus offers a dual concept with intrinsic tensions. Race in medicine provokes appeal and aversion, disassociation and solidarity, displacement and investment. In tracking the continuities and discontinuities of racialized heart disease discourses since the founding of American cardiology, we can see that the promise and danger heralded around BiDil tap into something deeper. Arguments over how to medicate race reveal fundamental tensions in democratic and unequal American medicine and society. Close attention to this particular story has implications for global scholarly and activist conversations about pharmaceuticals, race, and justice.

My argument is threefold:

1. *Heart disease has been enrolled in articulating Americanness, and so racial preoccupations were present at the founding of American heart disease research and have both endured and transformed since then.* Since its inception as a field, heart disease research has been grappling with the dangers of the "modern American way of life," access to which has been foundationally and fundamentally organized in terms of race. Also at stake has been access to cutting-edge medicine for both patients and practitioners. Articulations of inclusion and difference in cardiovascular research and pharmaceutical practices have been part of articulating democratic and racialized American ways of life.

2. *The durability of racialized disease categories—and the appeal of racialized drugs—does not rest on genetic determinism.* The appeal of race in medicine does not reduce to the appeal of genetics. Considerable epistemological eclecticism underlies notions of heart disease etiology, of which genetics is just one player. There are many ways to represent medically relevant racial difference besides genetics, and more important, medical practice is generally oriented around intervention. In order to give an accurate account of the role of race in medical research and practice and to gain new traction for critique, we need to move beyond situating genetics at the center and pay attention to how medicine not only arbitrates but also intervenes on difference.

3. *Medical treatment should be seen as a site of—rather than an alternative to—social and political contestation.* To understand mobilizations against health disparities, we should not assume that any particular action undertaken will fall cleanly into categories of biological or social, clinical or political. Paying attention to the complex and plural projects of clinician-researchers working in the area of race and medicine prevents any simple division between scientific reification, medical intervention, and social action. To understand the role of pharmaceuticals at this site, the context of market-oriented medicine should be a starting point for analysis rather than its end.

To lay out the book's argument more fully, I will attend to some of the key terms and topics, and describe the overall approach of the book in order to situate it within my scholarly field of science and technology studies (STS) and beyond. First, I will define and describe the processes that I am terming "medicating race," highlighting the specificities of medicine as a field of research and its particular value as a site for inquiry into race. Next, I describe the overarching approach, which is to track durable preoccupations with difference. I will then address the value and importance of the three constituent elements of my narrative: heart disease, pharmaceuticals, and black-white difference. Finally, I provide an overview of the chapters of the book.

Medicating Race

This book draws from critique of race and science, but it more specifically grapples with the distinct status of medicine as a field. Medicine is "not a coherent whole," but "rather, an amalgam of thoughts, a mixture of habits, an assemblage of techniques."[1] A central heterogeneity in medicine that interests me is medicine's duality as both a science and a practice—one that does not merely reify difference but also seeks to act on it. Philosophers of science have drawn our attention to the productivity of "representing and intervening" in knowledge-making,[2] and this tension is fundamental to medical knowledge. Medicine both represents and intervenes on racialized bodies. There is a rich polysemy in the word "medicating" that I am interested in mining for its theoretical insights. Attending to the immanence of *medicating* and *mediating*,[3] I argue that medicine is a field that *mediates* race, in the sense of arbitrating as well as intervening. Medical experts, disease categories, and pharmaceuticals all participate in *medicating* and *mediating* race.

The word "medicating" is in the present progressive tense because neither medicine nor its relationship with race is a settled thing granted by history or science. Medicine and race are emergent processes in motion in multiple spheres. Clinical medicine, like natural science that is the subject of much critical scholarship of race, cannot settle the debates about race at the nexus of the biological and the social. Race's relationship with medical practice remains messy both because medical data and efficacy are complicated notions that are hard to pin down and because clinical medicine is not independent from other biological and social discourses. This makes medicine a rich site for an STS analysis that seeks to abandon a priori distinctions between natural and social events, as Michel Callon has canonically argued.[4] To draw on Sheila Jasanoff's rich idiom, medicine is a site at which natural and social orders are *co-produced*.[5] When bodies and technologies come together in medicine, neither precedes the other. In medicating practices, both social and natural orders have the capacity to be bolstered and/or transformed.

This book considers "medicating" in a broad sense, as a verb that refers to actions taken in and about medicine as a field of social relations. "Medicating" importantly includes the most obvious meaning of the word, the administration of medicines, but it also encompasses much more. In addition to the prescription of drugs, "medicating" refers to other linked actions that medical practitioners engage in, including setting parameters around diagnostic categories, administering a range of diagnostic tests and treatments, conducting longitudinal studies, and writing clinical guidelines.

The concept of medicating is informed by, and in dialogue with, literatures of *medicalization*, but its emphasis on the emergent quality of medicine's relationship with social categories is central. Whereas medicalization can imply that there is some space essentially exterior to medicine that is being colonized and removed from other social spheres, such as morality or politics,[6] medicating race need not posit that a boundary is being crossed between the appropriately and inappropriately medical. The relationship between medicating race and, for example, politicizing race can be combinatorial rather than opposed. Medicating is not an alternative to a social movement, or an example of a nefarious political agenda, but a way to understand the process and progress of agendas and movements that are simultaneously moral and political, commercial and professional, and which play a role in how things came to be understood as racial and medical.

I do not presuppose that medicating is an inherently less moral way of addressing problems than other ways, as is commonly suggested in medicalization literature and in the medical anthropology that draws on it,[7] and in discussions of race and pharmaceuticals. The moral and the political are at stake in medicating as much as they are at stake in any other bio/social sphere. This becomes a particularly pressing issue in what Adele Clarke and her colleagues have termed the "biomedicalization era," in which "the focus is no longer on illness, disability, and disease as matters of fate, but on health as a matter of ongoing moral self-transformation."[8] In this biopolitics, as the sociologist David Skinner has argued, "confronting racism is not about the denial of biology but a struggle over it."⁹ Medicating race is not an *alternative* to taking moral and political action, but a high-stakes component of it.

Indeed, medicating is an excellent analytical framework for the STS critique of race because medicine intervenes on the boundaries between social and biological, material and semiotic. Race is at stake at precisely these boundaries. Thus, analysis of this intersection contributes to theories of race as well as to the history and social studies of medicine. Racial difference in heart disease is material: the premature mortality of African Americans as a group compared with white Americans as a group, which the leading black cardiologist Richard Allen Williams has called "the death gap,"¹⁰ takes place in actual bodies in the world and, no matter what caveats we make about the trickiness of data and etiology, the terrain is necessarily in part about biology. Yet racial difference in heart disease is also semiotic: the data cannot be extricated from lenses of difference-oriented preoccupations, and arguments about race and disease become ways to articulate difference in other aspects of society and individual identity. Social movements can seek to intervene on both symbolic and embodied registers—as Alondra Nelson has shown in her work on the health activism of the Black Panther Party, social movements can recontextualize medical ideas in diverse ways as they mobilize for health care and against medical harms, as part of a larger vision of racial justice.¹¹

I argue that in order to understand the productivity of race in medicine, race needs to be understood as a category that is always a subject of the dual aspects of medicine's mediation—bioscientific arbitration and pragmatic intervention. Race in biomedicine does not originate in the science and filter down to the doctors' offices; neither does it simply filter up. It does slightly different work in each sphere, but gains its durability through its capacity to travel between them. The task for critical scholars should not be to seek out a true or innocent science, attempting to purge the material-semiotic category of race from biology, but to track plural noninnocent discourses at the nexus of the biological and the social. Critique that rests only on scientific reification without attending to clinical intervention is both a failure to engage and contributes to the durability of the categories that it ostensibly critiques. Explaining racial disparities in heart disease through appeals to other social or biological phenomena does not free us from the task of addressing race, because it is precisely the relevance of race across heterogeneous ways of categorizing bodies in the context of social inequality that makes it particularly durable. Displacing race onto some supposedly more rigorously defined mode of accounting for difference—whether socioeconomic class, genetics, or something else—contributes to, rather than diminishes, the durability of race.

Medicating processes can become what the sociologists of race Michael Omi and Howard Winant have termed racial projects: "*A racial project is simultaneously an interpretation, representation, or explanation of racial dynamics, and an effort to reorganize and redistribute resources along particular racial lines.*"[12] To grapple with the accounts of those mobilized around race, pharmaceuticals, and heart disease, both the interpretive and the redistributive aspects matter. Interpretations, representations, and explanations for racial disparities in heart disease are mobilized in diverse ways, inseparable from demands for changing the distribution of resources such as pharmaceuticals and funding for longitudinal research and clinical trials.

Racial projects organized around disease categories and pharmaceuticals can take diverse forms, and pointing out that the discourse is racial is the start of the analysis rather than its end. Race is a dynamic and robust discourse that does not belong to those with a stake in perpetuating present inequalities alone, but rather to the terrain of the debate.[13] For example, pharmaceutical companies or disparities advocates can argue for or against any particular mechanism that offers hope (or provokes alarm), such as full integration of African Americans into mainstream American medicine's high levels of medication, or race-specific drugs. But we can tell that the discourse is a racial discourse, because no party in the conversation can talk about disease categories like coronary disease or hypertension, or drugs like thiazides or BiDil, without at least implicitly talking about race.

At the same time that medicine mediates race, it also mediates citizenship, and these processes are central to the constitution of biological citizenship in the United States. Whereas biological citizenship literature has generally focused either on rich countries in general or on particular resource-poor ones, this book attends to the distinctly American context. Some of the biological citizenship practices in the United States are like those in resource-poor settings. What Adriana Petryna has characterized in the Ukraine as "a massive demand for but selective access to a form of social welfare based on medical, scientific, and legal criteria that both acknowledge biological injury and compensate for it"[14] applies to demands for black hospitals in the early part of my account and to the demands for access to pharmaceuticals in the later part. These coexist with biosocial aspirations that Nikolas Rose and his colleagues have argued are distinctive of those in contemporary liberal democracies.[15]

Rose is right that contemporary biological citizenship as it emerges in direct-to-consumer genetic genealogy testing need not be seen as part of a trajectory with eugenics, and I am deeply sympathetic with the open-endedness of Rose's sensibility. However, if we are to grapple with biological citizenship in the United States, both our famously consumerist medicine and our infamously unequal access to it are fundamental. The diverse forms of biological citizenship overlap and coexist. As the legal scholar Dorothy Roberts has argued, race is as fundamental to the new biocitizen as it was to the old.[16] Paying attention to a broader historical terrain can give some texture to the continuities and discontinuities of how medicine has mediated race and citizenship in America.

The concept of medicating in this book encompasses, in addition to the processes of administering medicine and mediating biological and social orders, a valence of *meditating*. When doctors and others argue about how to medicate race, one thing that they are doing is *meditating upon* race, articulating emergent theories of the differentiated world through languages of medical terminology and data. In an elaboration of what the medical sociologist Stefan Timmermans has called a "second-order scientist,"[17] my project involves second-order meditating: meditating upon the meditations of historical actors to theorize race and medicine.

My methods for tracking these meditations were diverse. The earlier, historical chapters rely mostly on published materials from the first half of the twentieth century, as well as archival sources.[18] My understanding of these materials was enhanced by conversations with current and former researchers at the Framingham and Jackson heart studies. The later chapters draw from my main research process. I attended several conferences at which the intersection of race and heart disease was central, especially of the International Society for Hypertension in Blacks (ISHIB), and also the National Medical Association (NMA) and the Association of Black Cardiologists (ABC).[19] In addition to interviews with some of the key figures, my analysis was deeply informed by listening to conversations in progress. I found myself most interested in statements directed not at me as an individual, but between physicians—both from the podium to an audience and at less formal sites such as conference meal tables. I learned from the ways that the physicians were meditating upon race both in the sessions themselves, where the presentations on these topics were explicit, and in the in-between times. Approaching the field in this way, rather than principally through archival or oral history approaches, made some of the mundane practices visible. In a sense, this approach is an extension of what Warwick Anderson has highlighted as the need to explore "how ideas of race are deployed in the mundane practices of medical education,"[20] grappling with their role in *continuing* medical education. I did not get the chance to see how these doctors interacted with their patients, but I was able hear how they described their relationships with patients as they interacted with each other. Many were also very generous with me, explaining their field with enthusiasm and encouragement in ongoing conversations at, between, and outside these sites.

I also paid attention to invocations of race and pharmaceuticals that were happening outside medical contexts, enrolling these as sites of meditation upon intersections of race, pharmaceuticals, and heart disease. These range from a Coca-Cola Black History Month advertising campaign, to an episode of *Oprah*, to a cartoon by the incisive cartoonist Keith Knight. Attending to these kinds of sources is important because it picks up the broader salience of these issues of race in medicine. Including them is part of a co-productionist program for STS research that, as Sheila Jasanoff observes, "shifts our attention from *fact*-making (the traditional preserve of much work in science studies) to *sense*-making as a topic of overarching interest, with scientific sense-making as a particular, if highly significant, subcategory."[21]

Later in the project, I also became directly involved in organizing sites for these meditations on and at the intersections of race, pharmaceuticals, and heart disease. As a doctoral fellow of the MIT Center for the Study of Diversity in Science, Technology and Medicine, I was part of the organizing committee for conferences that emerged in the context of the hype and outrage about BiDil.[22] These conferences were sites of highly charged contestations among scholars from across the disciplines of history, social sciences, medicine, genetics, American studies, African American studies, and law, as well as pharmaceutical representatives and civil rights advocates. Exchanges that took place at these conferences became key sites for my own analytic engagement with the field.

Tracking Durable Preoccupations with Difference

In all of these mediations of and meditations on race and heart disease, I was struck by the *durability* of race. Durability is a concept that I use to capture the resilience of race in the face of critique. Compelling critiques of the use of race as a central organizing category from across the ideological spectrum—from conservative pundits who imagine a meritocracy that can be evacuated of its historical and current exclusions according to race, to the radical treatise

Against Race by the social theorist Paul Gilroy, which argues for a "planetary humanism"—have not weakened its appeal. Something is durable if it resists wear or decay, if it is resilient in the face of stress, age, attack, or changing circumstances. The very flexibility of race helps to make it highly resistant to destruction (yet amenable to deconstruction). Race is always changing and yet lasting and enduring, something that cannot be easily gotten rid of. This durability is the source of great frustration for many critics of race in medicine, who often operate as if race rises or falls on its scientific validity.

To grapple with the durability of race, it is essential to pay attention to it as simultaneously a central locus of power in the social world, and a site of discourse. Recent historiography of race has highlighted productive tensions within racial discourse, in which race is figured as both fixed and mutable, definite and unknowable. As Ann Laura Stoler has pointed out, "Ambiguity of those sets of relationships between the somatic and the inner self, the phenotype and the genotype, pigment shade and psychological sensibility are not slips in, or obstacles to, racial thinking but rather conditions for its proliferation and possibility."[23] Contradictions within notions of race contribute to rather than inhibit its durability. On this point, Waltraud Ernst argues that idiosyncratic and contradictory discourses about race do not weaken them but rather are part of what makes them "work": "Racial discourses work well not despite their logical inconsistencies, ambiguities and mixing up of premises but *because* of them. They are destructively all-pervasive precisely because they are overdetermined and multivariant, creating the possibility for different arguments or perspectives (moral, biological, cultural, etc.) to be accentuated within different contexts and depending on the aims pursued."[24] The ambiguities and plural registers, then, are generative. And so it should be no surprise that discourses of connections between racialized bodies and disease are not always coherent, or that pieces of them are sometimes mobilized in unpredictable ways.

Racial discourses also change over time. Because race remains so important across history, this can foster the illusion that race is outside history, but as Barbara Fields points out, race is a "historical product," not a "transhistorical" or "metaphysical" entity.[25] Moreover, even within any particular historical period, as the historians of race and science Evelynn Hammonds and Rebecca Herzig have argued, "even when race is the object of explicit study, its definition is rarely plain or stable."[26] That is why attending to *how* race becomes durable in each era is so important.

That race emerges out of a historical context is simple enough to assert;

how it does so is far more interesting. In tracking the continuities and discontinuities in racial discourses around one disease, my project complements recent scholarship in the history of race and medicine, including Jonathan Metzl's account of how schizophrenia "became a black disease,"[27] and, especially, Keith Wailoo's account of how cancer "crossed the color line." Wailoo argues that "the story of cancer and the color line therefore becomes the story of cancer's transformation *and* racialization—by which I mean, the processes by which scientists used the disease to create narratives of difference."[28] Like Wailoo's account of cancer over much the same period, my account of heart disease provides an opportunity to see how some ideas about the relationship between race and disease are rejected, some are inverted, and others stand the test of time. This repetitive rearticulation of race in heart disease constitutes its durability.

The durability of race in medicine does not come from any one source. Acknowledging the epistemological eclecticism that underlies race helps us to see why various debates over the etiology of racialized heart disease have not undermined racial reification itself. When debates over the past century have focused on whether the category at hand—syphilitic heart disease in the early twentieth century, or hypertension since the postwar period, or heart failure since the emergence of BiDil—is due to inborn characteristics or to social experiences, they have not disrupted the reification of racialized black heart disease itself. This is where my account diverges from most critical race studies and science and technology studies accounts of BiDil. Whereas many scholars argue that deciding whether the cause of disparities is biological difference or social inequality determines who is responsible for what should be done about it,[29] I do not think that race in the world operates on this kind of logic. Diverse actors can accommodate considerable epistemological eclecticism underlying what is recorded as status as African American, and that ambiguity is not a slip in racial discourses but part of what makes their proliferation possible. Ambiguity does not impede diverse medical and social response but facilitates it.

The approaches of science and technology studies have provided productive means to analyze the emergence of new scientific facts and technologies, and the concept of durability can bring an STS approach to bear on what might seem to be an old-fashioned topic such as race in medicine. In his essay "Technology Is Society Made Durable," Bruno Latour does not use "durability" as a technical term: his principal concern is actually with stabilization. Latour wants us to recognize that both human relations and mechanisms contribute to the relative stability of a particular assemblage, and that the dominance of particular humans or mechanisms is the result of the stabilization, rather than the cause of it. Despite Latour's own aversion to paying attention to any categories that exceed the network being analyzed—and he is particularly resistant to including race, class, and gender in any account—we might fruitfully apply this approach to the analysis of race and medicine. Insofar as claims about race and heart disease achieve stability, they do so in relationship with networks of physicians and researchers, which overlap with networks of activists and state actors, as well as particular pharmacopeias and configurations of bodies in the world. Racialized medicine achieves its durability not from the power of racist ideology on the one hand or mechanistic understandings of bodies on the other, but because many people—in government, in social activism, in medicine, and beyond—have coalesced around it as a way to articulate their visions of what to do.

These multiple imbrications are precisely why the durability of race need not be a source of hopelessness in a world of injustice. Durability is also flexibility. Recorded difference can be employed both to tell stories about existing inequality and to make demands for medical intervention and social change. Since the force of racial discourse becomes realized not in notions of fixity alone but in combustible combinations of fixity and fluidity, to understand the terrain of racialized pharmaceuticals and racialized medicine as a whole, we should attend to the ways that these debates render race both stable and malleable, both naturalize it and mobilize it. A conception of race as simultaneously resilient and changing is a better terrain for critique than one that merely decries its resilience, because it opens up possibilities for critical scholars to be part of articulating change.

Understanding durability in terms of a famous STS concept that Latour and others explore—the black box—can also be productive.[30] When race is operationalized as a variable—whether in the statistical reports of the early twentieth century, or more systematically in longitudinal health research, or in disease categories and prescription practices—it necessarily becomes for a fleeting moment what Latour would call a black box. In the Food and Drug Administration's indication of BiDil for heart failure in "self-identified black patients," all of the heterogeneous aspects that led to racially disparate heart failure are black-boxed. The prescribing physician may believe that black heart failure is caused by genetics, or by a high-salt diet, or by psychosocial stress, or by inadequate treatment of hypertension, but etiology can be black-boxed and the diagnosis itself used for action. That so few physicians do prescribe BiDil shows that the statements of the FDA or the pharmaceutical company do not have the power to dominate on their own. And yet, racialized disease categories are importantly different from the types of claims that Latour tracks, such as "the structure of DNA is a double-helix."[31] Racialized disease categories—from "diseases of modernity" at the beginning of the twentieth century to "heart failure in self-identified black patients" at the beginning of the twenty-first—never become fully stabilized. The black box keeps on being reopened, sometimes even by the same people who use it as a step stool.

Durability is not an inevitable state of affairs, and it must be constantly propped up and sustained. One thing that can feed durability is preoccupation. Together with physical objects in the world (such as pharmaceuticals and bodies), and facts (such as the results of clinical trials), *preoccupation* can prop up durability. *Durable preoccupations* are where fact and affect come together, and are particularly important for understanding medicating as a site of accounting for and protesting inequality in society.

The concept of preoccupation offers a way to consider not merely the facts of a disease, but how the mind becomes engrossed, how the attention and the intellect can be commanded in debates over disease categories and identities in a way that is viscerally charged. Preoccupations are *affective*: they require us to grapple with how "activities of the body and mind are simultaneously engaged," and "reason and passion, intelligence and feeling are employed together."[32] Affect refers to "bodily capacities to affect and be affected," and yet it is not presocial, because, as Patricia Clough evocatively argues, "there is a reflux back from conscious experience to affect."[33] Since both cardiovascular events and pharmaceuticals to reduce cardiovascular risk can induce sensations of "reflux" in a physiological sense, preoccupations with heart disease are a rich site at which to consider Clough's proposition that affect is not only in human bodies and consciousness, but also in technologies.

Much of this book addresses the ideas of physicians for whom engagement in these practices is part of their daily work, and so preoccupation is also connected with *occupation*, both as a term for a profession and as a way to label the tasks that fill the day. The emergence of cardiology as an occupation and heart disease as a preoccupation have always been intertwined.

At the intersection of a disease category and a social identity, we have the opportunity to think through both the material and the semiotic aspects of our lived experiences. Ideas become our preoccupations when they engross our attention, to the exclusion of other ideas and in a way that is viscerally charged. This visceral charge, more than the metaphoric language per se, is what Susan Sontag's classic *Illness as Metaphor* most valuably alerted us to.

For example, as I have argued elsewhere, breast cancer gives American women at the turn of the twenty-first century an opportunity to talk about how many children we've had, or haven't had, our sexuality, our beauty, our ethnicity, our mothers, our toxic environments, and more.[34] Breast cancer is not somehow naturally or inevitably available for narration in this way, but came to be so in the wake of feminism's second wave.[35] Many women have followed the lead of such public figures as Audre Lorde in telling stories of their bodies and their lives through this disease.[36] Yet preoccupation is not a matter of direct personal experience, which is neither necessary (as the appeal of breast cancer activism for those without breast cancer has shown)[37] nor sufficient (not every disease experience will become narrated as central to a life story). Indeed, as the sociologist Kate Weiner argues, heart disease may be less conducive to identity practices in part because of its perceived ordinariness and ubiquity.[38] This book attends to the ways that stories of identity and difference have been told through heart health and heart disease.

A key aspect of preoccupations is that they precede any particular piece of data. Data do not determine preoccupations, and mere prevalence does not make a disease relevant for politicization or for cultural or identity practices. Rare diseases, such as bird flu, often attract considerably more viscerally charged energy than common, and deadly, ones such as pneumonia. In fact, preoccupations precede data. For example, a long-standing preoccupation surrounds masculinity and heart disease, and so its toll on women is consistently framed as new or surprising, regardless of the data. In the insistence that "women get heart disease, too," it is worthwhile to linger on the "too." It points to preoccupation with the implicit masculinity of the category, and articulates the preoccupation even as it contests it.

There is a generative tension in the framing of the leading cause of death as an exception. In the insistence of such actors as the founder of the Association of Black Cardiologists that "African Americans get coronary heart disease, too," it is similarly worth lingering on the "too." It points to preoccupation with the implicit whiteness of the category, and articulates the preoccupation even as it contests it. Throughout the period I describe here, racial preoccupations are both articulated and contested in diverse ways—in physicians refusing in the early twentieth century to recognize the African American cardiovascular disease in front of them, in longitudinal investigators both claiming and disavowing representation of a larger body politic, in arguments over disease categories and drugs that are variously understood as genetic or social, cheap, or cutting-edge.

One question that is central to this book is how difference comes to make a difference. Two aspects of racial difference are pertinent: that racial difference is amenable to durability because it is *recordable*; and that preoccupations with racial difference cannot be understood as separate from lived experiences of racial inequality.

Categories of difference need not be *measurable* to be operationalized in medicine, and many differences that are central to medical practice are recorded rather than measured, such as age, gender, family history, and more. The durability of racial difference draws on its *recordability*—not its measurability or elusive lack thereof. Attending to ways that difference is recordable, as opposed to measurable, is also a way to grapple with another dual aspect of difference: difference suggests diversity, but codifying difference according to discrete characteristics narrows the scope of the definition of diversity. That is, difference is about othering, but the othering is not so total as to exclude some common ground on which degrees of difference between things can be judged.

I am attentive to what the parameters of difference are imagined to be. Throughout the century of research that I discuss, there has been a tension in the idea of inclusion: whether African Americans should be included because they are part of an American public, or because they are distinct. One meaning of difference is *distinguishing characteristic*, and various types of heart disease have been held up as corresponding to various types of Americans. The construction of those distinctions has increasingly drawn on statistics from longitudinal research and clinical trials. By attending to some of the same issues that Steven Epstein, a sociologist and science and technology studies scholar, characterizes as the "inclusion and difference paradigm,"[39] I track ways in which participation in medical knowledge and pharmaceutical practice have become part of articulating inclusion and difference in American ways of life. These articulations emerge in the context of a society that is at once unequal and democratic. The historical trajectory of constructing and contesting difference in the United States is distinctly rooted both in slavery, and in its abolition —in both the perpetuation of white supremacy, and its contestation.

When difference occurs in the context of inequality, difference becomes disparity. This book is in dialogue with the interdisciplinary literatures of disparities, including those of historians, health professionals, civil rights activists, and policy makers. The medical historian David Jones, writing about American Indian epidemics, has pointed out that the meaning of disparities is not transparent: "Disparities can be seen as proof of natural hierarchy, as products of misbehavior, or as evidence of social injustice."[40] There has been tension in critiques of racialized medicine between the tendency to emphasize the severity of racial disparities to call for justice and the tendency to try to remove race by drawing on other factors to explain the disparities in a less socially loaded way.

Differences provide fodder for preoccupations when they correspond with situations of dominance. As the feminist legal theorist Catharine MacKinnon has pointed out, any observations of difference are not separable from conditions of dominance.[41] Attention to the relationship between difference and dominance helps one to see why, for example, though ethnic difference among whites was recorded early in the Framingham Heart Study, it came to be no longer so. Preoccupations with racial difference in medicine—especially black compared with white—have remained durable not because of the compelling statistics about difference but because of the continued social reality of conditions of unequal access to power. This is why this recordable difference becomes not only an opportunity for taxonomy but also a mandate for advocating action against present inequalities.

In order to track durable preoccupations with difference in medicine, I have chosen to organize my analysis around a series of intersections of three elements: heart disease, pharmaceuticals, and black-white difference. This is a choice among many potential paths of inquiry. I will now explore each of the three elements to highlight how they have distinct value, in their own right, and in combination.

Why Heart Disease?

As historians and sociologists of heart disease have argued, the category of heart disease is itself multiple and elusive, exceeding objective and subjective grasp.[42] And yet heart disease is an apt venue for critical studies of medicine because it offers an opportunity to critique medicine not at its fringes but at its core. Critical race feminists have drawn attention to the ways that reproductive medicine participates in and perpetuates racial discourse,[43] and this kind of analysis should also be applied to the traditionally masculine category of heart disease. For all of its demographic and medical research import, heart disease has been generally understudied by STS and critical studies of medicine more broadly. In the long-standing productive interest in genetic topics, and the current flourishing of neuroscientific ones,[44] there has been relatively little interest in heart disease as a field, but there should be. The literature attending to identity practices around heart disease is small relative to that investigating reproductive, psychiatric, and genetic disease, but it is rich—especially attending to gender, and also to race and class.[45] Part of my project is to interrogate how heart disease articulates individual and social bodies in ways that are both like and distinct from other disease categories.

Like all disease, heart disease has been the subject of existential debates, that is, the extent to which it actually exists. For example, there has been debate about whether risk factors such as hypertension should properly be considered diseases and/or be so widely treated with pharmaceuticals. In a medicalization framework, a diagnosis of "elevated blood pressure" can be seen as an example of "defining a naturally occurring attribute as a medical problem."[46] However, in contrast to psychiatric disease, critiques of medicalization of heart disease do not extend to challenging its very existence, to denying that problems with our hearts can make us sick and die. As well, in contrast to such disease categories as sexual dysfunction, heart disease is also not vulnerable to claims that it belongs only outside medicine. Thus, heart disease poses a worthy challenge. In the words of the physician and historian Robert Aronowitz: "A physician colleague of mine, wanting to stress the absurdity of relativist arguments about disease, thought she might deliver the coup de grâce by saying, 'Now you're going to tell me that heart attacks are socially constructed.'"[47] It is precisely because no one can deny the existence of some biological reality to heart disease that thinking through the nature of social construction here can be particularly productive.

Where discussions of psychiatric diseases can too often be bogged down in polarized exchanges about whether or not they have a biological existence, discussions of heart disease can begin in the nexus of biological and social realities. Where arguments for the social construction of psychiatric diseases can be misinterpreted as suggesting their spontaneous invention or unreality, arguments for the social construction of heart disease foreground the real embodied experience of social construction. The challenge Aronowitz accepts, to explore the ways that coronary heart disease "has been as much negotiated as it has been discovered" and the way that its "name, definition, classification, and ultimate meaning . . . have been contingent on social factors as much as strictly biological ones,"[48] is inspiring to those in the emerging field of history and social science of somatic disease. This book is deeply indebted to Aronowitz's call. By considering the social construction of heart disease together with that of race and of pharmaceuticals, this book elaborates and extends his attentiveness to the contingencies in the social and biological.

Organizing my analysis around heart disease is a way to make it more tangible, even as it elides considerable heterogeneity within the term. In some sense heart disease has always existed—atherosclerosis has been described in Egyptian mummies, and efforts to understand the heart in health and disease have ancient roots[49]—but it is also distinctly modern. A symptom profile recognizable as angina pectoris was first described in Georgian England, and fifty years later in Europe and the United States.[50] Heart disease came to prominence in both the United Kingdom and the United States in the first half of the twentieth century, and the modern specialty of cardiology becomes recognizable in both countries by the 1920s;[51] that is the period in which this book's story begins.

Since the stabilization of heart disease as a field of research, heart disease has been an umbrella disease category that includes heterogeneous phenomena of a few major types that increase the burden on the heart and/or cause it to fail.[52] Of course, as Joel Howell has argued, "the structure and content of cardiology, like that of all specialties and subspecialties, is historically mediated and constantly changing."[53] In the chronological presentation of the chapters of this book, different categories of heart disease alternate as a focus of attention. In early cardiology, coronary heart disease was primary, and it was principally contrasted with infectious heart disease. Indeed, coronary disease has remained the principal focus of cardiology, and refers to those disease categories that are related to hardening and physical blockages of arteries, including arteriosclerosis, coronary thrombosis, and ischemic heart disease. In the Framingham study just after the Second World War, coronary disease was still the focus, but, through the study, hypertension became defined as both a risk factor for coronary disease and as its own etiological model of heart disease. Hypertension as a disease category and African American hypertension as a disease category emerged together, in the 1950s, 1960s, and 1970s, and the "slavery hypothesis" that emerged in the 1980s and 1990s has become a theory of differences in hypertension. The distinctions between heart disease categories have been enrolled in racial discourses—coronary heart disease has been associated with whiteness, and infectious heart disease and later hypertension has been associated with blackness.

The drugs that I consider are for distinct forms of heart disease. The first, a class of drugs called thiazide diuretics, is for hypertension (in all patients, and as we will see, especially in black patients). The second, BiDil, is for heart failure in "self-identified black patients." Heart failure can be understood as the end stage of heart disease, whether hypertensive or coronary in etiology. In the evolution of what heart disease has been understood to encompass, there has been both continuity and discontinuity in articulations of race in heart disease, and in its medical approaches and treatments.

Heart disease has long been a particularly prominent and lucrative site for pharmaceutical development. Drugs to reduce heart disease risk played a key role in the historical development of the blockbuster drug model, which as Joseph Dumit has pointed out, generally operates on a logic not of curing illness but of making normality dependent on drugs.[54] Amid the growing interest in the role of pharmaceuticalization in transformations of health,[55] this makes heart disease a rich site for inquiry.

Heart disease also has promise as a site for inquiry into bioscience, because it has long resisted geneticization.[56] As we grapple with an increasingly postgenomic biology,[57] race and heart disease can provide a distinctive site. As Evelyn Fox Keller presciently argued in 2000, "Genes have had a glorious run in the 20th century," but "these very advances will necessitate the introduction of other concepts, other terms, and other ways of thinking about biological organization, thereby inevitably loosening the grip that genes have had on the imagination of the life sciences these many decades."[58] Sickle cell anemia has been a particularly rich site for analyzing race in what Keller called "the century of the gene"; the historian of medicine Keith Wailoo, for example, has used that disease to anchor his account of the politics of race and health in the ascendance of, and disillusionment around, genetic medicine.[59] Scholars working in contemporary bioscience areas such as epigenetics have shown that models in the life sciences are shifting from conceptualizing genes as deterministic, to understanding them as necessarily contextual,[60] and the sociologist and STS scholar Jenny Reardon has considered "the postgenomic condition" with particular attention to race.[61]

Heart disease provides a useful taking-off point for analyzing race in the postgenomic era. There is already a glimmer that the intersection of race and heart disease is a fruitful site: Anne Fausto-Sterling, a biologist and STS scholar, has provided an intriguing discussion of how developmental systems theory matters for understanding race and hypertension.[62] If science and technology studies analysis of race does not move beyond genetics as deterministic, it will be stuck in nature/nurture frameworks out of step with contemporary work both in biomedicine and in the historical and social studies thereof. Starting from a focus on heart disease, rather than on genetics or even postgenomics per se, can provide a fresh route to bring race into conversation with current medicine, cutting-edge science, and critical scholarship.

Why Pharmaceuticals?

Pharmaceuticals are objects that are very readily recognized as material-semiotic, where it is easy to make the case for the capacity of objects to carry both matter and meaning. Race is also a material-semiotic category, one that takes on a peculiar ontological status at its intersection with heart disease and pharmaceuticals. Racial disparities could conceptually be medicated away, in the sense that differences in such biomarkers of risk as blood pressure could be eliminated with medications. Yet racial difference cannot quite be medicated away, in the sense that preoccupations with racial differences always exceed the data itself. Using disease categories and pharmaceuticals to think through race is productive if we accept that race, too, is irredeemably material-semiotic, and cannot be purged of either aspect.

A key insight of the burgeoning focus of science and technology studies scholarship on pharmaceuticals has been the creative productivity of the intersections of human identities with pharmaceutical practices, and it is therefore no surprise that the investigation of psychopharmaceuticals has been particularly rich.[63] The development of and contestation over the Pill on the one hand, and antiretrovirals on the other, have also provided fodder for these issues, and work on gendered diseases and especially HIV/AIDS is an important model for my work because it provides insight into mobilizations of identity-based social movements embracing and resisting disease categories and pharmaceuticals.[64] Historians within science and technology studies have attended to the reconfiguring connections between research science, marketing, and distributions of pharmaceuticals for both psychological and somatic disease through the twentieth century.[65] The anthropologist and STS scholar Joseph Dumit has highlighted the role of pharmaceutical advertisements in constituting new grammars of identity in health and disease,[66] and as the cultural studies theorist Kane Race has argued, all medicines are "re-creational," sites for re-creating ourselves and our world.[67]

Of course, as for example Alondra Nelson's subtle account of race and genetic ancestry testing has shown, genetic facts can also be fodder for creative identity practices.[68] And as scholars interrogating the particular implications of genetics research on indigenous peoples have shown, the stakes for identity can be very high: the stories told by geneticists matter not only for the individuals involved, but also for group identities and relationships with nation-states.[69] Forensic DNA has tremendous power, in imprisoning and freeing from prison, and in the adjudication of human rights claims and postconflict states.[70]

Yet pharmaceuticals are a distinctive site for the analysis of race, because of the primacy of intervention simultaneously on the social and the biological. Paying attention to pharmaceutical practices can highlight the ways that medicating is not isomorphic with geneticizing or biologizing. In too many critical studies of race and medicine, the terms "genetic," "deterministic," and "biological" are treated as synonyms. However, if we put pharmaceuticals at the center of the analysis and take their material and semiotic aspects seriously, we have the opportunity to foreground the ways in which biological bodies are shaped by social experience and amenable to medical intervention. That is why pharmaceuticals are key to my analysis, not only in the later chapters, which specifically analyze particular pharmaceuticals, but also in chapters about the durability of African American hypertension as a disease category, and about a genetic theory for the cause of African American hypertension. The immanence of the categorization of African American hypertension, and the therapeutic intervention of thiazide diuretics, is vital for understanding why and how diverse antiracist actors invoke distinctly African American disease.

The "thinginess" of pharmaceuticals is also crucial to understanding their appeal; they operate on the symbolic order at the same time that they "make dis-ease concrete."[71] Paying attention to the ways that pharmaceuticals become sites of exchange of both commerce and meaning-making gives us the opportunity to see how markets and meanings are coproduced. Rather than participating in nostalgia for a less commercialized medical era, we have the opportunity to interrogate profit-driven medicine. Because analytical attention to the commodity fetishism of drugs has overwhelmingly focused attention on highly profitable blockbuster drugs, profit has been given too much explanatory power. Attending to a generic drug class (thiazide diuretics) and a commercially unsuccessful drug (BiDil) provides fresh terrain to consider both the possibilities presented by and the resistances to market logics.

Notes on Terminology: Why So Black and White?

Readers may notice some slippery terminology and anachronistic framing in my account, on two levels: using current terms such as "African American" even when describing early cardiology, and using a bifurcated black-white framework in a multicultural America.

The first anachronism can be addressed quite succinctly: because I am centrally interested in how arguments about the past are enrolled in arguments in the present, I do not change quotes that describe ideas like "Negro health," but, in addition to putting them into historical context, I also bring them into contemporary terms. Moreover, overattention to fidelity to terminology of a historical period can create the false sense that the definition of race was more stable and circumscribed in the past than it is now—that everyone mobilized around "Negro health" shared a coherent understanding of what "Negro" signified—whereas I want to emphasize that the meanings of race have always been unstable and contested in each period.

The second potential anachronism is more complicated to address. Although the word "America" can refer to an entire hemisphere, in the discourses I track and in my own use, "America" refers to the United States. The U.S. context is central to why I focus on black-white difference. Of course, even within the United States, not all notions of racial difference are black and white. The articulations of Asian immunity and risk throughout the period—from a 1931 invocation of "the calm, accepting Chinaman" by one early cardiologist,[72] to the inclusion of a special session on Japanese populations parallel to the special session on African Americans at the 2005 American Society for Hypertension Meeting—could be the site of a comprehensive analysis of its own. Such an analysis would capture different aspects of American citizenship and disease than mine does, because the citizenship of Asian Americans has been constituted so differently from that of African Americans.[73] Attention to Hispanic/Latino heart disease is increasingly prominent, and, as Michael Montoya has demonstrated in his account of diabetes research, a fertile site for scholarly analysis.[74]

And yet, because the discourse of race and cardiovascular disease in the United States has overwhelmingly been one of black-white differences, those are justifiably central. Indeed, the racial preoccupations of articulations of heart disease, especially in the earlier period being described here but also today, reflect a broader situation. As Michael Brown and his colleagues argue, the "relationship of African Americans to whites therefore remains fundamental to any analysis of racial inequality."[75] They write of racism: "It persists, in large part, because 'whiteness' has always been important in defining who is and who is not an American. The original legislation that specified who could become a naturalized American was unequivocal: naturalization was restricted to white males. To further complicate matters, whiteness in the United States has never been simply a matter of skin color. Being white is also a measure, as Lani Guinier and Gerald Torres put it, 'of one's social distance from blackness.' In other words, whiteness in America has been ideologically constructed mostly to mean 'not black.'"[76]

As we will see, in discourses of race and heart disease, Americanness has often been at stake. As Warwick Anderson has argued with regard to whiteness in the history of racial science and medicine in Australia, "the clinic and the laboratory should be added to those sites where the nation—any nation—may be imagined."[77] In the early period when degenerative forms of heart disease were defined as typical of modern Americans, that was imagined to apply to whites, and—sometimes implicitly and sometimes explicitly—not to blacks. In the middle of the century when the Framingham Study longitudinally tracked a "normal or unselected" population, the whiteness was originally plural and attentive to the possibility of differences among white ethnic groups, but reflected a broad sense that coronary disease was something that affected "the white population." If that was understood as something that excluded "nonwhites," both longitudinal research and pharmaceutical practice has at the same time and increasingly since been centrally interested in the category of "nonblacks."

In all of this, my definition of race is purposely imprecise. Indeed, I believe that precision in definition is the wrong goal for any account of race in a society in which race is so complicatedly bound up with access to resources and power. For my purposes, the term "race" is a common noun that appears on census forms and on the medical histories that are so central to medical practice, a word with wide circulation in medical spheres and well beyond. If this seems a rather simplistic definition, it is because I am less interested in how race is defined or ascertained than in how it is mobilized. (As Teresa De Lauretis asks with regard to gender: do you tick the box or does the box tick you?)[78] I am looking at race as *discourse* (in a Foucauldian sense),[79] which is of course not to say that race is merely discursive—not in a context in which race plays such a central role in access to resources and broader lived experience.

I do not put the term *race* in scare quotes, even though I am sympathetic with many who do. I do not think that what Catherine Eagan has called "undermining quotation marks" do any such thing.[80] Such quotes, in the words of one linguist, disavow responsibility: "What the writer is doing here is *distancing* himself from the term in quotes. That is, he's saying 'Look, that's what they call it. I'm not responsible for this term.'"[81] But my goal in this book is not to create distance from medical invocations of race, but rather to engage with them. Many scholars who use scare quotes in reference to race do so to posit something of a straw man: some other who "really believes" in the racial categories that antiracist scholars know better than to believe in.

This illusion that scare quotes can distance the speaker from responsibility for terms is similar to what the theorist Slavoj Žižek describes in Lacan's lectures on atheism: since the true site of beliefs is not in conscious acts but in the unconscious—not just "deep in me" but "out there" in "my practices, rituals, and interactions"[82]—professing not to believe becomes much more complicated. And indeed, division between those with critical notions of race and those with uncritical ones does not correspond with any particular terminology choice, and straddles any medical/social science line. I am interested in tracking both the mobilizations of and retreats from characterizing disparities as *racial*.

The fear of being responsible for race is one better addressed directly than disavowed. As Jacques Derrida reminds us, we are guilty insofar as we are responsible.[83] As I argue most explicitly in my conclusion, innocence is not a possible moral stance for anyone participating in discourses of race, and so our subject position must be, in Donna Haraway's terms, "noninnocent."[84] We should not try to shirk responsibility.

Overview

The structure of this book is roughly chronological, beginning early in the twentieth century. Chapter 1 considers preoccupations with coronary heart disease, race, and modernity of the founders of cardiology and their contemporaries in the period between 1910 and the Second World War. I suggest that existing explanations of cardiology's rise can be both enriched and problematized by analyzing the ways in which these accounts are imbued with the racial frameworks of the period. I read founders of cardiology as theorists of a cardiovascularized modernity, in which both cardiovascularity and modernity are racialized. Claims of racial difference in heart disease etiology were present at the founding of heart disease research. The taxonomy of differential etiology by race of the period—that posited whiteness as connected to (noninfectious) coronary disease and blackness as connected to (infectious) rheumatic and especially syphilitic heart disease—was part of broader narratives about white degeneration and progress, and black infectiousness and uplift. Thus, ongoing contestations that African Americans *do* get coronary disease are part of laying claim to participation by African American patients in the modern American way of life, and by African American physicians in modern American medicine.

Chapter 2 analyzes the contingent and emergent racialization of the Framingham Heart Study, an extremely influential longitudinal study that began in a Massachusetts town just after the Second World War. The chapter argues that the homogeneous whiteness of Framingham emerged only as its early investigators both disavowed the imperative to representation and maintained their embrace of extrapolation, and as intrawhite ethnic difference was becoming less salient in describing difference among Americans. The chapter also draws the Framingham Study into comparative relief with the all-black Jackson Heart Study, which began in 2000 and continues into the present. The latter study does not merely repeat Framingham in a new population, but is rather a self-consciously postmodern repetition with a difference. The Jackson Heart Study both supplements and fragments notions of who can stand in as a typical enough American from whom to extrapolate.

Chapter 3 grapples with the durability of African American hypertension as a disease category. Hypertension has been a principal site of disparities research, and physicians and many others have used African American hypertension as a way to both articulate difference and advocate intervention. The chapter is centrally interested in why it is that clinician-researchers in the area of African American hypertension alternate between opening up the disease for scientific inquiry—asking wide-ranging questions about the etiology of disparities—and setting aside the ambiguities to advocate treatment. It describes the historical emergence of African American hypertension in the 1960s and '70s at the confluence of the emergence of hypertension as a risk factor, rearticulations of older, racialized infectious-versus-coronary distinctions, and civil rights discourses. It was appealing as a site of physician mobilization, both because it allowed them to participate in cutting-edge medical research and practice, and allowed them to use newly available pharmaceutical treatments to decrease the heart disease risk of their patients. The chapter also outlines ongoing etiological debates, and shows that doubts about the relative role of socioeconomic class, psychosocial stress, and other factors, do not undermine the durability of race, but rather bolster it. Amid alternative ways of understanding the etiology of disparities, the *recordability* of race makes it more durable than any alternative, distinctly amenable to being enrolled in demands for action.

The fourth chapter focuses on one particular theory of African American hypertension that has drawn particularly vociferous critique, the slavery hypothesis, and argues that it should be understood in the context of epistemological eclecticism and interventionist medicine, rather than genetic determinism. It provides close readings of invocations of the theory in diverse venues, ranging from epidemiology journals to the *Oprah Winfrey Show*. The chapter unpacks these invocations of the slavery hypothesis both to illustrate the heterogeneity of ideas about race and about medicine that can be enrolled in racialized invocations of disease, and to argue that although the evidentiary basis for the theory is indeed weak, efforts to stamp out the theory may be a misplaced use of antiracist energy. The chapter attends particularly closely to an invocation of the theory outside of a medical or clinical encounter, in which Henry Louis Gates Jr. responds to a presentation of the theory by reporting his own consumption of hydrochlorothiazide and identifying himself as a "salt-saving Negro." This provides a bridge to the next chapter, which brings attention to that drug class to the fore.

Chapter 5 moves the focus more centrally to pharmaceuticals by attending to medical debates about thiazide diuretics, a class of antihypertensive drugs that has been linked to African American hypertension as a disease category. Recent government-funded research has promoted thiazides as an affordable and efficacious way to treat hypertension in everyone, and especially in black patients, and I describe a debate in which that research is contested. Because thiazides are generic, attending to the commodity fetishism around them provides the opportunity to see that drugs' relationships with preoccupations with difference exceeds their role in narrow economic interests. Attention to the commodity aspects of thiazides—especially the inextricability of their use value (efficacy) and their exchange value (price)—shows that the appeal of (or aversion to) drugs is not limited to marketing. Because of the confluence of the drug for blacks and the cheap drug, it becomes a site for diverse articulations of racialized American biological citizenship. In the debates about the particular appropriateness of thiazide diuretics or of brand-name alternatives, African Americans are betwixt and between pharmaceutical grammars of basic care and consumerist freedom. Consideration of these drugs that are at once racialized, proven, old, and cheap, provides an opportunity to consider how debates over drugs can articulate debates over the nature of inclusion and difference in American ways of life.

Chapter 6 turns to the drug that has been a focus of renewed interest in race and medicine among science and technology studies scholars: BiDil. This chapter tracks the contingent development of this branded combination of two generic drugs at the intersection of race and heart failure. When it won the FDA's approval in 2005, BiDil became the first drug ever approved for use in a specific race, bearing the indication for heart failure in "self-identified black patients." The blatancy of its racialization has attracted considerable scholarly critique, and yet much of the critique has leaned too heavily on old arguments about race and genetics on the one hand, or about blockbuster drugs on the other. Neither of these lines of critique is up to the task of deconstructing a drug that is simultaneously effective in treating symptoms and delaying death, supported by diverse epistemologically eclectic actors, and commercially unsuccessful. The chapter highlights the divergent goals of the various actors that aligned around BiDil's approval. For the Association of Black Cardiologists, the FDA, and the pharmaceutical company NitroMed, BiDil was a means to address different problems, and these actors should not be analytically collapsed. The chapter foregrounds the specificity of heart failure as a disease category, and critiques assumptions that drugs inevitably reach their markets. It also argues that BiDil has undecidabilities: the drug is irredeemably *pharmakon* (remedy and poison), and it is material-semiotic. Attempts by some of those mobilized for and against the drug to purge either side of those undecidabilities are unsuccessful. Drugs, like race, are both material and semiotic, and there is an inescapable polyvalence of a "black drug" in this current historical moment.

The conclusion highlights the relevance of this book's account for race and medicine and for medical ethics, as well as reviewing the continuities and discontinuities in the intersections of race, heart disease, and pharmaceuticals recounted in the book. It is organized around a close reading of a juncture at which a debate about race and medicine broke down, after positions on BiDil were framed as an opposition between those "down with the people" and those "up in the academy." I argue that race and medicine is best characterized as plural noninnocent discourses, rather than as racists versus antiracists. Race is a topic about which neither activists nor academics should feel comfortable, and discussion would better proceed by acknowledging that all engagement with it is noninnocent. I frame the book's relevance for broader questions in medical ethics by exploring the ways that BiDil fit into, and failed to fit into, traditional quandary ethics. I argue that our project should be to make medicine answerable to justice, not to provide answers to narrowly framed ethical quandaries. Attention to generative dissonance should be a resource for scholarly engagement, and I hope that race seems more difficult to come to terms with after reading the book than it had before. Closing with contemplation of the myth of the hydra, I argue that any decrease in the durability of race in medicine can only follow its decreased importance in broader preoccupations with difference, and that if we ever leave an account of race and medicine feeling satisfied that we have understood it, debunked it, or even staked out an innocent position on it, we are in error. Inspired by prophetic pragmatism, and committed to ethical noninnocence, I suggest that although there is no place of engagement above the fray, there is, nevertheless, hope.

CHAPTER 1

Racial Preoccupations and Early Cardiology

At a special symposium of the American Society for Hypertension in 2005, the founder of the Association of Black Cardiologists (ABC), Richard Allen Williams, told an anecdote from his training.[1] When he was a bright young student at Harvard in the 1960s, his mentor Paul Dudley White asked what his interest was. When Williams answered that he wanted to study coronary heart disease in blacks, his mentor was dismissive, and said that he hoped that the sharp young student would not waste his time—White told Williams that a "full-blooded Negro" never got coronary disease. This story got a laugh from the audience, and their reaction merits analysis.

On one level, Williams's anecdote is a performative gesture of laughing at the ignorance of forefathers. Laughing at the naiveté of the great thinkers of the past is a frequent narrative device among physicians, and I observed it at many conferences. References to Paul Dudley White, a central figure in the founding of American cardiology in the 1910s and '20s and a prolific leader in the field until his death in 1973, are particularly popular. The laughter shared by Williams and his audience could foster camaraderie among the physicians in the room, who could feel flattered that they had access to knowledge that visionary founders lacked. Perhaps emphasizing how far the field has come can also assuage anxiety about how small contemporary contributions can feel in a mature field like cardiology. Yet jokes about the ignorance of cardiology's founders evoke both distance from the field's founders and a connection to them. Williams's joke both enrolls Paul Dudley White in the lineage of the Association of Black Cardiologists, and stakes a claim for the importance of ABC's distinct contribution. But there is another important element here: how could it have been so clear to White that African Americans should be excluded from the population affected by coronary heart disease, and yet so clear to Williams that they be included—indeed, so clear to Williams's contemporary audience that White's error on that front becomes humorous? What has been at stake in debunking the notion that African Americans do not get coronary disease?

In this chapter, I argue that in Williams's commitment to prove White wrong, we can see a dialectical response to the theses of the founding of cardiology. I suggest that existing explanations of cardiology's rise in the period between 1910 and the Second World War—disease demographics shifting from infectious to degenerative disease, lifestyle changes in which mental strain replaced physical strain, and the professionalization and standardization of medicine—can be both enriched and problematized by analyzing the ways in which these accounts are imbued with the racial frameworks of the period. I read White and other founders of cardiology as theorists of a cardiovascularized modernity, in which both cardiovascularity and modernity are racialized. At the intersection of race, cardiovascular disease, and the modern American way of life in the early twentieth century, there was a freedom to exclude blacks from the attention of cardiology because of an idea that they didn't get heart disease—or if they did, it was not in the same ways as modern whites, which was emblematically coronary heart disease. There has been continual contestation ever since—especially by black cardiologists—that blacks *do* get heart disease, and *both* in precisely the same ways and in ways of their own. Williams's preoccupations are in this sense continuous with the physicians and statisticians writing in the 1910s, '20s, and '30s, because even today the facts of black coronary disease still keep being both important and surprising. The existence and prevalence of coronary disease among African Americans, and its relationship with other etiologies of heart disease, especially hypertension, remain unsettled. Data have not and cannot resolve the issue, and racial difference in heart disease remains a durable preoccupation.

Degenerative Disease and the Boundary Work of Early Cardiology

Heart disease is conventionally understood as a disease that becomes more important in an aging society that has a decreasing infectious disease burden. This shift has been characterized as the "demographic transition" (initially described in 1929 as a shift from high birth and death rates to low birth and death rates),[2] and as the "epidemiological transition" (initially described in 1971 as "degenerative and man-made diseases displace pandemics of infection as the primary causes of morbidity and mortality").[3] Historians of cardiology have also invoked this to explain the field's rise.[4] If medical needs were a driver of medical specialization, a change in population makeup and disease prevalence would cause the rise of cardiology.

However, as we will see, although cardiology has long been described as a medical specialty that would address the needs that humanity would face after infectious disease was eradicated, the succession turns out to be complicated. Explaining the rise of cardiology through the decreasing prevalence of infectious disease takes for granted that cardiology was, at its inception, focused exclusively on noninfectious disease. This ignores how common infectious heart disease was in the early twentieth century. Narration of cardiology by both its founders and its historians as postinfectious is not an observation but rather a preoccupation-laden claim about which kinds of heart disease characterize modernity. Heart disease was subcategorized into infectious and degenerative heart disease, and this categorization was racialized. Infectious heart disease, especially syphilitic, would come to be more associated with blacks, and degenerative heart disease, especially coronary, would come to be more associated with whites. This taxonomy of two types of heart disease for two racial types does not simply end once the etiology of heart disease becomes overwhelmingly noninfectious population-wide. Rather, as we will see, it is renewed in associations between whiteness and coronary disease and blackness and hypertension.

In an important sense, infectious heart disease led to the founding of the field of cardiology. One reason that Paul Dudley White took a fateful internship in England to study cardiovascular physiology in 1913 was that his sister had died of rheumatic heart disease, which was a common form of infectious heart disease.[5] The technology that White would bring back to the United States would become important in defining degenerative heart disease, but his motivation was infectious heart disease. Heart disease had not yet become a major focus of medicine, and White describes being warned that study of heart disease would relegate his work to the "back few pages of textbooks" in which typhoid fever, pneumonia, diphtheria, and tuberculosis were "the infections [that] held the limelight."[6] Thus, White narrates the founding of cardiology as preceding the ascendance of degenerative disease over infectious disease:

> As I returned to the Massachusetts General with my electrocardiograph, I felt like a lonely adventurer entering an unexplored and unknown country, planning to spend my life in a new and as yet unrecognized specialty limited to the heart and blood vessels, both normal and diseased. This was the decade before a handful of us founded the American Heart Association and

two decades before we were permitted by our elders and even by most of our contemporaries to call ourselves cardiologists. It was the dark days B.C. (Before Cardiology), when the great White Plague, tuberculosis, was still the main cause of death, and rheumatic fever was responsible for the majority of our heart patients.[7]

In cardiology's first decades as a specialty, organizers around heart disease would model their efforts on campaigns combating infectious diseases, and infectious heart disease would remain a numerically important component of the field. As Joel Howell argues, the American Heart Association "arose directly from the antituberculosis movement, both conceptually and organizationally."[8] The landmark professionalizing events in the founding of cardiology—the 1915 founding of the Association for the Prevention and Relief of Heart Disease in New York City, and the 1924 founding of the American Heart Association—incorporated efforts to combat infectious forms of heart disease.[9] A 1928 review comments, "It is fairly well established that there are three common types of heart disease: rheumatic, syphilitic, and arteriosclerotic,"[10] and describes many local studies, all of which ascribed roughly half of the cases of heart diseases to infectious causes.

Early heart disease researchers did not so much claim that degenerative disease was already dominant, but that it was becoming so. In the 1928 review, we read that although half of heart disease was infectious in etiology, the *increasing* rate of heart disease was due to degenerative causes. Moreover, because "the possibility of prevention and cure remains open in the infectious group" but not in other heart disease,[11] the latter category was promoted as where the field should direct its attention. In this declaration not of its dominance but of its ascendance, degenerative disease becomes emblematic of the future.

Cardiology's founders were among the many physicians and others talking about the decline of infectious disease and bringing their focus to the degenerative diseases of aging. Here is how one important practitioner, Stewart R. Roberts, described the situation in 1925:

> The outstanding fruition of the last fifty years of medicine is the increase in the length of the average life from 35 to 58 years. . . . The prevention and cure of acute infectious diseases, the wider range of a scientific surgery and a scientific sanitation are the chief influences. Typhoid fever, yellow fever, and diphtheria are nearly blotted out from civilization, and yet heart disease is on the increase. Organic heart disease is today the greatest cause of

death. No more could John Bunyan call tuberculosis the "Captain of the men of death," and no more could Osler apply the title to pneumonia.[12]

Roberts staked out prevention of heart disease as the next project of medicine: "Science and medicine have well attacked the acute infectious diseases. Vaccinate and there is no smallpox. The problem of heart disease is far more complex. The task of properly studying and preventing the cardiac is before us."[13] Physicians in popular media, too, emphasized the rising importance of degenerative disease over infectious disease. For example, a lecture by Dr. Haven Emerson at the Massachusetts Medical Society was reported in a 1921 *Boston Globe* article in this way: "He insisted that heart disease must be attacked as tuberculosis has been for the past 20 years, by creating a public consciousness in regard to the menace and by taking it in the incipient stages."[14] In the article, this demand is explicitly racialized: "The white race is more susceptible to heart disease than the colored race." Similarly, a University of Pennsylvania physician, C. C. Wolferth, told the *New York Times* in 1930 that "degenerative diseases of the heart and blood vessels comprise what is probably the most important problem facing the white race."[15]

Although the racialization of a postinfectious paradigm was mostly implicit rather than explicit, staking the future of the field in degenerative disease should be read as part of racial discourse. To draw on Priscilla Wald's evocative elaboration of Benedict Anderson's terms, articulation of the population affected by degenerative heart disease configures an "imagined immunity" of the "imagined community" of modern Americans.[16] Since, as we will see, blackness was so associated with infection, the imaginary of a postinfectious medical specialty was in an important sense articulating a field that did not concern African Americans. Thus, the idea of cardiology as a field that emerged once infectious disease was held at bay was not descriptive, but deeply ideological. The sociologist Thomas Gieryn coined the foundational STS term "boundary work" to describe the ways that science is demarcated from nonscience,[17] and the concept is useful for understanding how privileged categories within science are constructed as well. Interest in noninfectious diseases of the heart preceded their majority in the caseload, and much thinking through relationships between heart disease and a racialized modernity was done in the boundary work between infectious and noninfectious disease. Ideological and cultural resonances of degenerative diseases and coronary disease in particular became ways to think through the American way of life before the diseases themselves dominated morbidity and mortality.

In this period, there was a discrepancy between what we might imagine to be the *paradigmatic pathologies* of blacks and of whites. While fears and hopes about black disease and health were focused on infection, an emerging discourse of heart disease would bring fears and hopes about white degeneration to the fore. In Donna Haraway's charting of racial discourses of the twentieth century, she has suggested that the "paradigmatic pathology" of the first three decades of the twentieth century was "decadence, rotting, infection, tuberculosis," whereas the "paradigmatic pathology" of the decades between 1940 and 1970 were "obsolescence, stress, overload."[18] In this sense, cardiology can be read as part of a transitional apparatus, starting to address white obsolescence and stress in a period in which blacks remained characterized as infectious and tubercular. Cardiology was coalescing in the first decades of the twentieth century, but it became a site for thinking through the paradigmatic pathologies of the future.

Modern Medicine for a Modern Way of Life

Heart disease was imagined to be characteristic of white Americans not only because their burden of infection was decreasing, but also because they lived a modern life of "stress and strain." The physician and historian of medicine Robert Aronowitz has given a rich account of the centrality of racialized conceptualizations of the modern way of life to the emergence of the disease category of coronary heart disease, and Paul Dudley White is a key figure.[19] Paul Dudley White was a particularly rich witness to the emergence of modern understandings of coronary heart disease because "for more than a generation," he was "America's most influential academic cardiologist," an articulate witness to the transformations.[20] For White, a key aspect of the strain of modernity was that it was characterized by speed, which has resonances with the Fordism of the period—the modernity of industrialization, with a pace set by machines rather than on a human scale. White argued in his 1931 textbook that "even allowing for missed diagnoses in the past, angina pectoris is evidently increased in frequency, and is encountered more in communities where the strain of life is great and a hurried existence the habit than in leisurely parts of the world. The situation is appalling and demands some action on our part. Almost certainly the most effective move that we can make is to call a halt on the war of mad rush today."[21] White was describing a very particular kind of strain, unique to a life considered to be fast-paced. Through his conflation of speed and strain, it became possible for White to articulate preoccupations with the strain caused by the perceived startling loss of leisure experienced by urbanites in prosperous countries.

Stewart R. Roberts is less remembered than Paul Dudley White, but was a successful elite physician at the time, a professor of clinical medicine at Emory from 1915 to 1941, and widely published on topics in internal medicine including pellagra and heart disease.[22] He was a leader of professional medicine in his time, serving as president of the Southern Medical Society in 1924–25 and president of the American Heart Association in 1933–34,[23] and merited an obituary in the *New York Times* that characterized him as "a diagnostician and a specialist in internal medicine and heart diseases."[24] He was also part of the leadership of "the New South," connected to the movement for race reform.[25]

Like Paul Dudley White, Roberts connected increasing heart disease with the era, writing in 1925: "We have come to the period in which heart disease is the chief cause of death in civilization."[26] In a 1931 piece, he wrote in particular about the stress of civilization: "Civilization as we know it in Western Europe and America, the ambition, effort, and community state of mind of these areas, the increasing responsibilities that come with age, and an aging circulation, apparently are the foundations for the increasing prevalence of angina."[27] This characterization is implicitly racialized, and Roberts's argument becomes more explicitly racialized later in his piece. The Western civilization that Roberts describes is not imagined to encompass African Americans. His description of the distribution of angina pectoris provides a succinct articulation of the racial archetypes that preoccupied the elite white, Anglo-Saxon Protestants who claimed for themselves the label "American": he writes that it "occurs usually in the sensitive, nervous type, as the Jew, or in the tense, efficient American, rather than in the dull, happy negro or the calm, accepting Chinaman."[28] Roberts speculates about etiology:

> The white man, particularly those living lives of stress in urban conditions of competition, work and strain, makes his little plans and lays up cares and riches and takes much thought of the morrow; the negro knows his weekly wage is his fortune, takes each day as it is, takes little or no thought of the morrow, plays and lives in a state of play, hurries none and worries little. What must it be to live unhurried, unworried, superstitious but not ambitious, full of childlike faith, satisfied, helpless, plodding, plain, patient, yet living a life of joy and interest?[29]

In part, Roberts based his racial taxonomy on twenty years of clinical experience, claiming that during that time he never saw angina in an African American.[30] But he is epistemologically eclectic in his meditation, and includes insight from his own intimate experience as well, introspectively describing his resentment toward his "Ethiopian maid," who is not disturbed by the ringing phone nor by his scolding her for not having answered it: "I strain, she lives with the day. She illustrates the advantages of being uneducated, untutored, unambitious, just one who has by nature been born with 'an internal adjustment—to change her soul into an attitude of acceptance.' But I meet difficulties every day, and many times a day, and try much or little to change and correct the difficulty externally rather than to adjust myself to it internally."[31] In the context of angina's association with such positive traits as responsibility toward oneself and others, ambition and hard work, this disease disparity becomes a way to argue that whites' increased predisposition to coronary disease had a positive valence—in Aronowitz's terms, "an ambivalent honor."[32]

Roberts's narrative thus resonates with that of late nineteenth-century musings about "neurasthenia" among highly civilized "brainworkers."[33] It also has much common ground with cancer awareness in Roberts's own era, as richly recounted by historian of medicine Keith Wailoo: Roberts's explanatory model for what he sees as a distinctly white disease is imagined to mark the bodies of people with complex inner lives.[34] Yet where Wailoo's account shows that the characteristic anxieties of cancerous bodies were feminine and focused on the past and regrets, the characteristic anxieties of anginal bodies were masculine and focused on the future. Cancer and heart disease could thus be complementary ascendant degenerative diseases, each demarcating the civilized from the primitive, cancer being distinctly feminine, and heart disease distinctly masculine.

While some diseases stigmatize their sufferers, angina in this period sometimes marked its sufferers as good modern citizens. And if germs gathered toward the bottom of social hierarchies, coronary disease collected up, and claiming coronary disease was staking a position at the top of social hierarchies. Roberts concludes his piece:

> The internist can bear witness to the increase in the number of cases of angina, hypertension, and nervous indigestion among the white races of Western Europe and North America. . . . The psychology of stress, strain and struggle in the white races is in sharp contrast to the humorous carelessness of the musical negro or the placid acceptance of the gentle Chinaman. The white race talks of speed and records, domination and colonization, drives, rallies, sales and sales-resistance, estates, trusts and results, it

increases its effort and income to gratify its desires, and then multiplies its desires. We call it progress and western civilization. The Chinese and the negro accept and, perhaps far more than the white man, conquer both their spirits and their nervous systems. In this sense the white man's burden is his nervous system.[35]

Importantly, the price of "progress" that is the "white man's burden" is paid by its *agents*, and its agents are only a small part of the population of "North America." Roberts portrays white suffering in the service of their heavy responsibility as tragic, and the notion of white disease as evidence of responsible white sacrifice for the sake of progress is itself a characterization of the biopolitics of the period. In an important sense, Roberts is articulating the contours of white sacrifice for modernity. We can read the distinction between the diseases of whites and those of African Americans in the early twentieth century as analogous to Georgio Agamben's distinction between those who can be killed and those who can be sacrificed.[36] African Americans, for Roberts, remain in the category of what Agamben has understood as "bare life." At stake is boundary work between (in Agamben's terms) "the citizen" who is white, and the not yet civilized "bare life" which is black. It is through this maneuver that blacks are not the ones paying the price of progress in Roberts's framework. African Americans are not full citizens, and only citizens of modernity can be sacrificed to it.

Blacks' death rate in the period was higher, but that did not make their deaths carry a valence of sacrifice for modernity. The rhetorical exclusion of black embodied experience in a modern age points to preoccupation. We might imagine that those who have the higher death rate in the modern world would be framed as the ones being sacrificed to modernity. If these matters were data-driven, it would seem to be blacks and not whites who were bearing the disproportionate weight of modernity's "burden." But by denying black agency, Roberts also denies blacks the role of heroes in tragic tropes. As Cornel West points out in his distinction between the "tragic" and "mere suffering," "the notion of the tragic is bound up with human agency."[37] The ongoing suffering of African Americans in the early twentieth century is in these terms not "tragedy" but "mere suffering."

When other observers in the period produced data that contradicted Roberts's claim about black immunity from heart disease—Edward Schwab and Victor Schulze, for example, argued that blacks actually had more heart disease and greater mortality from it—the disparity was still used to argue for black inferiority: "In view of the facts that heart disease in the negro compared with the white race is of greater incidence, occurs at a younger age, pursues a more rapid course, and has a higher mortality rate, the opinion is offered that the cardiovascular system of the American negro of the South is inferior to that of the white race, and is more vulnerable to insult whether this be applied as an infection, a degeneration, a toxemia, or in the form of the stress and strain incident to the complexities and modes of modern occidental civilization."[38] We can see here that claims about differential racial susceptibility do not by themselves determine relationships between disease rates and racial superiority. Arguments can be framed in both ways. For Schwab and Schultze, African American heart disease demonstrated black racial inferiority. They explicitly cite and engage the work of Roberts, for whom white heart disease (especially angina) demonstrated white racial superiority, and read their opposite data in an opposite way to reach the same conclusion: white superiority. Differential prevalence of disease does not by itself then force any particular conclusions about the value of the patients suffering from it.[39]

Not all who made "price of progress" arguments to explain this white disease of modernity made such explicit cases about racial differentiation, yet there is an important implicit racialization in this very framing. Notions of the strains of modernity were notions of white middle-class masculinity. Indeed, the founders of cardiology were elite American-born white men of ambition who saw their way of life as epitomizing modern American life, and their clinical study of and personal experiences with coronary disease—they believed themselves to be particularly prone[40]—became emblematic of the price paid for that way of life. Although much of this writing was appearing during the Great Depression, when many Americans were struggling with real scarcities, these physicians imagined their sedentary lifestyles full of ambition as quintessentially American. The erasures necessary to maintain this narrow vision of Americanness show how racialized their project was.

A Time of Racial Contestations

The context in which cardiology would emerge between 1910 and the Second World War was a vital time for the working out of race in the United States. The historian of medicine David McBride has identified the "sociomedical racialism" of the period as constitutive of the genealogy of contemporary black experience of AIDS.[41] By reading these debates about race and infectiousness as a contrastive case, we can see within them implicit claims about whiteness and noninfectious disease, which constitute part of the genealogy of heart disease. In the widespread observations that African Americans had much higher rates of infectious disease and much earlier mortality than white Americans did, it was not clear how to make sense of the disparities or what should be done. Key grounds for the debate were black *constitution* and black *infectiousness*.

One discourse in which black disease and health was being worked out was with regard to constitution. It was becoming clearer that the black extinction predicted by Frederick Hoffman's influential 1896 tract *Race Traits and Tendencies of the Negro* would not come to pass, but apt ways of understanding black bodies in freedom, poverty, and uplift were still up for grabs.[42] As David Jones, a historian of medicine, points out, when confronted with disparities, observers have an "overabundance of potential explanations"—disparities might be seen as "proof of natural hierarchy, as products of misbehavior, or as evidence of social injustice"—and those explanations can "motivate or undermine interventions, influencing whether observers prevent an epidemic's spread, treat its victims, or exploit its opportunities."[43] When W. E. B. Du Bois documented the African American condition, he was clearly aware of how fraught the documentation of disparities can be: "What the Negro death rate indicates is how far this race is behind that great vigorous, cultivated race about it. It should then act as a spur for increased effort and sound upbuilding, and not as an excuse for passive indifference, or increased discrimination."[44] For Du Bois, closing the disparity would require both black self-help and their greater inclusion in social institutions.

Black advocates' efforts to separate out the environmental factors from the constitutional factors contributing to high rates of black disease were part of their contestation of Hoffman's dire predictions, and they generally concluded that the environmental or social factors were more important than the constitutional or racial ones.[45] Du Bois argued that "even in consumption [tuberculosis] all the evidence goes to show that it is not a racial disease but a social disease."[46] Debates in venues such as the *Journal of the National Medical Association*, the leading black physicians' group's main organ, considered whether poor black health in urban areas like Philadelphia should be solved by a return to the rural South "appropriate" to the race; or by improving urban conditions; or by implementing "disciplinary training" on blacks.[47] Even if constitutional factors were generally minimized by black health advocates, the terms were not completely rewritten in their venues: "The law of 'The survival of the fittest' holds as true today as ever before, and is indeed applicable to the Negro race; for, with the rapid changes in conditions due to the progressive march of civilization, the race will more and more be brought to the test as to its physical, mental, and moral status."[48] Musings on racial constitutions would continue to bear the residues of the ethnological, Lamarckian, polygenist, and evolutionist traditions that informed turn-of-the-century understandings of race, and would be enrolled in diverse calls for action throughout the era.[49] Advocates would continue to contest suggestions that blacks' constitutional differences were an excuse to do nothing to include them in public health efforts.[50]

The other discourse in which black disease and health was being worked out was with regard to infection. Of course, infectiousness has continued to be mobilized in demarcating racial others, especially with regard to AIDS both within the United States and globally, and policing a racialized divide between what Charles Briggs and Clara Mantini-Briggs have called "sanitary citizenship" and "unsanitary subjects" remains a central organizing principle of many public health efforts.[51] But at the start of the twentieth century, infectiousness was at the foreground of articulations of black disease both by racist theorists and by advocates for black health. As Haraway points out, in the early decades of the twentieth century, "race—and its venereal infections and ties to sexual hygiene—was real, fundamental, bloody."[52] Attempts to mete out the relative importance of constitution and environment in the infectiousness of blacks[53] did not contest the deep imbrications of blackness and infectiousness. Both medical literature and the social movements around black health in the period were preoccupied with black sickness as infectious, and enrolled notably double-edged slogans such as "Germs have no color line."[54]

Diverse political narratives and agendas could draw on this preoccupation with blacks as infectious. It might be a justification for white paternalism, on the grounds that only by making sure that blacks lived in sanitary conditions could whites be safe from infection passed on by them.[55] The figure of blacks as an infectious menace was profoundly stigmatizing,[56] yet the connection between blackness and infection cannot be simply dismissed as an invention of white supremacists. Evelynn Hammonds and Rebecca Herzig, both historians of race and science, have emphasized how entangled racial fears and hopes can be,[57] and this was certainly true at the intersection of blackness and infectiousness in the early twentieth century. Those who sought to fundraise for black public health efforts and black hospitals also appealed to white self-interest. One appeal enrolled "constitution" in a different sense than the embodied one, by using terms from the Fifteenth Amendment to the U.S. Constitution, adopted after the Civil War: "Disease germs are the most democratic creatures in the world; they know no distinction of 'race, color, or previous condition of servitude.' The white race and the black race will continue to live side by side in the South, and whatever injuriously affects the health of one race is deleterious to the other also. Disease among the negroes is a danger to the entire population."[58] This framing is central to the work of the Rosenwald Fund, which would be a philanthropic center for black hospitals and a source of claims such as "Bacteria have a disconcerting fashion of ignoring segregation edicts."[59] Of course black uplift and white philanthropy could work together. The National Negro Health Week Movement, which Booker T. Washington had founded shortly before his death in 1915 as the "National Health Improvement Week" and which grew through the 1920s into an influential mass movement, played up dire assessments of black poor health in order to spur both black mobilization for sanitary uplift and white philanthropic support.[60] This is a particularly American form of what Adriana Petryna terms *biological citizenship*, in which "the damaged biology of a population has become the grounds for social membership and the basis for staking citizenship claims."[61] The citizenship claim here is at once explicitly democratic and deeply racialized.

In the context of mass mobilization around black infectious disease, there were glimmers of interest in black degenerative disease. Although most of the articulations of degenerative disease as paradigmatic of the future were either explicitly or implicitly white, even by the 1930s advocates for black health started to suggest that African Americans were making the same transition away from infectious and toward degenerative disease. For example, noting that blacks' syphilis rates were declining, physicians at Howard University argued for "increasing attention to the diseases of metabolism, 'wear and tear,' of degeneration."[62] Staking a claim for African Americans as suffering from degenerative disease was part of articulating a place for that population in the future.

Contesting Scientific Medicine's Exclusions

One reason that it was important to posit a place for African American patients in modern disease experience was that doing so would posit a place for African American physicians in modern medical practice. The way that lines around the profession of scientific medicine have been drawn is crucial to understanding the terrain into which cardiologists such as Richard Allen Williams are intervening.

As a widely shown Coca-Cola advertisement for Black History Month in 2007 publicized, the first person to perform successful open-heart surgery, in 1893, was a black man.[63] He was Daniel Hale Williams, who had founded

Chicago's Provident Hospital two years before. He would go on to be a founding member of the National Medical Association two years later. In 1913, Daniel Hale Williams was inducted into the American College of Surgeons, which was the sole body that conferred specialist status for surgeons at the time. It took another two decades before another black man would be admitted (Louis T. Wright in 1934). The demographics of cardiac surgeons was contingent, deliberate, and exclusive. As late as 1945, a would-be applicant to the American College of Surgeons received the response "Fellowship in the College is not conferred on members of the Negro race at the present time," and though the decision was reversed, a requirement to be a member of the local American Medical Association branch continued to effectively close access for many black physicians in the South.[64] Cardiac surgery, insofar as it became white and male during the ascendance of the fields of both cardiology and surgery, did not become so because white men were the only ones with ambitions or interests in the area. Cardiac surgery has been a site of the racialized historical processes of technology, standardization, and professionalization that shaped the unequal access to training and practice of modern medicine in the United States.

Access to the machines and specialized training of emerging specialties such as cardiology depended on access to specialized technology, and to modern hospitals. As the historian of medicine Christopher Lawrence has argued, the electrocardiograph was important in distinguishing heart disease from other disease and cardiology as a specialty.[65] Historians of cardiology in a more celebratory vein have also emphasized the role of the electrocardiograph in contributing to the "mystique of the new specialty."[66] The increasing role of technology in defining disease generally and heart disease in particular might be seen as progress of the rational over the irrational, or loss of a more human practice of medicine,[67] but access to technology became a prerequisite for the practice of modern medicine. If Foucault crucially alerted us that changes in medical knowledge should be understood not simply as an increase in knowledge but as a reorganization of what is thought to be knowable,[68] these transformations also have implications for *who* can make knowledge. The intertwined aspects of that technology and the professionalization of the field of cardiology are part of a broader professionalization and standardization of technologically sophisticated medicine that effectively excluded most African American physicians from cardiology.

These modernizing processes set exclusionary boundaries around who could practice specialized medicine in scientific hospitals, and black health movements responded in plural ways. Here we can see another way in which boundary work is operating, between those diseases requiring merely hygienic or well-established basic medical interventions and those providing a mandate for professional, scientific medicine. At stake was whether blacks could be included among the elite doctors of the American hospital system, whether a black physician could be what Rosemary Stevens has described as "the modern doctor, associated with the new hospitals, [who] was—and is—a master engineer, a hero in the American mode, fighting diseases with twentieth-century tools."[69]

Professional, scientific medicine was increasingly exclusive. In the wake of the 1910 Flexner Report, a landmark in the professionalization of medical education in the United States, five of the seven medical schools that had trained blacks closed. Flexner himself did think that there was a role for black physicians, but that it was not as full members of the modern medical community, but as humanitarian servants of their "own race" and as sentinels against black infection seeping into white communities. Flexner thought black physicians' role would be limited in two key ways: they would serve only blacks, and their mandate would be to protect whites from black dangers. He argued that although "medical care of the negro race will never be wholly left to negro physicians," "the negro must be educated not only for his own sake, but for ours."[70] The public health scholar David Barton Smith encapsulates Flexner's take this way: "Germs may not have a color line, but medical practice should."[71] The ideological model Smith describes here is one that will continue in the later periods described in this book: white doctors are framed as having access to knowledge about all groups and types of diseases, while black doctors are imagined to only have more limited knowledge of their own community which is neither scientific nor generalizable. Because black doctors were conceptualized as only treating black patients, part of what is at stake in the discursive intervention that African Americans, too, get coronary disease, is an argument that African Americans are appropriate practitioners of fully modern medicine.

Flexner's framing of the limited scope of black practice spurred social movement responses. A central part of the black hospital movement and nascent movement for civil rights in medical care was the fight for access for black physicians to practice fully modern medicine in fully modern hospitals. Some efforts aimed to set up and support black hospitals that would meet the new accreditation standards, where black physicians could be trained; and others sought to integrate mainstream institutions, where black physicians could be trained alongside whites.[72] Uniting both of these efforts was a sense that the needs of black patients and those of black doctors could not be separated.

Those who built black hospitals were put on the defensive for "fostering seg-regation" by vocal integrationists such as Louis T. Wright.[73] Wright thought that any efforts to make distinctions between the needs of black patients and those of white ones would hurt the claims to equality of black practitioners and of the whole community.[74] On the other hand, as the historian Vanessa Worthington Gamble describes, many physicians thought that "separate in-stitutions were necessary because integration was a slow process and the ill health of the race demanded immediate solutions."[75] No matter which avenue was pursued, although the emphasis on black infectiousness had been useful for gaining funds for black hospitals, it was not as useful for demanding sufficient resources to engage in scientific medicine.

Whether they were advocating improvements in black hospitals or integra-tion into mass institutions, as black physicians sought to expand their scope beyond hygiene, it became important to argue that black patients required the same advanced treatments that white patients did. Black physicians and their supporters emphasized that a black doctor needed access to hospitals in order to have access to the advances of "medical science" and "keep abreast of the times, in order to enable his patients to enjoy the advantages of modern meth-ods of treatment,"[76] in a "modern hospital" that "affords wonderful oppor-tunities for physicians to develop a special knowledge of the several branches of medicine,"[77] and that it was important that they be "modernly equipped."[78] Thus, as Gamble argues, when black physicians mobilized around a black hospital reform movement, they sought to improve black hospitals and train-ing both in service of "the black masses" and to promote "their own profes-sional interests."[79]

The symbolic subordination that critical race theorists have suggested was deeply intertwined with material subordination for the black masses had an impact on black elites as well.[80] In the privileged zone of scientifically minded physicians, the symbolic subordination of excluding black physicians from the most modern hospitals threatened to exclude them from the entire sphere. Jim Crow deeply constrained the ability of those that a 1924 article in the *Journal of the National Medical Association* described as the "goodly number of men" who strove to be "a worthy asset to any group of medical scientists."[81] The demands that black patients and black doctors needed access to technologically ad-vanced hospitals were deeply intertwined.

Preoccupation Endures amid the Rise in Statistical Thinking

Physicians and public health advocates were not the only ones making arguments about which diseases were relevant for African American patients and practitioners. It was also a time of the ascendance of a modern mode of statistics from the life insurance industry, which would work through ideas about racial differences in distinctive ways. Life insurance methods would play an important role in the shape of heart disease research to come (for example, in the Framingham Heart Study, the subject of the next chapter).[82]

First, a caveat: the early data about black-white differences in heart disease rates are not at all reliable. Among other problems, unequal access to health care meant unequal representation in health data, diagnostic categories were unstable, and bias among those making diagnoses led them to see the racially differentiated rates they expected to see. But the drive toward what Jones has called the "rationalization of disparities" is a symptom of preoccupation with racial difference in concepts of disease.[83] Like Jones, I focus "not on diseases themselves but on beliefs about diseases and disparities,"[84] and the durability of the beliefs that there must be a difference between blacks and whites at the level of heart disease says more about the continued importance of race in America than it does about bodies past or present.

In the same period as the emergence of cardiology, a growing body of data was emerging from the life insurance industry that would both lay the foundation for heart disease research to come and articulate race in particular ways. Louis I. Dublin, a statistician for Metropolitan Life Insurance, was particularly innovative epistemologically, developing approaches to observational study that were methodologically sophisticated enough to resemble studies performed decades later.[85] He wrote several articles about race and disease, starting with "Factors in American Mortality: A Study of Death Rates in the Race Stocks of New York State, 1910," published in 1916, which found that the death rate of immigrants of various European groups was much higher than that of native-born whites.

Dublin became increasingly focused on black-white difference later, in articles that both speculate about racial adaptation and innovate in mathematical modeling. In a 1928 piece, Dublin described tuberculosis as the leading cause of death among black policy holders and noted that heart disease was a close second.[86] He would develop these ideas further, and his 1937 article titled "The Problem of Negro Health as Revealed by Vital Statistics" is a particularly interesting window into emerging articulations. On the one hand, Dublin suggests that the excessive deaths for each age and sex group of blacks is related to their poor adaptation to the North American environment. And yet, he notes progress that seems to contradict that constitutional claim. He notes that in the two decades before his report there had been a striking decline in black death rates such that "there would have been almost ten thousand more deaths of colored policyholders than actually occurred, in 1935, if the 1911 rate had prevailed."[87] Describing the statistics in terms of an average black person, the statistician also broke down the numbers in this way: "His expectation of life in 1930 was the same as that of the white man about thirty years earlier."[88] "The Negro death rates for practically all diseases in which care and sanitation are of paramount importance are much higher than among whites. It is probably that their higher death rate is due more than anything to ignorance, poverty, and lack of proper medical care. Pulmonary tuberculosis, tuberculosis, typhoid fever, pellagra, malaria, and puerperal conditions are examples of such diseases in which the mortality rates are much affected by unfavorable or insanitary environment—or by low economic status—and all of them have higher death rates among Negroes."[89] This situation was held to be in contrast with whites, whose diseases were of the mind and nerves, including heart disease with nervous etiology, rather than the lungs. Dublin bolstered his own data with an army study in which blacks had "only half as many cases of functional cardiac disturbances of nervous origin" as whites. Even though Dublin wrote that in 1935 "organic heart disease was the leading cause of death among the colored Industrial policyholders of the Metropolitan Life Insurance Company," and their rate was at 1.5 times that of whites, tuberculosis is highlighted in this report as "an outstanding cause of death among Negroes."[90] Thus there is a disconnect between what was an "outstanding cause of death" and what was merely the current "leading cause of death." Preoccupations with racial difference permeated even insurance, a field that is iconic for its rationality, such that the principal contributor to high death rates in blacks was still seen as atypical of them.

Dublin's study and others like it were taken up by others interested in articulating racial difference in disease. For example, S. J. Holmes, a zoology professor from the University of California, quoted Dublin when he included heart disease in his long list of black illnesses. In a 1937 article otherwise dominated by discussion of infectious diseases such as tuberculosis, he included one paragraph on heart disease. He noted that the black death rate was higher than the white one, and included diverse etiologies of organic heart disease to account for the disparity, yet he highlighted infectious cases within the heart disease category: "According to Dublin, 'it is especially among the colored patients that syphilitic heart disease is prevalent; in this group it accounts for about a third of the cases.' Davidson and Thoroughman, as a result of their studies, find over 25 per cent of positive Wassermanns in Negro heart cases conclude that 'syphilitic heart disease causes the greatest amount of disability next to the arteriosclerotic group.'"[91] The phrasing here around syphilis is seductive, but it is peculiar. Holmes's source acknowledged that syphilitic heart disease was the *second* biggest portion of heart disease among blacks, "next to" the category that was actually the biggest, and yet did not undermine the suggestion of syphilis's centrality. It was already considered established that blacks had a higher rate of syphilis in general, and of syphilitic heart disease in particular.[92] That the now-infamous Tuskegee Syphilis Study documented heart disease among the array of pathologies resulting from untreated syphilis[93] illustrates the association between blackness and syphilitic heart disease, and statistics about other heart diseases would not jar that preoccupation. This is of a piece with what Ann Laura Stoler has called "imperial dispositions of disregard": "'ignorance' versus 'acceptance' fails to capture the complex psychic space, tacit ambivalences, and implicit ambiguities" of historical actors grappling with difference.[94] Here, the preoccupation with infectious disease and sexual hygiene allowed the numerically greater killer to be simultaneously acknowledged and disregarded. Data cannot solve this problem of racial difference at the center of cardiological taxonomy.

Debating the Past in/and the Present

On November 15, 1915, a front-page obituary in the *New York Times* reported the death of Booker T. Washington, the most prominent black leader of the turn of the twentieth century: "Booker T. Washington, foremost teacher and leader of the negro race, died early today at his home here, near the Tuskegee Institute, which he founded and of which he was president. Hardening of the arteries, following a nervous breakdown, caused his death."[95] Yet in the weeks that followed, rumors circulated questioning the diagnosis of arteriosclerosis. One of Washington's physicians publicly stated that his illness and death had in fact been caused in part by "racial characteristics," a phrase that was widely perceived to be insinuating that Washington had died due to syphilis.[96] Both the indiscretion of his doctor and the facts of the case were contested at the time, and have provided fodder for historical analysis.[97]

In 2006, a review of Washington's medical records was conducted by a team that included a historian, a hypertension specialist, and an infectious disease specialist, with the support and cooperation of Washington's descendants.[98] What was the appeal of such a project? Arguments about racialized medical narratives in the past matter for racialized medical narratives in the present. As Hannah Landecker has elegantly shown in her account of the retellings of the origin and nature of the HeLa cell line, stories about the woman whose cells are now immortalized, Henrietta Lacks, become ways to tell contemporary stories of both bioscience and race.[99] In the reopening of Booker T. Washington's file, there was no compelling immortal line to grapple with, but it might analogously be an opportunity to reopen inscriptions of race in century-old medicine as a route to telling stories about contemporary medicine.

In the report of their reinvestigation, published in the *Journal of Clinical Hypertension*, the investigators reviewed the facts from Washington's medical files in light of today's methods of diagnosis. Among the highlights included were his history of increasingly severe indigestion, fatigue, and headaches; his physical exam description as "a middle-aged African American man variously described as having the 'medium brown skin of a mulatto . . . luminous eyes . . . a rather Irish face . . . and the odd look of an Italian'"; eye and heart abnormalities; very high blood pressure; and a negative Wasserman (syphilis) test.[100] They reached the conclusion: "Mr. Washington did not have syphilis. His negative Wasserman test proves that. Rather, as indicated in the hospital record made public for the first time in this conference, he had malignant hypertension, which destroyed his kidneys, damaged his heart, and eventually killed him."[101] In one sense, this article settles the debate. It uses data to claim a definitive diagnosis of hypertension in place of a suggested one of syphilis. But with regard to the larger question of whether Washington's death was related to "racial characteristics," it renders the debate unsettled: "Were 'racial characteristics . . . in part responsible'? The data reviewed by Dr. Wright suggest that, indeed, there might be endogenous factors peculiar to African Americans that are responsible, at least in part, for the common occurrence of hypertension and its adverse consequences."[102] Thus, the article both settles and unsettles the relationship between Booker T. Washington's race and his death, as well as the relationships between African American race and morbidity today. The authors did not reject racialized diagnosis per se, but replaced one outdated and highly stigmatized racialized diagnosis with a current less stigmatized one.

From this refashioned sense of "racial characteristics," the authors considered connections they saw as relevant today: implications for treatment, and the role of genetics. The new diagnosis was performed by a prominent black hypertension specialist, Jackson T. Wright, who took the opportunity both to consider the case at hand and to expound upon the challenge of African American hypertension generally. Noting that in 1915 there was neither effective treatment for hypertension nor even the awareness of the need for treatment, Wright pointed out that despite our increased knowledge and tools, blood pressure control remains a challenge today, "especially in black populations." Wright took the opportunity to promote intervention in the present to decrease heart disease risk among African Americans today: he offered pragmatic advice for effective treatment through multidrug therapy, weight loss, exercise, and salt restriction. Wright offered an array of possible explanations for the disparity, such as socioeconomic status, environmental factors, biomarkers, and "a yet-to-be-characterized genetic susceptibility."[103] Wright's focus was on the facts of disparities and treatment avenues, remaining agnostic on etiology: "Hypertension arises more often and at an earlier age, is more severe, and causes more target organ damage in African Americans than whites, for reasons that are nearly as uncertain in 2007 as in 1915."[104] He concluded: "Hypertension shortened the life of Booker T. Washington, just as it continues to do in poorly treated hypertension patients."[105]

Of all of the possible etiological factors Wright described, his coauthor Mackowiak singled out genetics for further comment, considering and then rejecting it as an explanation for African American hypertension. He noted the poor correlation between racial variation and genetic variation and then elaborated:

> Mr. Washington was the product of an African (slave) mother and a white father. If his "rather Irish face" or "odd look of an Italian" were indicative of his father's heritage, would he not have been as Irish American or Italian American as an African American in terms of his genetic composition (ie, his "racial characteristics")? In view of such ambiguities, it is no wonder we are not much closer today than we were in 1915 to understanding why hypertension singled out this prominent American or why it continues to be so severe a problem for African Americans.[106]

There is an absurdity in the suggestion that mixed parentage could possibly make Washington—who was born into racial slavery and became a major black leader in the early twentieth century—"as Irish American" as he was African American. It reveals the way in which race is ideological, in Barbara Fields's sense, emerging in a "context that tells people which details to notice, which to ignore, and which to take for granted in translating the world around them into ideas about that world."[107] In the incommensurability between Washington's context and Mackowiak's context, we can see the ways in which race, despite its durability, is not a single transhistorical thing.

I am more interested in what happens next: the positioning of "genetic composition" and "racial characteristics" around an "ie" in this analysis is a tantalizing construction of a transhistorical synonym. The preoccupation with "racial characteristics" has not changed, but what holds the place opposite "racial characteristics" has changed: infection, related to hygiene, constitutional susceptibility, and immorality, has been displaced by hypertension that is somehow related to genetics.

The time span between Booker T. Washington's death and its reinvestigation is the same as that of this book, and the intervening space serves as my terrain. The changing assessment of his cause of death and its meanings has a similar trajectory to that of my book's narrative. The concept of racial characteristics remains durable even as the content of those characteristics has changed, and Booker T. Washington remains "racially characteristic." In this awkward transformation we can see both the malleability and the durability of preoccupations with race in diagnosis. The diagnosis is durable enough to allow Wright to use it as a basis from which to advocate for treatment in the present, even as it continues to harbor unsettled epistemological quandaries. As we will see in later chapters, Wright's commitment to treatment of hypertension, with a special emphasis on black hypertension, is his life's work. Attention to the intervening space between the 1915 attempts to diagnose the death of Booker T. Washington and the recent reinvestigation provides an opportunity to map out new and renewed arguments about racial difference in heart disease and the contested ramifications thereof for medical practitioners and for other social spheres.

Continuing Contestation

Debunking black immunity to coronary disease has been part of the mission of antiracist cardiologists for decades,[108] and it has long been part of Richard Allen Williams's project. In his landmark 1975 *Textbook of Black-Related Diseases*, Williams refuted claims of a white monopoly on angina in the early literature of black-white disparities in heart disease. He attributed earlier underdiagnosis to poor patient-history gathering from black patients, and flagged the frequency of "indigestion" as a cause of black deaths as particularly specious. Referring to the 1965 National Health Survey, he noted, "It is interesting to note that the National Health Survey indicated that angina pectoris may actually be *more* common in Blacks than in Whites."[109] Williams was confident that new research was righting past errors, yet he too used a rhetoric of surprise when noting that angina was more common in blacks. His use of the word "actually" and the italicization he puts onto *more* marks preoccupation, signaling the embedded idea that blacks have less angina than whites even as he refutes it.

Writing their mammoth history in 2002, physicians Michael Byrd and Linda Clayton mark the 1980s and '90s as the era when "medical myths about coronary heart disease (CHD) in Blacks were dispelled conclusively for the first time." They cite the findings of *The Report of the Secretary's Task Force on Black and Minority Health*:

1 Instead of CHD being uncommon in Blacks, CHD is the leading cause of death in U.S. Blacks;
2 Instead of acute myocardial infarction (AMI) being rare in Blacks, AMI hospitalization rates are high in Blacks with higher case fatality rates than Whites.
3 Despite the myth of angina being rare in Blacks, they have high prevalence rates of angina in the United States.
4 Despite the myth of a White preponderance of CHD compared to Blacks, U.S. CHD mortality and prevalence rates are similar in Black and White males, with Black females having higher CHD mortality and prevalence rates than White females.
5 Despite the myth that Blacks are immune to CHD, they proved to be relatively susceptible in the United States.[110]

The grammar of "myths" in these protestations is revealing. Byrd and Clayton use "myth" in the sense of falsehood, but their text also carries a valence of "myth" as founding story of a people. As ordinary as they insist that black coronary disease is, they call attention to the whiteness of the diagnosis in the minds of many clinicians. The grammar of exception is a symptom of preoccupation, and reinforces whiteness as the original model of the diagnosis of coronary disease.

Racial profiling in medicine has become for the most part statistical rather than universalizing—few self-respecting medical scientists today would claim the nonexistence of any given disease in this or that population, even as it is commonplace to use differences in prevalence to make arguments that function in much the same way. Even the most ardent BiDil believer never suggested so strong a binary that would perfectly and neatly segregate the races as easily as Paul Dudley White did in his comment to his student Richard Allen Williams. And yet knowledge generated in the postwar period did not *replace* that from early cardiologists such as Paul Dudley White—indeed, White himself was an early advisor to the Framingham Heart Study. White has been said to have brought the idea for the study back from Britain, where his teacher Sir James MacKenzie had envisioned a longitudinal study in order to find "the beginnings of illness."[111] Framingham would take the field in these more statistical directions. But as new forms of knowledge were added to old ones, overlapped with them, modified them, arguments about the nature of difference remain salient in heart disease research.

In an important sense, Williams's 1960s aspirations for black inclusion as coronary heart disease researchers and patients are continuous with those that inform more recent projects by black cardiologists, including the Jackson Heart Study and the study that led to BiDil. Staking a claim for the existence of African American coronary heart disease patients has been intertwined with staking a role for African Americans as cardiologists. Williams's intervention simultaneously rejects the exclusion of black patients from a central site of modern medicine, and the exclusion of black experts from the scientific inquiry into black disease. The racialization of modern American medicine's *subjects* and that of its *objects* need to be understood together. Ambitious African American physicians have long strived to be the *subjects* of medical progress, which is to say, practitioners of scientific medicine that contributes to the knowledge of the profession as a whole. One way they have bolstered that project is by claiming African Americans as the appropriate *objects* of medical progress: patients whose disease experiences are relevant for current research, and who should receive cutting edge care. Although the audience of physicians at the 2005 symposium laughed at earlier doubts that these things are true, the issues remain unsettled.

CHAPTER 2

Making Normal Populations and
Making Difference in the Framingham
and Jackson Heart Studies

I n June of 2006, the International Society for Hypertension in Blacks (ISHIB) marked its twentieth anniversary with a set of lectures during its annual conference. Charles Curry, then president of ISHIB, introduced the program with genial informal comments about how far the community had come, in terms of understanding how to prevent heart disease through intervening on risk factors. He pointed out that the risk factor was a concept that came from the Framingham Heart Study, before warmly introducing the next speaker, with a grin: "Our next speaker is Dr. Herman Taylor from the Jackson Heart Study. I usually call it the black Framingham."[1]

This introduction was well received, and warm applause welcomed Taylor to the stage. And the phrase is evocative. If there is a "black Framingham," then what is the original Framingham Heart Study? Does the landmark study that has become a touchstone for heart disease research in the second half of the twentieth century lack race, or is it white? How was its racial identity constructed historically, and how has it been negotiated as the study has become invoked as a standard in evidence-based medicine?

When Herman Taylor laid out the context for his own study in Jackson, Mississippi, he described the Framingham Study in a familiar way: "The Framingham Heart Study was ingenious. It took a very simple idea and ultimately resulted in a change in our approach to cardiovascular disease. It took a typical American town, mostly at that time it was second-generation immigrants, but a typical American town to look at in a microscopic way, at what might be the underpinnings of this unchecked epidemic. The concept of the risk factor that we all use commonly every day was actually developed at Framingham, [and] led to the golden age of cardiology."[2] But as he reviewed the familiar historical trajectory of cardiovascular mortality, which rose from the beginning of the twentieth century to its peak in the immediate postwar period and then declined, he noted that this "golden age" only seems like a global success story. It hides what he called a "critical subplot," that there are portions of the population that do not share in this turnaround in mortality—particularly African Americans, especially in Mississippi. He described these disparities as "an embarrassment to us as a nation," and a mandate for his own study. He continued: "I always enjoy comparison to the Framingham, because Framingham has done so much for understanding of the cardiovascular disease epidemic. We can only hope to approach that kind of record. The future of the Jackson Heart Study, I believe is in this local and global idea."[3] In Taylor's invocation, Framingham emerges as both a particular kind of place—a typical one, a white one, an immigrant one, a 1950s one—and a particular kind of knowledge—local with global implications.

By going back chronologically to attend to Framingham's early racial frameworks, we can see the work that was put into constructing Framingham's racial and ethnic identity as a window into its epistemological innovation. Its unmarked whiteness was not inevitable or natural. Rather, it was a contingent and emergent aspect shaped by intersections of old racialized diagnoses; old and new notions of whiteness; and new notions of how to manage difference in epidemiological research. As I will show, the investigators did not simply start with an undifferentiated standard white human sample from which to extrapolate, but rather constructed one through two moves: (1) the disavowal of the concept of representation and (2) the use of within-group differences as a way to produce scientifically useful knowledge that could be extrapolated beyond the group. They articulated changing concepts of whiteness in each of those moves, articulating new and renewed relationships between whiteness and cardiovascularized modernity.

Part of the story that I am telling is a democratizing one: the expansion of the purview of the field of cardiology from elite men in the founding of cardiology, to a larger multiethnic white population of men and women in the Framingham Heart Study, and on to a simultaneously fragmented and inclusive notion of the population that includes a diverse black population in the Jackson Heart Study. Through these moments in the history of heart disease research, we can see the expansion and fragmentation of the idea of who lives a modern American way of life. In this changing scope of coronary disease, one thing that has been at stake has been who could stand in as "typical," "normal," and "American" enough such that they could serve as a population from which to extrapolate a field of research.

Seeing Framingham in relief with the Jackson Heart Study allows us to see how Framingham and Jackson both posit their populations not necessarily as "typical," but as "typical enough"—or, as we will see, in the terms of an early Framingham investigator, "not grossly atypical." At their inception, both were framed as simultaneously racialized and yet sufficiently relevant to provide a basis for broadly applicable knowledge. Both studies rely on the insight that no single population can tell everything, but that any population studied in sufficient detail can tell *something*.

Yet I will also attend to the ways in which Jackson is not a simple repetition of the Framingham Study. Jackson's study design opens the question of the relationship between representation and extrapolation further. Jackson has not replaced Framingham, which continues, but is adding to it. It also is a self-consciously postmodern innovation taking off from it, a repetition with a difference that is not simply derivative. The Jackson investigators are theoretically engaged and making striking epistemological interventions, at the same time that they stake out terrain for African Americans as objects and subjects of an iconic form of medical study. For Jackson, observation is enrolled in intervention, and "typical," "normal," and "American" are each plural concepts.

Making Framingham "Normal"

The Framingham Heart Study was begun in 1948 under the auspices of the U.S. Public Health Service before transferring shortly thereafter to the National Heart Institute (now the National Heart, Lung, and Blood Institute, NHLBI). It ambitiously sought to follow a large population of residents of Framingham, Massachusetts, for two decades, and has continued well beyond. Originally recruiting 5,209 middle-aged Framingham residents, it expanded in 1971 to add a similarly sized cohort of their children, and is now adding a third generation to the biannual research visits.[4] Its goal has been to find connections between lifestyle (including diet and smoking), test results (including blood pressure and cholesterol), and heart disease incidence. In the immediate postwar period, heart disease was increasingly prominent as a cause of death and as a preoccupation, and together with other studies that used a range of other approaches,[5] Framingham grappled with how to answer the questions that had been raised in the interwar period but could not yet be answered, developing new ways to ask and answer questions about the challenges of modern strain, modern lifestyles, and modern medicine. It has come to be a landmark in longitudinal research, epidemiology, and concepts of heart disease.

The 1947 proposal is still recognizable as what the project would become: "This project is designed to study the expression of coronary artery disease in a normal or unselected population and determine the factors predisposing to the development of the disease through laboratory experimentation and long-term followup of such a group."[6] The terms "normal" and "unselected" refer to the status of the population as "free of disease." The Framingham Heart Study is iconic of an approach that arose in the early 1950s, especially impor-tant in the study of coronary heart disease: looking longitudinally and pro-spectively at "normal" populations.[7]

Yet normality is an elusive concept in medicine, even though the binary between normal and pathological is foundational to medical thinking.[8] Study-ing healthy populations—rather than ones selected because they already had a particular disease of interest to investigators—was an innovation that reversed the lens of pathology. One part of understanding the kind of knowledge claims made by the Framingham Study is as an early iteration of what Joseph Dumit has described as a shift from seeing the body as inherently healthy with need of occasional intervention to restore that natural health, to one always at multiple risk for disease and in need of preventive health care.[9] The principal biostatistician of the early study would go on to define "free of disease" as a locution of convenience, but a state fundamentally impossible to prove given its reliance on the limitations of the technologies of surveillance.[10] For both epistemological and practical reasons, the investigators in practice did not strictly exclude those found on examination to have disease.[11] In an important sense, defining "normal" as "free of disease" meant defining "normal" as "at risk for disease."

From the start, there was a slippage between normal as healthy and normal as representative of those at risk. In an early undated draft of a description of the Heart Disease Epidemiology Study (which would become Framingham), its founding director, Gilcin Meadors, wrote: "There is of course no ideal or per-fect sample of the population in this country. Such a population would have the same distribution of such characteristics as race, sex, occupation, economic status, rural and urban location, and age as the general population. It is of less importance to have such a sample than to record rather accurately the charac-teristics of the group studied. To simplify the interpretation of results, how-ever, a community with fair representation of the main characteristics would be desirable."[12] What are the bounds around concepts such as "fair representation" and "main characteristics?" Who is eligible to be "normal?" Here, we can see a slippage between what is meant by "normal and unselected": between being "free of disease," and being a "fair representation."

One thing that made Framingham a "fair representation" of "main characteristics" is that the town's population was imagined to be at risk. Observation of a healthy population made the study more time-consuming, since investigators would have to wait longer for events of interest to occur in sufficient numbers to be reportable. And so even at Framingham, subjects who were considered to be at risk for coronary disease were the ones selected: the city was overwhelmingly white, and only the middle-aged were recruited. It is notable here that although race was routinely mentioned as a characteristic that might matter, the fact that the population chosen for the study was all white would not be understood as an important limitation. This point connects to the racialization of coronary heart disease discussed in the previous chapter. Infectious causes of heart disease were included in the scope of Framingham, and hypertension as etiology was included as one of many hypotheses, but the focus was squarely on the heart disease category understood as white: coronary heart disease. This would not by itself preclude investigators from studying blacks or others imagined to be at lower risk for coronary disease—after all, investigators included women in part to see what it was that might be protecting them. Yet it does set the scope of the relevant subjects of study.

The sense of the "normal" that was particularly relevant for early investigators was the sense of familiar and convenient. The selection of the town was made less for representation than for stability and the amenability of the population—as well as easy commuting distance from Harvard. This description from an interim report by the early Framingham investigators Thomas Dawber and Felix Moore describes the sample selection characteristically:

> The town of Framingham cannot itself, of course, be regarded as a sample. It was picked with the advice of Dr. Vlado A. Getting, Health Commissioner of the Commonwealth of Massachusetts and Dr. David D. Rutstein, Professor of Preventative Medicine, Harvard University Medical School, because it was of the desired size to yield the required number of persons; it was close to a medical center; it contained both industrial and rural areas, and some assurance had been received that the townspeople, both lay and medical, would be willing to cooperate. In short, it was a place where such a study could be done, and it was not grossly atypical in any respect that appeared relevant.[13]

This concept of *not grossly atypical* was an innovation in understanding the applicability of biomedical knowledge, and can be read as a precursor to what Steven Epstein has described as the "creation of the standard human."[14] It provides an example of the phenomenon that Epstein observes, as well as extending it to consider how much work it takes to get people to look "not grossly atypical" before they can plausibly stand in as "standard."

Thus, aspects of "normal" at the study's inception included: free of disease, demographically relevant to the disease in question, and familiar and convenient to investigators. Yet the "normal population" studied in Framingham would be posited not so much as already standard, but rather as *standardized*. Once a subject was in the study, a change in status along any of these axes did not disqualify a participant from the "normal." Onset of illness, shifts in assessment of the subject's demographic risk categorization, or relocation far from investigators—none of these caused a subject to become excluded. Whether the participants in the Framingham Heart Study were ever normal in the sense of either "representative" or "ideal" would remain unsettled. The Framingham sample was never representative even of the town in which it was situated—undercounting the sick and the uncooperative, for example[15]—much less the whole country or world. By creating an epistemological model that contrasted cases and controls according to set characteristics, the risk factors identified at Framingham have turned out to hold up very well in studies in other populations around the world. But once the Framingham subjects had been charted according to established characteristics, they would become "normal" in the sense that they could be a standard from which to extrapolate.

The disavowal of "normal" as "representative" was never complete, however, and in the historiography of Framingham the tension between normal and representative is often lost as Framingham stands in for 1950s nostalgia. Framingham's popular historiography invokes it not only as normal in the senses I have discussed, but also as a *representative* American town. For example, a 1973 *New York Times Magazine* article described it this way: "In the history of the growing awareness that heart attack is associated with certain traits and habits characteristic of affluent civilization, there stands one great scientific landmark—the Framingham study. Framingham, Mass., is a gray factory town surrounded by pleasant suburbs 21 miles from Boston. As a town whose 28,000 residents in 1949 were ethnically and sociologically representative of the American population, it was a logical candidate for the Heart Disease Epidemiology Study of the National Heart Institute."[16] Descriptions of postwar Framingham ring familiar because of their conformance with 1950s stereotype. Daniel Levy, the study's current principal investigator, and his coauthor Susan Brink describe the town in these terms: an independent town, with a largely middle-class population who had become homeowners through the GI Bill, a GM plant, a shopping mall, and a "typical" ethnic mix of (Euro-)Americans, of average weight and diet.[17] There was even a Hostess factory, turning out Twinkies and Wonder bread.

The way Levy and Brink describe this postwar environment is of a piece with 1950s white Americana. For Levy and Brink, a "middle-class" town is "typical," and their account has a palpable nostalgia for an era in which it was possible to imagine that we were all in it together, before the civil rights movement and the War on Poverty exposed American society's ongoing fissures. If there were particular dangers imagined to lurk in the town they did not consist of its inequities, but in the lifestyle made possible by its "life-threatening prosperity."[18]

Many have been critical of the notion of Framingham's status as representative of the United States, precisely because life in the town was of a piece with postwar Americana rather than typical of a complicated society amid transition. For example, the psychologist James Lynch has written that although in "its ethnic, social, and economic mixes it appeared to be mainstream American—a model city, so to speak, for medical research," Framingham only "seemed average."[19] According to Lynch, Framingham's population of "hard working, mostly white, mostly middle class" "churchgoing, nondivorcing type people"[20] was extraordinarily settled and stable. This stability was both something useful for the researchers and atypical of America.

Levy and Brink highlight ethnicity in their account, rendering Framingham as "representative of latter day demographics."[21] They describe the "ethnic mix" of Framingham—"including roots in Poland, Ireland, Italy, Greece, French Canada, and England"—as "a reflection of European ancestry at the time."[22] Histories of whiteness have documented this consolidation of white American identity as simultaneously expanding the category of whiteness and solidifying the line between it and other categories.[23] Even though the Framingham cohort is not representative *now*, Levy and Brink imply, it once was. But this is an assertion that becomes easier to make in retrospect, and ignores the disavowals of representation by those who preceded Levy as Framingham investigators. Claims of representativeness might be easier to posit in the past than in any given present. Historical descriptions of Framingham become very much descriptions of *America* at a point in time, a place that is considered to be both specific and spreading, both through the assimilation of immigrants and the spread of the modern American lifestyle through globalization.[24]

Insofar as early investigators paid attention to the ethnic makeup of the town, it was not to ensure representativeness. An early manual of operation of the Framingham Study provides evidence that the investigators recognized the importance of understanding the demographic makeup of the town for logistical reasons, emphasizing that "in order to secure the active participation of people in a research program" it was necessary to ascertain "sociological and psychological factors" such as "economic status," "nationalities represented," "historical background," "superstitions," and "how . . . people feel about being part of a research program."[25] In print, the investigators put it this way: "As a start, a health educator was placed in the Health Department with the assignment of studying the community. This meant not only learning about the history, resources, and government of the town but, more important, getting to know the people—their national origins, economic conditions, and lines of social stratification; their religious, fraternal, and civic organizations; and their recognized and potential leaders."[26] The investigators were concerned about the specifics of the racial and ethnic makeup of the town, but after acknowledging these community aspects, they argued that these would not hinder the applicability of their findings to American whites at large. They were making a conceptual division between representation, which they disavowed, and extrapolation, which they embraced. Of all of the definitions of normal in play— free of disease, at risk for disease, convenient to investigators, representative of some larger whole, and coded according to standardized characteristics— the most fundamental was normal in the sense of a standard from which to extrapolate.

This distinction between representation and extrapolation would become critical in epidemiological research. Thomas Royle Dawber, who took over leadership of the study in 1949 and remained its director until 1966, participated in sharpening distinctions between representation and extrapolation. In a published report in 1951, the investigators suggested that while it might be optimal to do the study in many cities and across groups, it would be too expensive. Writing in the *American Journal of Public Health*, they pointed out: "Ideally, perhaps, epidemiological investigations of cardiovascular disease should be set up in a number of widely separated areas simultaneously, so that various racial and ethnic groups will be represented, and a variety of geographic, socioeconomic, and other environmental factors can be considered."[27] The two words that frame this sentence—"ideally" and "perhaps"—are both worth meditating upon, because it is in the space between them that the Framingham Heart Study takes place. These words acknowledged the ideal of an infinitely expansive notion of sample population that was circulating in the period. And yet, at the same time, they questioned the assumption that such a sample would be ideal, independent of whether it was realistic. They suggested that even if it were possible to have a purely representative sample, the data produced would not necessarily be better.

In this 1951 piece, the investigators defended their limited scope on practical grounds, but their scientific grounds for defense were not quite as well developed as they would become. Explaining that a smaller town was preferable to a big city "for the type of community approach required to secure full cooperation and coverage," they left open the possibility that until their findings were verified elsewhere they would not be generalizable: "This limitation in geographic coverage clearly limits the generality of conclusions which can be reached."[28]

Yet, in the very same 1951 article, the Framingham researchers suggested that their findings might be capable of being extrapolated after all—but only as far as "the white race." The investigators used the term "community" to describe Framingham rather than the more scientific-sounding "population" or "sample" used earlier by Meadors, but made a statistical argument for extrapolatability to all those of diverse European ancestries included in the postwar definition of "white": "There is, however, reasonable basis for the belief that the distribution of arteriosclerosis and hypertension *in the white race* in the United States is such that within-community variance is greater than between-community variance, and a wide range of type-situations influencing development of these diseases may be found in any community."[29] After an article that had considered difference along many possible axes—regional, socioeconomic, "other environmental"—the only axis of difference that remained worthy of mention was whiteness. The fact that they were using an argument that is familiar in form to arguments about interracial and intraracial difference today should alert us that it is not that mode of argument itself that is effective or not in closing the debate, but that its effectiveness depends on its alignment with other modes of defining racial difference. Yet this homogeneous whiteness of the Framingham study was not a given at the outset of the study, but a conceptualization of the population that emerged and became stable over the 1950s and '60s.

Dawber would continue to caution throughout his career against overconcern about the ways in which a sample population is not representative of a whole, including in his 1980 book, which he meant to be the definitive summary of the study. He emphasized that a representative sample was both impossible and unnecessary. He argued that finding "absolute incidence" of disease in the "entire selected sample" had "limited applicability" in part because of ethnicity "since the population of this New England town was in itself not totally representative of the United States. There were virtually no blacks or Orientals, and the composition of the white population was not necessarily that of white populations elsewhere." However, he argued, using scientific approaches to make comparisons within the group by well-defined characteristics would render random sampling superfluous: "Random sampling is not essential if the purpose of an epidemiologic study is to compare subgroups of the population determined by specific characteristics."[30]

Later in the same text, however, Dawber went further. He suggested that not only could risk factors found through scientific comparison between groups of Framingham participants be imagined to apply to Americans generally, but even their incidence of heart disorders could be extrapolated:

> In spite of these uncertainties, there appears to be good reason to accept the Framingham findings as a reasonable estimate of the actual incidence of the various disorders, with some obvious exceptions: there were too few black residents of Framingham to provide sufficient incidence data; the makeup of the white population was not completely representative of the U.S. white population; and there were more participants of Italian extraction than would be found in most communities in this country. However, unless national origin plays an important role (which apparently it does not), the data may be considered reasonably representative of the North American white population.[31]

In this quote, it was taken for granted that blacks (among other nonwhites) were not within the scope of extrapolation. And yet there is also something tantalizing in the brief mention of white national origin. When Dawber mentioned that national origin "apparently does not" play an important role, he glossed over the emergent processes that made that white functional homogeneity "apparent."[32]

Opening Framingham's Ethnic Black Box

In the invocations of connections between heart disease and race in the first few decades of the twentieth century tracked in the previous chapter, it seems clear that heart disease investigators thought they knew who they were talking about. But by the time of the founding of the Framingham Study, heart disease investigators were not quite as sure. There was a fracturing of whiteness in their categorization, as well as an embrace of its inclusivity. Both fracturing and inclusivity are part of articulating the intersections of race and heart disease in the period. In the historiography of the Framingham Heart Study, much has been made of how limited its collection of social data was—the historian of medicine Gerald Oppenheimer describes a "short shrift to the social dimensions": "Framingham limited social items in its baseline exam to subjects' names, addresses, educational attainment, and nationalities."[33] I want to suggest that on such a tiny list of social characteristics, the inclusion of "nationalities" of these U.S. residents demands further analysis. It provides a route to opening the black box around Framingham's whiteness.

It mattered that the Framingham sample was white in the sense that it would be a study of coronary disease, but at its inception the question remained open whether it mattered which kinds of whites they were. Unsettled racial imaginaries were encoded in the Framingham Heart Study's early intake forms. Analysis of them shows that the homogeneity of the whiteness of the sample was not simply a given, but was rather constructed iteratively in particular moments in time. An active and contingent process of simplifying and flattening makes the population legible, in James Scott's sense,[34] in its whiteness as much as in its other characteristics.

Between 1947 and 1951, the racial and ethnic coding on the subject intake forms was not stable. An early form marked "Set used April 1949—June 1950 for volunteers to clinic" had questions about both race and national origin.[35] Options for race had two checkboxes and a blank: "W, N, or OTHER (Specify)." Options for national origin had a simple fill-in-the-blank. One set of proposed codings for the race question looks similar to today's racial categories: "Race: 1-White, 2-Negro, 3-Other, 4-Unknown."[36] On the other hand, another proposed coding sheet in the same file has extraordinarily complex combinations for the race and national origin questions (see figure 1). This handwritten "personal history sheet" is extraordinarily eclectic. It codes race and sex together, but has separate lines for age, marital status, and education. Its national origin coding is very elaborate, with a high degree of specificity for describing not only the subject—who might be counted as a combination of nationalities — but also the national origin of each of the subject's parents and grandparents.

These coding practices seem never to have been actually implemented. The elaborate attempts suggest that it was not obvious how to fit something as complex as race and national origin into new modes of data recording; at a time when many medical publications were based on a few cases or a few hundred, it was not yet clear how to manage complex information on thousands of subjects. The Framingham Heart Study was extending the technological scope of medicine and heart disease by means mechanical and then computational.[37] The iterative process of charting and recharting coding options can be read as part of an emergent methodology. As Jon Agar has written with regard to the mechanical and then computational systems in British botany, the limited capacities of data storage necessarily simplify and distort representation and distribution—and even as data capacity increases, "the effect remains."[38]

A coherent order for recording national origin was arrived at by 1951. This might have been because a new researcher joined the Framingham team in 1949—Felix E. Moore, a quantitative sociologist with a talent for applied statistics and a veteran of the Census Bureau.[39] Yet Moore did not use census categories. On the new forms (see figure 2), there was no longer a question about race,[40] and categories of national origin were much less expansive and elaborated than those on the census forms of the same period.[41] The new forms would survive the 1950s and be coded onto punch cards for the multivariate analysis that would become so important in how Framingham would make its claims.[42] Race may have dropped out because the whiteness of the study population had already been established. With data processing as onerous as it was, there was some disincentive against including variables not expected to vary much. There was only one question about national origin, and it allowed for combinations to be punched in a much less unwieldy way than the one proposed above, even if it lost a great deal of detail by having the multiple punches entered "without specification as to which is which."

I will come back to the handwritten annotations, but for now want to think through what this manual instructs the coder to do. This column is noted to be "multiple punch," because the "National Origin" question was designed to accommodate more than one answer. First, the interviewer entered a number for the subject's place of birth. For most of the participants, that meant entering a "1" in the box, which indicated United States and Alaska, because the question was understood to be one not of indigeneity but of nativity. Then, if

Code For Data on Personal History Sheet

Col. 1-4   actual record number (0001 – 6000)

Col. 5-6   Race and sex :

     01 White male   02 White female   03 Negro male
     04 Negro female   05 Yellow male   06 Yellow female

Col. 7-8   actual age (29 – 59)

Col. 9   marital status

     0 Single   2 Married   3 Widowed
     4 Divorced   5 Separated

Col. 10   Education

     1 Grade school   2 High school   3 College
     4 Professional   5 ?   6 ?

Col. 11-12   national origin

     01 all U.S.
     02 U.S. and Gt. Britain
     03 U.S. and Ireland
     04 U.S. and Italy
     05 U.S. and Scandinavia
     06 U.S. and Germany or Holland
     07 U.S. and France
     08 U.S. and other
     09 all Gt. Britain or Ireland
     11 all Italy
     12 Gt. Britain or Ireland, and Italy
     13 British Isles and Scandanavia
     14 British Isles and Germany
     15 British Isles and France
     16

1. "Code for Data on Personal History Sheet." From the file Coding—First Examination. Framingham Heart Study, Framingham, Mass.

Col. 13   Place of birth of father

       0   U.S.
       1   Canada
       2   Gt. Britain
       3   Ireland
       4   Italy
       5   Scandanavia
       6   Germany or Holland
       7   Belgium, France, Spain or Portugal
       8   other European
       9   Other

col. 14   Place of birth of mother

       0
       :
       9

col 15   Place of birth of father's father

       0
       :
       9

Col 16   Place of birth of father's mother

       0
       :
       9

Col. 17   Place of birth of mother's father

       0
       :
       9

Col. 18   Place of birth of mother's mother

       0
       :
       9

```
Col 14      National Origin (multiple punch)
            This column is multiple-punch to include info on subject, parents
NOTE:       and grandparents--but without specification as to which is which
Col 14 is     1 - United States and Alaska
              2 - Great Britain, England, Scotland and Wales
blank on      3 - Ireland
Tape          4 - Italy
              5 - Scandinavia (includes Finland, Denmark, Norway, Sweden and
                    Iceland)
              6 - Germany
              7 - France
              8 - Canada (includes Nova Scotia, New Brunswick, Prince Edward
                    Island and Newfoundland)
              9 - Other
```

2. "Deck 05 Coding Manual." From Tape Coding Manual Book 2 (of 3).
File 06 in Papers of the NHLBI, Bethesda, Md.

ancestors were from a different country than the subject, a number correlated with that place was entered as well. There was no limit on how many numbers could be checked, so mixed ancestry could be accounted for.

Pre-U.S. ancestry categories from the coding sheet are limited to eight choices plus an "other." Remarkably, there were no options assigned here for Eastern Europeans. Many of Framingham's Eastern European immigrants were Jewish, and it may be that the postwar aversion to questions about religion led to the exclusion of the whole category. Another possibility is that the categories at Framingham were simply taken from somewhere else with a different demographic range.

In early coding, it was clear that the main interest was in "Native U.S." versus "Foreign Born," which is how an early spreadsheet filled in by hand breaks down the data.[43] Even though early coding showed that the group was heavily British (1,315 with British ancestry and 182 British born) and Irish (859 ancestry and 100 born), interest was strongest in Italian (400 ancestry and 235 born). I would speculate that interest in Italians was disproportionate to their representation in the sample because a relatively large portion was foreign born compared with other subgroups as well as with the United States at large.[44]

In the early 1960s, there were some comments about the Italianness of Framingham's sample in publications from the study. For example, a report about nutrition noted: "The foods called 'Pasta' collectively are important in the Framingham Study because about 20 percent of the population is of Italian ethnic origin."[45] There is something absurd about this note, since the table in that report also features an important American pasta-based food staple: macaroni and cheese. It suggests that the Italians of Framingham still seemed a bit exotic to these researchers.

In 1964, in response to questions about the "Environmental Factors in Hypertension," Dawber, the principal investigator, talked about the Italians in the study with a most generous assessment of their numbers, even as he discounted the difference between them and the rest of the Framingham population:

Q: Thomas: Have you compared the ethnic background and the number of generations in America between your college people and the high school and grade school people? In view of the waves of different nationalities arriving in America, I should think there might be differences in ethnic origin which would be worth looking at.

A: Dawber: About 40 per cent of the population in Framingham is of Italian extraction, mostly from Southern Italy. The educational level in these two precincts where they live is somewhat lower than in some of the other precincts. We could not get any clear relationship of national origin to coronary heart disease.[46]

Dawber's focus on Italians may reflect the simultaneous foreignness and prominence of Italians in Framingham in the period. On the one hand, a high proportion of the Italians were foreign born compared to people of other national origins. On the other hand, Italians were prominent in the city. Before the study began, the only board-certified cardiologist in Framingham had an Italian surname—Cornicelli.[47]

National origin did not remain a parameter in the findings of the Framingham Study. Interrogating this is an opportunity to add nuance to STS theory of categorization: whereas Ted Porter, for example, has brought our attention to how "impressively resilient" categories can be once created and collected, "scarcely vulnerable to challenge except in a limited way by insiders,"[48] how can we understand situations in which a parameter withers away?

Looking at earlier publications from the Framingham Heart Study, we can see a transition in preoccupations with national origin around 1960. Two different publications had the subtitle "Six Years Follow-Up Experience." The 1959 version, "Some Factors Associated with the Development of Coronary Heart Disease," discussed national origin at length and provided tables comparing different groups, even though it concluded that differences according to national origin were "not statistically significant."[49] In the 1961 version, "Factors of Risk in the Development of Coronary Heart Disease,"[50] national origin as a category of analysis had disappeared. A negative result on national origin was originally reported as a result nonetheless, but its declining relevance rather than its statistical power contributed to its disappearance.

One reason that analysis of the national origin question disappeared in the 1960s was explicitly technological. Because it was a "multiple-punch" question, data from it was lost when the NHLBI moved the data from punch cards to tapes in 1969; certain types of multiple-punch responses could not be easily transferred to data tapes, and so, as a result, the ancestry codes were left blank.[51] Instructions for coders were annotated for data conversion, and "National Origin" was crossed off and "Blank" was written in the corner.[52] This is an illustration of the role of data storage in shaping this large medical study.

It is as important to understand how categories become erased as it is to understand how they become inscribed. If attention in science and technology studies has productively addressed the ways that racial (and other) categories have a power to shape knowledge,[53] this approach can bear the same problems that Wendy Chun has identified in software studies: privileging software as "readable text," ignoring the significance of hardware and effectively erasing instances when inputs and outputs do not correspond.[54] The increasing availability of more powerful computers encouraged exploration at Framingham of multivariate models of risk,[55] but the new machines had constraints of their own. The limitations of data recording and storage don't exactly preclude any given questions from being asked or pursued. These limitations only create an uneven terrain, in which some questions become easier and others more difficult to ask. This requires that the threshold of motivation be higher to make the harder-to-ask questions worth asking.

The disappearance of this intrawhite ethnic parameter from the Framingham data set was not inevitable. Two things might have led investigators to preserve the data on the national origin questions. First, it might have remained of interest to investigators if early analysis had found more striking differences in cardiovascular disease by national origin. Alternatively, if differences by national origin, no matter how statistically insignificant, had remained something that seemed to resonate with post-1960s preoccupations with differentiated American identities, the investigators might well have transferred more national origin questions to binary "working decks" and thus preserved the data.

A couple of questions related to ethnicity do survive in the data set because they had been put into binary working decks before the data transition: whether foreign born or not, and whether Italian or not. This may provide insight into which preoccupations with intrawhite difference remained vital in the 1950s. Other questions along these lines could have been maintained/preserved in the later data had they remained salient to the researchers. As Geoffrey Bowker and Susan Leigh Star, STS theorists of classification, have pointed out, "Any information system that neglects use and user semantics is bound for trouble down the line—it will become either oppressive or irrelevant."[56] Part of the resilience of the Framingham approach is the way that its data analysis methods can accommodate irrelevance of portions of its data set even as many of its vectors of difference, such as lipid and blood pressure levels, have become entrenched in that study and well beyond. The specifics of national origin have not remained durable preoccupations in the way that black-white racial differences have; they have faded into the haze of 1950s pan-whiteness.

Over the 1960s, '70s, and '80s, the Framingham Study has provided the concept of the "risk factor" and evidence about some of the most foundational factors such as smoking, diet, hypertension, and lipid levels. It has had an impact on evidence-based medicine and conceptualizations of risk categories of heart disease that is larger than can easily be estimated. Although this study was made by and about the explicitly and then implicitly white middle class, and can be understood to tell a story about American health and life in the middle of the twentieth century, it has also provided tools to tell stories of other categories and communities—including, as we will see in the next chapter, defining African American hypertension as a disease category.

Framingham's Racial Framework since the 1990s

The tremendously influential 1993 NIH Revitalization Act, which reauthorized the National Institutes of Health and required that women and minorities be included in research studies,[57] has had an impact on the Framingham Study. Like other studies that receive federal funding, Framingham has had to address the requirement to include "diverse" populations in its sample. Though the study had always included women, it did not include a population that was ethnically diverse in the terms of the 1990s.

In the process of complying with the act, Framingham has obscured the diversity of its own original cohort. A pamphlet celebrating Framingham's fiftieth anniversary describes the changes in Framingham this way: "Once a homogeneous, white middle-class suburb, this town had become more like a city, with an ethnic patchwork that included African Americans and new immigrants from Latin America and Asia." Overstating both the scientific sampling and the heterogeneity of the original sample, the pamphlet continues: "When 5,209 people were chosen for the Study in 1948, a random sampling was taken. Because few minorities were living in the town at the time, no conclusive information about specific groups could be culled."[58]

Having to comply with the new inclusion requirements was not an easy fit for a long-standing study never designed to be representative. It also revealed the entrenchment of Framingham's racialization. Although the slipperiness between the city's name and the study's name can mislead on this count,[59] participation in the Framingham Heart Study has not since the first generation of participants been determined by residence in Framingham. Rather, only descendants of the original participants have been eligible to join the new cohorts of the main study. Citizenship in the Framingham Study is thus hereditary. Unlike a model of citizenship determined spatially, kinship is a mode of relatedness that is presumed to necessarily preserve races of the past in the present. As such, the Framingham Study is particularly unsuited for this historical moment that Epstein has characterized as the "inclusion-and-difference paradigm."[60]

The Framingham Study has complied with new NIH guidelines by starting the Omni Study in 1994, which looks at a new cohort comprised of minorities in Framingham itself. The fiftieth Anniversary Pamphlet describes the Omni Study in a way that epitomizes the inclusion-and-difference paradigm:

> The Omni Study, with its narrower focus, would help health officials understand how and if heart, lung, and blood diseases exist disproportionately in some groups, see if risk factors associated with these diseases are the same or different for minorities than among the other two cohorts, and find out if the so-called Americanization of some minorities had become detrimental to their health.
>
> "It is important that the Study reflect the diversity of Framingham," says Levy. "This diversity gives us a chance to observe, and compare, the risk factor levels and unfolding of certain diseases in various groups."[61]

In this public relations pamphlet, the reason to include minorities is conceptualized in a very narrow way—for the purposes of comparison against whites —rather than reconceptualizing community in a way that includes minorities as primary members. However, in less celebratory venues, even the investigators suggest that the numbers are too small to make any claims about racial/ethnic comparisons—there are only a few hundred participants in Omni, from all minority groups, chosen without any attempt at randomization. And indeed attempts to include the whole of the community have been half-hearted. Portuguese speakers, who are a sizable community in Framingham and highly visible through the signs on the storefronts that have rejuvenated downtown,[62] are not included because the study staff lacks the language capabilities to include them.

In discussions of the addition of the Omni cohort, funding considerations appear widely. Language from a 1994 memo included a line that would continue to appear in many more memos over the later 1990s: "To assure that the Framingham Study population will be representative of the U.S. population, and to be competitive for future NIH funding, it is essential that the Omni Cohort become an integral part of the Framingham Study. An Omni Cohort even larger than 300 will undoubtedly be needed."[63] In 1998, a memo from an investigator to others read: "The feedback on my grant was very direct and critical about the lack of minorities. Whether it is scientifically sound, as both of you have pointed out, recruiting minorities will be critical for funding of ancillary studies."[64]

Thus, the Framingham investigators have added the Omni Study to comply with new funding regimes, but do not incorporate the minority study comprehensively on the scale of the Framingham Study itself. However, this does not suggest lack of commitment to the principle of including diverse populations in longitudinal research. Rather, the investigators have focused their energies on providing support for comprehensive study of diverse populations elsewhere. The Framingham investigators have been invaluable consultants on the most ambitious longitudinal research project to date that focuses on cardiovascular disease in minorities, and does so with sufficient resources and attention to make it valuable: the Jackson Heart Study.

The Jackson Heart Study as "Black Framingham"

The founder of the Association of Black Cardiologists, Richard Allen Williams, cites the Framingham Heart Study many times in the cardiology chapter in his 1975 *Textbook of Black Related Diseases*. Yet he was skeptical of its full applicability to black patients: "The data collected in predominantly White Framingham may not be applicable to predominantly Black Watts, Hough, Roxbury, Newark, or Washington."[65] He made a plea for a Framingham-type study of a racially diverse population: "In order to know exactly what the characteristics of Black coronary-prone persons are, it should be obvious that Black persons at risk must be tested. This has not been done on a prospective basis. Ideally, a longitudinal Framingham-type study should be structured for a community consisting of Blacks, Whites, and other racial and ethnic groups. . . . It is hoped that such a study will be assembled in the near future. No better application of epidemiological principles to cardiology can be conceived."[66] The Jackson Heart Study would be, in part, an answer to Williams's plea. Yet whereas Framingham defined a white northeastern town as "an American town," the Jackson Heart Study, begun in 2000, has defined the large black population of a southern city as its foundational population.

Questions of branding are paramount in this sort of grammar of the "black Framingham," invoked by Charles Curry in the vignette at this chapter's opening. To point out that associative branding work is being done is not necessarily to criticize it. We might map the grammar of [black] [Framingham] as [a new kind of] [known thing]. When I asked Framingham investigator Daniel Levy what he thought about the Jackson study's moniker, he described it without derision as a "brand name that physicians know."[67] Indeed, brand extension does not diminish the value of the original brand, but raises its status as referent. The emergence of Jackson does not reduce the funding or other resources available for Framingham, but rather increases the size of the field of its type of large-scale longitudinal research. And Levy, himself, together with others involved in Framingham, are proud of the work that they have done supporting the Jackson Heart Study.

The research designs have changed in the fifty years between the two studies, and that is just one part of the discontinuity. Although the labeling of Jackson as "the black Framingham" does not capture it comprehensively and is one that some investigators are trying to "get beyond" so that the Jackson study can come into its own,[68] the discourse of "the black Framingham" does interesting work with regard to concepts of American typicality, normality, and representation. I argue that the Jackson Heart Study can be read as a double postmodernity. First, both its population and research design are beyond modern/typical. Second, its epistemological framework is beyond observation, to an emergent epistemology that interrogates the ways of knowing of both the investigators and the participants in ways that shape the science.

When the Jackson Heart Study's principal investigator, Herman Taylor, speaks in laudatory terms about the Framingham Study, as at the conference I described in this chapter's opening, his rendering of its role as a "typical American town [of] second-generation immigrants" is of a piece with its common historiography. Yet unlike Richard Allen Williams, Taylor does not suggest that the people of Framingham were too white to be representative.

Instead, he suggests that looking at any group "microscopically" would help to understand all people. As with Framingham, the high risks that the population is believed to face are a reason that situating the study in Jackson is particularly worthwhile, but it is hoped that the knowledge will help both that community and humanity.

In this vein, the Jackson Heart Study does not necessarily aim to show the distinctiveness of African Americans. On the contrary, many of the findings have emphasized the similarities between blacks and whites. Taylor mentions, for example, that there are higher rates of coronary disease among blacks than many physicians think, since physicians have the erroneous idea in their "memory banks that blacks have only hypertension."[69]

It is not, then, only (or even primarily) an interest in the distinctiveness of their population that drives the researchers of the Jackson Heart Study, but rather a belief that they, too, can represent "humanity." The Jackson Heart Study design does have distinctive questions. Jackson's scientific goals include further study of known heart disease risk factors with a focus on hypertension-related disease, as well as sociocultural risk factors such as stress, racism, and coping strategies, and it also hopes to study intraracial genetic factors and identify novel risk factors for cardiovascular disease.[70] The investigators believe that looking closely enough on the local level can help to shed some light on the global level. They make the same disavowal of representation of an American whole that Dawber made. Like him, they stake a claim that attentiveness to intragroup difference will be extrapolatable to that group and beyond.

The Development of the Jackson Heart Study

The Jackson Heart Study emerged out of the multicommunity study called Atherosclerosis in Communities (ARIC).[71] In an effort to reach decent levels of African American participation for the four-site ARIC study overall, which was mostly taking place in white-majority areas, Jackson was chosen as an all-black sample. It began in 1987, seven years before the NIH guidelines mandating the inclusion of minorities in research. Yet the promise that the "all African-American cohort" at Jackson would "provide answers for the excessive cardiovascular disease burden of this ethnic group" shows that it was part of the trend that would lead to those guidelines.[72] The racial and ethnic categorizations used in ARIC, as in NIH-funded studies generally, are the current census categories. Interviewers filling out the forms chose how to categorize the patients by race, and the possibilities were limited to white, black, Native, or

Asian: "Race: Record the participant's race as White, Black, American Indian or Alaskan Indian, or Asian or Pacific Islander. This may require asking the question verbally if it is not obvious."[73] This looks very different from the multiple-punch Framingham model. When the time came to evaluate the ARIC study, it was decided to expand its Jackson site. Thus emerged the terrain for the Jackson Heart Study. Only those ARIC participants who self-identified as black were invited to return for the Jackson Heart Study, and an expanded pool was also recruited.

The decision to make Jackson an all-black study, rather than merely black in proportion to the city's population, was made in the context of concern about the difficulty of recruitment and retention. It was hypothesized that recruiting and retaining a high enough level of black participants might be easier to do if the study were completely focused on that population. Key here, as with Framingham, was that the capacity to do the study well was more important than the sample's representation of some whole.

One reason that it is productive to make comparisons between the Framingham and Jackson studies is to show the common ground they have. For example: why were these populations chosen? For Framingham, emphasis was on a stable but varied population that could be tracked for a long time; proximity to investigators; and amenability of the population to research. Efforts to make each of these true shaped the design of the Framingham study, for example by including whole families as units rather than individuals, and having a role for volunteers as well as for randomly selected subjects. A sense of civic duty fostered by identification with the small city was both sought out and bolstered by the investigators, and investigators cultivated a sense that the study "belongs to" the community of Framingham, in the service of the world.[74] Similarly, in Jackson, the choice was made to make it an all-black study because it was felt that the community would be more likely to rally around it if it were all-black rather than merely reflective of the demographics of the city (in the manner of the other ARIC populations).[75] Making the study all-black was a way to help the community to identify with it and take ownership of it, thus making the study itself feasible.

As the Framingham Heart Study population compares with the general white population, analogously, the population studied at the Jackson Heart Study is more middle-class, more educated, and living a better lifestyle than the African American average. But this is part of how each becomes "normal." They are a norm in the normative sense of the word, not in the sense of an average. Unlike in Framingham, poverty is explicitly represented in the Jackson

Heart Study population—but so is the college-educated black middle class, with the disproportion to the latter, and this atypicality is invoked to suggest that the study is uniquely comprehensive.[76]

Another point of common ground is the relationship between the researchers and participants, for example in terms of racial identity. When I asked Bill Kannel, a former head of the Framingham Study and longtime investigator, what he thought about the Jackson Heart Study's moniker as "the black Framingham," he responded that "everybody tends to want to understand their own group."[77] He explained that Framingham investigators had done an all-white study of this kind, and suggested that it was logical that blacks would also want to do an all-black study of this kind. But there is both identification and elision in this concept of "their own group." Most of the Framingham investigators were not, of course, from Framingham. Kannel himself was from New York City, Meadors was Southern, Dawber was the Canadian-born child of English immigrants raised on Massachusetts's South Shore. They need not identify with its population in any demographic or other sense in order to find the New England town an appropriate object of study. Moreover, Framingham came to be their "own" as they developed the real, concrete connections of extended engagement with the community.

At Jackson, too, it is both true and a misrepresentation to say that the investigators are studying "their own group." As in the Framingham Study, there is some slippage in whether the community being studied is "the same" as the investigators. It is important that it is black investigators studying black patients, and that they frame their particular expertise and mission in these terms. The investigators are overwhelmingly black, and indeed an important part of the process has been increasing the pipeline of black health professionals and building connections between two historically black colleges (Jackson State University and Tougaloo College) and the medical campus of the main state university (University of Mississippi Medical Center).[78] At the same time, most of the investigators are not from Jackson and have been trained elsewhere; the investigators are very conscientious about the gaps between themselves and their research participants.

Relatedly, a striking contrast between the two studies is that whereas Framingham excluded much of the explicitly social, Jackson foregrounds it. In Framingham, questions about class and psychological state were considered to be "too sensitive." Jackson, in contrast, attends to these issues in interesting ways: there is attention not only to socioeconomic status generally, but to variations in socioeconomic status over the life course.[79] This is a particularly

American way to conceptualize class—not as a fixed category, but as a state that is simultaneously real and in flux. There are also careful measures of stress, focused on stressors of racism and of daily life.

One question that was not considered to be "too sensitive" in Framingham but was considered to be "too sensitive" in Jackson was skin color. Where Framingham asked investigators to include their assessment of "skin color" as "normal," "pale," "ruddy," "sallow," or "jaundiced," as well as degree and location of freckling,[80] in Jackson "including a direct or indirect measure of skin color was given substantial consideration and ultimately abandoned for reasons of cultural sensitivity."[81] On the other hand, while questions about religion were specifically excluded from Framingham, "organizational and private religiousness; spiritual experiences; religious coping" are all specifically included in the Jackson data, as measures of the construct of religion as a potentially important psychosocial resource.[82]

One way that the relationship between investigators and participants is contrastive is in the promises the investigators make to the community. Framingham's observation-only approach made no claims to benefit the participants in the study themselves or to take their questions and concerns to heart in the study design. Although the Framingham investigators recognized that their study was not really a "natural history study" in that the participants were not impeded from seeking medical care, and saw themselves as facilitating treatment by participants' own physicians,[83] that narrow framing is no longer acceptable. Since Jackson was conceptualized in a black community a generation after the exposure of the abuses at Tuskegee, where African American men were denied treatment of syphilis for decades so that the "natural history" of the disease could be ascertained,[84] a "natural history study" is no longer framed as an unachievable ideal: it is unacceptable. Indeed, in local press coverage in Jackson, it has been described as "the Un-Tuskegee Experiment" because it combines its research component with education and community outreach.[85]

The modernist ideal of passive observation that the Framingham investigators acknowledged failing to reach is now one that is rejected. Now there is a need to help the actual community of study, while studying it and beyond, and to incorporate community concerns in a way that reaches beyond "recruitmentology" in Steven Epstein's terms, and changes the way that the science is done.[86] Relatedly, there is an explicit aspect of *capacity building* in Jackson: part of the purpose of the study is not only its own findings, but building a cadre of future minority investigators.[87] Including two historically black institutions among the three running the study is a way of putting African Americans into the pipeline of a major economic engine of biomedical research.

Jackson as a Model City, Posttypical

If the presence of the Shoppers' World mall in Framingham was part of what made that town emblematic of the age in which the study arose, the location of the Jackson Heart Study's facilities is also fitting. The Jackson Heart Study is attached to a building called the Jackson Medical Mall, because it was a mall that was defunct for some time and then became a clinic and medical center of sorts. The Jackson Medical Mall is technically separate from the Jackson Heart Study, though spatially they are indistinct. The Jackson Medical Mall includes a few retail shops and eating facilities as well as health care centers and clinics, some independent and some under the auspices of the University of Mississippi Medical Center.[88] It is in one of Jackson's black neighborhoods, and the building was neglected before being reclaimed as "one-stop shopping" for nonprofit medical care. This edifice of the shopping-mall-turned-medical-area captures a postmodern moment that is postindustrial in its organization of labor and of consumption.[89]

Jackson, like Framingham, disavows representation and yet still operates on valences of a "typical American town." If America of the 1950s was plausibly a New England small town, it might today be southern sprawl. When the Framingham investigators found something "not grossly atypical" in 1948, it was a New England town with second-generation European immigrants adding to the old white mix. In an atypicality that is no longer afraid to be blatant, the Jackson investigators found their model population in 2000 in a Sun Belt city in which it is African Americans who are added to the old white mix, but considered separately. In terms of immigration, Jackson is not "typical"—indeed, ironically, if Framingham were to be studied in a fully inclusive way today, it would be more emblematic of the current historical moment in terms of immigration and its contestation.[90] And yet Jackson is pulling on some considerable valences of its own historical moment in America: postindustrial, sprawling, Sun Belt, diffuse. In the words of its principal investigator: "The scientific questions and the population on which the JHS focuses make it a study for our time."[91]

The Jackson Heart Study does not pretend to represent its city's entire population; it is nonwhite by design. Unlike in Massachusetts, where Framingham's Omni Study included whites who were involved in minority communities because of concerns that they would feel excluded,[92] there do not seem to have been such concerns from whites in Jackson. In the context of studies that claim to represent the "whole" while routinely failing to represent the African American part of that whole, claims to be able to study a whole no longer seem tenable in quite the same way. Like Framingham, but more convincingly, Jackson articulates its project as a valuable contribution to a field, rather than as a lone study that will answer all questions. In the context of huge amounts of data and what appear to be particular gaps, selecting the African Americans alone comes to make sense.

Emergent Epistemology

In understanding Jackson as a postmodern project, I am using a framing that is in alignment with that of the investigators themselves. The researchers consider themselves to be making contributions to interpretive phenomenology.

One epistemological challenge of which the Jackson investigators are well aware is the influence that the questions asked have on the data. In their report *Community-Driven Model of Recruitment*, they discuss Heidegger and the epistemological challenges of quantum physics before expounding: "Whether researchers are attempting to model complex interactions between subatomic particles, physiological control systems or constructs like hostility and cardiovascular disease the basic conceptual tools of measurement and inference are similar to those outlined above. The question to be asked here is: How do we bring to the process of questioning the phenomenon we seek to study in terms of setting it up to respond in certain ways? What is closed down, invisible or outside the gaze of the researcher when a particular question is tested?"[93] They go on to "contrast basic sciences with social sciences" on the basis of "the extent to which meanings and interpretations for both participants and investigators hold sway for the phenomenon being studied." In the encounter between investigator and participant, the identities of investigators might distinctly matter first for building trust and second for shaping results.[94] They see their contributions as not limited to science in the sense of data, but also to "interpretive methodology":

> Hermeneutics, or interpretation, as an approach to research acknowledges the situated temporal nature of both the researcher and the participants. The hermeneutic method works to uncover how humans are "always already" given as time. That is to say, humans are always already in their own

worlds, living in particular spaces, times and ways. Hermeneutics has no beginning or end that can be concretely defined, but is a continuing experience for all who participate. The work of the interpretive phenomenologist moves beyond traditional logical structures in order to reveal and explicate otherwise hidden relationships. The descriptions of what *is*, are interpreted to show what *could be*.[95]

The investigators quote Cornel West, suggesting that "vigilance is necessary to guard against systems of domination and control in cultural studies where research practices may serve to 'highlight notions of difference, marginality, and otherness in such a way that it further marginalizes actual people of difference and otherness.'"[96] And they explicitly set out to do a different kind of science. The Jackson investigators' primary interest in the lives of their subjects is distinct from Framingham's initial focus on identity, which was essentially limited to recruitment. Jackson's approach combines this interest in recruitment and retention with a sense that the value of the research is at stake. It is not a mere repetition of Framingham, but a repetition with a difference.

Heart Disease Research as a Site for Inclusion in American Ways of Life

As described at the chapter's opening, the Jackson Heart Study's principal investigator asserts that the study is necessary because this population has been left out of the "golden age of cardiology" that was ushered in by Framingham and related therapeutic advances. While other populations have benefited greatly and seen a reverse in the increasing cardiovascular disease mortality that they had been experiencing in the first half of the twentieth century, there has been a plateau among African Americans. This sense of being left out of a progressive narrative of history is an interesting one in the context of the history of cardiology.

Even though the investigators hope that Jackson can tell us something not only about black people in Mississippi but about people in general, as Framingham did, that is not a seamless proposition. It is an open question whether the reception of Jackson will ever be read to suggest anything for "America," or for "people." The mimicry of Framingham in Jackson is ambivalent, in a way that is sympathetic with Homi Bhabha's meditation upon the simultaneous resemblance and difference between the English and the Anglicized,[97] and its hybrid knowledge forms have an uneasy relationship with universal applicability. It is the durability of racial preoccupations, not data per se, that may make the results too inextricable from their markedness with the racial Other to be broadly accepted as universally applicable. This is the sort of question with which I will reengage in my discussion of pharmaceuticals, in particular the African American Heart Failure Trial (A-HeFT), which was the trial that led to the approval of BiDil for "heart failure in self-identified black patients." There has been frustration, both among some black cardiologists and among social science critics, that the Food and Drug Administration could not see that A-HeFT showed that BiDil works in people including blacks, not just in people who are black. One issue that is at stake is which study subjects can stand in as universally applicable sources of data.

Robert Mitchell and Catherine Waldby see Framingham as part of the gene-alogy of national biobanks, pointing out that the Framingham Heart Study, like other large-scale epidemiological studies in the United States and else-where at the same time, was "strongly linked with the idea of national public health and the administration of a discrete national population."[98] After the Second World War, there was a rapid democratization of conceptions of who was at risk for heart disease, which was connected to ideas about American solidarity in the postwar period. Though heart disease has sometimes been framed retrospectively as a disease that struck people from all sectors of soci-ety—"paupers and presidents"[99]—there had been considerably more attention paid to presidents. The Framingham Heart Study can be read as the democrati-zation of attention to heart disease that shadowed the democratization of a sense of who was at risk: extending from elite white men to a broad, albeit not fully inclusive, American middle class—including "new" Americans (immi-grants and their children) and women. The Jackson Heart Study can then be read as a simultaneous extension and fragmentation of that kind of project. As many scholars have observed, demanding inclusion of diverse populations in genomics research has become part of demanding inclusion in cutting-edge science—both among scientists of color in the United States, and among post-colonial scientists.[100] The Jackson Study can be seen as of a piece with this trend, at the same time that it is continuous with the older model of longitudi-nal research in nation-making.

Framingham and Jackson thus have continuity with early cardiology, in that heart disease research is again a site of representing modern American dis-ease, and who counts as fully American is expressed through the populations that become the focus of heart disease research. In the previous chapter, we saw that coronary disease was considered in terms of the racialized modern life of the elite. This chapter has explored two more periods, each with attendant racialized populations at risk for cardiovascular disease. Framingham has attended first and foremost to the coronary disease of the white middle class resulting from combined risk factors. Jackson attends to the burden of morbidity and mortality on people of color who are characterized as having been left behind by America's postwar medical advances. Medical knowledge about the diseases of the heart comes to include an expanding notion of who counts as American: from elite white men, to multiethnic white men and women, to African American men and women—and in parallel from high socioeconomic status to middle class and then socioeconomically diverse.

In each expansion, we can see an expansion of modern medical practice. If predictions of a decrease in the infectious disease burden were part of defining early cardiology, the introduction of penicillin bolstered a sense that noninfectious heart disease was the disease of the age that demanded new tools of investigation and new solutions.[101] The practitioners in Framingham were from the newly professionalized, certified, and standardized portion of medical practice that emerged between the wars,[102] and these "highly cooperative" and "well-informed" physicians were crucial to the decision to locate the program there.[103] The Jackson Study, too, becomes a site of modern medicine in this sense, particularly focused on developing a cadre of African Americans pursuing biomedical research at the highest level.

In some senses, Framingham is a fulfillment of the modernizing aspirations of the founding of cardiology. Framingham reaches the standardization of research and diagnosis identified as goals in the earlier period and does so in a larger community understood as modern and American. Framingham stakes out a space between racial representation and racial normality as it grapples with how to answer questions about normal pathologies of normal life—and Jackson both extends and fractures the normal.

Longitudinal studies are heir to both early cardiology and to life insurance, and Framingham can be seen as a key site for the construction of what Dorothy Nelkin and Laurence Tancredi have characterized as "the actuarial mindset" and "reductionism" in matters of health.[104] In its attempts to standardize, the Framingham Study was an extension of the modern endeavor of early cardiology, and it provided the rationalizing concept of the risk factor. And yet the study and its risk factor concept would pave the way for the postmodern fracturing of epistemologies of disease.[105] The risk factor concept pushed beyond a focus on etiology, and moved the relationships of study beyond the causal. Along the way, the Framingham investigators innovated in scientific epistemology through multivariate analysis. The epistemological innovations of the Jackson investigators can be seen as both extending the rationalism of longitudinal research and posing fundamental challenges to the promise of rationalism.

"The black Framingham" is not Framingham with merely a tonal difference. The differences in its parameters due to its racialization are not separable from its historical location a half-century after the former began. It is also the socioculturally aware Framingham, the genomically savvy Framingham, the southern Framingham, the urban-sprawl Framingham. Each of these differences are intertwined with its racial difference, as are its double postmodernities of posttypical and postobservational. The Jackson Heart Study, I have argued, is a postmodern repetition with a difference that both elaborates and fractures the enterprise of early cardiology and the Framingham Study. It simultaneously represents innovations in and limits of the concepts of systematization and of normal population.

CHAPTER 3

The Durability of
African American Hypertension
as a Disease Category

I n May 2005, the American Society of Hypertension (ASH) had its twentieth annual meeting at the San Francisco Marriott.[1] As a new and special feature, the proceedings dedicated the first day to "special symposiums" that addressed "special populations." Parallel six-hour-long programs addressed concerns of treating hypertension in African American, Hispanic, and Japanese populations. The symposium "Hypertension in the African American Population" consisted of wide-ranging presentations by prominent figures in the field. The talks raised several fundamental issues—debunking genetics as an explanation of disparities; describing long-standing barriers to care and brand-new clinical trials; and promoting new evidence-based guidelines for treatment in that group. Most of the speakers emphasized the complexity of African American hypertension.

Then there was a change of tone. Looking precisely the elder statesman that he is in the community, Elijah Saunders—a charter member of ASH, a founder of the International Society for Hypertension in Blacks (ISHIB), and organizer of the day's sessions—took the stage and talked about the practical implications of African American hypertension. He spoke with an authority that projected an above-the-fray sensibility, saying that there is a lot we don't know about mechanisms, but we do know that blacks are dying and that we need to save lives. He suggested that although research into genetics or worrying about who is really black should continue, there was a more pressing issue. He advanced his PowerPoint slide to a picture of an older African American couple and said: "But we are talking about people who look like this picture." This brought a warm laugh. He said that for people like those in the picture, we know that dietary modification works, and that no drug class should be eliminated from their treatment.

The panel continued, but I want to pause at this moment. Saunders's discursive intervention here is an instance of a tactic that is common in the field of race and medicine: a call to clinical pragmatics after expositions of the complexity of the social and scientific terrain. There are two rhetorical moves happening within this panel. First, there is a call to open up fundamental questions about race. Second, there is a call to close the conversation to allow implementation of operational answers. These are not actually opposed rhetorical moves, as we can tell by the fact that they are made by the very same people. Elijah Saunders himself had participated in organizing the symposium. Indeed, he saw the event as something of a vindication of his long advocacy for more attention within ASH to African Americans as a high-risk group.[2] As we will see, ideas about racial difference have been present in hypertension research since its rise to prominence in the 1950s and especially the 1960s, and attention to African American hypertension in particular has often been tied to calls for raising awareness and treatment of the risk factor in order to diminish disparities. Both in his career and in this particular symposium, Saunders participates in both opening the debate on the definition and role of race in hypertension and moving to close it, at least sufficient to mobilize response to African American hypertension.

The symposium Saunders had pulled together used an array of approaches to try to open up conversation on the complexities of race. They invoked genetics (albeit to reject them), history, humanistic moral claims, pathophysiology, subgroup analysis, and focused clinical trials. And yet Saunders made the rhetorical move here of saying that the epistemological debates and cutting-edge research were beside the point: we know who we are talking about and that they are not getting well-established, good care. Here we can see a tension between epidemiology and clinical medicine, even among research-oriented physicians. Where epidemiology strives for the establishment of scientific facts about the causes and distributions of disease, clinical medicine always also strives to determine the course of action to be pursued at the patient's bedside.

In the context of their work in organizations like the International Society for Hypertension in Blacks and beyond, clinical practice is often understood as one component of a broader project for social justice for people of color. For the most part, these physicians are well aware of the limitations of what medical practice can achieve to ameliorate disparities in a society in which inequality is structural and deeply entrenched. However, in their capacities as researchers and clinicians, it still makes sense to organize a panel that focuses on research into and administration of medication. These clinician-researchers are interested in participating in scientific debates at the highest level, which is necessary for producing the publications to achieve their professional goals. But they are also civil rights–oriented physicians, in the tradition of earlier black physicians' organizations, who see their most fundamental goal as intervening to improve the health of African Americans.

How can we understand the simultaneous drive for further research, and the assertion that sufficient therapeutic intervention is already possible? Why does the format of presentation of African American hypertension alternate between opening up the status of the disease category and then moving to close and operationalize it? I argue that this vacillation is central to medicine, as a field that is both scientific and therapeutic. In order to understand the productivity of medicating race, the status of race as a category needs to be recognized as *simultaneously* one of bioscientific inquiry and one of practical clinical taxonomy. I argue that critiques that address only scientific reification without attending to clinical intervention fail to engage medicine. By tracking the historical emergence of African American hypertension as a disease category and ongoing etiological debates that contribute to the durability of the category, we will see that race's productivity in medical data and practice relies not on its measurability, but rather on its *recordability*. Race is inscribed in the photo on Saunders's PowerPoint slide, and routinely recorded on everyday physicians' medical history charts. The flexible gap between immeasurable race and recordable race is vital for understanding its power.

Notes on the Historical Emergence of African American Hypertension

The 2005 ASH Symposium on Hypertension in the African American Population represents a particular moment in the status of African American hypertension as a disease category. How did we get to this point, such that it makes sense to set aside a day of a hypertension conference for "special populations," African Americans among them? How did this disease category come to have these tensions in which arguments about the social and biological causes of disease are raised without quite intersecting, and bioscientific arguments remain parallel to clinical medical practice?

"Hypertension" and "high blood pressure" are interchangeable terms referring to pathologically high levels of blood pressure in the arteries. Whether or not blood pressure is considered "high" is determined numerically, and what is considered to be the "normal" range has narrowed over time. Some blood pressure is of course necessary to survive, and the boundary between normal and pathological has remained contested even as hypertension has stabilized as a risk factor and come to be treated like a disease.[3]

African American hypertension as a disease category emerged at the same time that hypertension as a disease category did, in the 1950s and '60s. It can be read as the intersection of multiple trajectories: the hypertension that had long been observed to be high in African Americans emerged as a key modifiable etiological risk factor for heart disease; earlier cardiology's racialized distinctions between coronary and infectious heart disease could be mapped onto new distinctions between coronary and hypertensive heart disease; and black and other civil rights–oriented physicians mobilized and professionalized around the prevention of nonepidemic disease, especially heart disease.

Claims that African Americans have high rates of hypertension are long standing, extending back to the era in which hypertension was generally conceptualized as only a rare and immediately malignant condition. So are claims that blacks have higher mean blood pressures than whites, even in nonpathological ranges. Michael Byrd and Linda Clayton, physicians and historians of race and medicine, have described physician attention to racial differences in hypertension in the antebellum period, and in their account, this is one of the few physiological observations from the period that has withstood scientific scrutiny.[4] According to the epidemiologists Jay Kaufman and Susan Hall, the first instance of racial comparison of blood pressure was in a 1932 report in the *American Journal of the Medical Sciences*, in which blood pressure was the "most striking difference noted in physical examination."[5] The morbidity tracked in the article, however, had nothing to do with blood pressure, but rather spanned the gamut of infectious diseases (tuberculosis, influenza, malaria, venereal disease), appendicitis, home injuries, and degenerative diseases. Through the 1950s, racial differences in blood pressures continued to draw great interest and debate about the relative role of civilization versus inheritance,[6] even as blood pressure was a physical characteristic without—yet—clear connections to morbidity.

Even before biomedical research understood hypertension to be an etiological factor in coronary disease, extremely high hypertension was known to be a danger and considered to be particularly common in blacks—according to one 1940 study of heart disease at a black hospital, "hypertensive heart disease is one of the deadliest of all cardiac ailments for Negroes."[7] A 1943 report suggested that "hypertension is twice as common among Negroes as among whites."[8] Moreover, although academic medicine was not focused on hypertension, it was already emerging as a correlate of risk in the sphere of insurance, an industry that was an important source of nonetiological correlative work that would inform thinking about both risk factors and race more generally.[9]

Yet in the first half of the twentieth century, elevated blood pressure was still not generally considered to be a problem on its own, but rather an epiphenomenon of other problems. As the prominent early hypertension researcher Irvine Page noted in his memoir: "As late as 1945, there appeared to be only a handful of true hypertensive individuals, and to most people, 'hypertensive' was an adjective meaning 'high strung.' "[10] Elevated blood pressure was a clinical sign that suggested underlying pathology, but not a disease in itself. Luminaries such as Paul Dudley White were skeptics on the danger of hypertension, suggesting in this period that it was either not worth treating for itself or potentially dangerous to treat because lowering it might interfere with a necessary compensatory mechanism.[11] This made hypertension very different from coronary disease, the category of heart disease that was so central to early cardiology (and so connected with whites). It was not until after the Second World War that hypertension emerged as a risk factor that could be understood as physiological and etiological.[12]

Hypertension as a disease category in the sense used today—a generally asymptomatic pathology of risk for cardiovascular disease—and African American hypertension as a distinct form thereof emerged contemporaneously, in the 1950s and '60s. The demonstration of hypertension as a risk factor by the Framingham Heart Study, and the availability of drugs such as thiazide diuretics that had a low toxicity profile,[13] turned hypertension into a focus of medical attention. Although the Framingham Study did not include African Americans, its investigators speculated about racial difference as they speculated about this new site of disease. The Framingham investigators themselves participated in the simultaneous constructions of hypertension and African American hypertension in the 1950s and '60s. Addressing "environmental factors in hypertension" in a 1964 paper, the investigators wrote that "blood pressure distributions" were "similar" among "such diverse groups as: Caucasians living in Europe, the United States, and the West Indies; among Chinese living in Taiwan, and among Japanese in Japan," but that

Negro populations have higher blood pressures than whites living in the same areas and studied by the same investigators, particularly among females and in the older age groups. Distributions of blood pressures among Negro populations living in the United States and in the West Indies, whether rural or urban, high or low salt eaters, are similar. Their blood pressures are higher than those of Negroes in Liberia, a principal source of Negro migration to the Western Hemisphere. Admixture of the Negro races in the Western Hemisphere makes the interpretation of this data difficult. It is in this general background of unencouraging experience that the study of particular environmental factors, which could conceivably affect the blood pressure level, must be approached.[14]

Here, we can see the distance between direct evidence and the invocation of commonsense racialization of cardiovascular disease. Although their phrasing evokes neutral grammars of data, there are no citations or evidence for these assertions about "Negro populations," suggesting that the authors conceive of these statements less as arguments than as reflecting the consensus of the field. Unable to grapple with the embodied admixture that is not merely genetic but also historical and cultural, much history is paved over in word choices such as "migration" to describe the slave trade and "admixture" to describe oppressive sexual relations under slavery. Paucity of data is not actually the problem. The investigators make an odd claim about the source of the difficulty of research into environmental causes of racial disease disparities: that "admixture" gets in the way of interpretation. Logically, assimilation would be the kind of mixing that would pose a problem for separating out environmental causes of disease by race, but the investigators lacked a language for cultural, in addition to biological admixture. The peculiarity of the investigators' framing should alert us to the fact of racialized hypertension's existence at the nexus of the biological and the social.

In the simultaneous articulation of both hypertension as a risk factor and racial difference, long-standing preoccupations with racial difference in heart disease were, in Ann Laura Stoler's terms, both "new and renewed."[15] By the 1960s, early cardiology's racialized bifurcation of heart disease into coronary versus infectious was no longer relevant. In the ascendance of hypertension as a risk factor, a new bifurcation between coronary disease and hypertensive disease could step into a similar role.

At the same time, civil rights and Black Power movements made illnesses of African Americans a focus for physicians, community organizers, the government, and society as a whole. Professional black organizing around hypertension and related diseases was emerging in a context of black health and black power: the Black Panther Party included blood pressure screening, along with screening for sickle cell anemia and sexually transmitted diseases, in their People's Medical Centers.[16] At the fringes, the Afrocentrist psychiatrist Frances Cress Welsing situated hypertension within her theory of melanin and white supremacy.[17] More broadly, framings of African American hypertension in the period were resonant with the larger civil rights indictments of poor African American health. For example, one *Washington Post* article from 1971 described high blood pressure as occurring "four or five times more often in blacks than whites," and a "mass killer in Washington's inner city." The etiology was portrayed as ambiguous: "High blood pressure may be hereditary, it may be due to 'socio-economic stress' and other pressures that are especially severe on persons growing up in the slums and, lastly, it may be due to excessively salty diets common in low income areas."[18] In the article, the urgency of the issue was framed as part of addressing the urgency of urban issues generally. In the same era in which black protest was being pathologized as a mental disease,[19] *high pressure* put the broader social crisis into somatic terms.

As a foundation for a social movement, hypertension had some appealing qualities that sickle cell anemia—a much more prominent racialized disease— did not. In particular, hypertension had the possibility of quick and effective intervention. Whereas sickle cell anemia had captured the imaginations of a generation, promises for treatment through molecular medicine were always in the future and ultimately unfulfilled.[20] In contrast, African American hypertension could be treated, with medications and lifestyle interventions that were at hand if only they could be made properly available. There was good treatment upon which to improve, a welcome reason for optimism amid the hopelessness that came to characterize sickle cell anemia.

Moreover, as risk factors superseded Mendelian diseases as the paradigm of cutting-edge research, asymptomatic hypertension became an appealing site for physicians keen to participate in up-to-date science and practice. With protodiseases such as hypertension increasingly defining the object of medical research and intervention,[21] participating in hypertension research and treatment became an opportunity to participate in the major medical trend of the day. The 1970s were a time of ascendance of evidence-based medicine and systematic clinical guidelines. The 1976 clinical guidelines that would become the first in a series produced by the Joint National Committee on Detection, Evaluation, and Treatment of High Blood Pressure exemplify this emerging genre. Right from that first JNC report, race was enrolled in the category of hypertension: "Special efforts to detect high blood pressure in black populations should be made since the prevalence is much greater in that group,"[22] and calls for special attention to black populations have continued in later iterations.

The JNC guidelines are an example of expert discourse, and yet it is easy to overstate the contrast between what the medical anthropologist Edwin Greenlee has characterized as erudite versus subjugated knowledges in the discourse of hypertension.[23] When African American hypertension captured the interest of new and renewed civil rights and medical communities, it often took specifically community-minded forms. In initiatives such as church-based blood pressure screening programs that combine the promotion of physical health with that of spiritual health, it becomes apparent that there is no essential "outside" to medicine: the medical screening becomes a site of rather than an alternative to community action. Indeed, interventions organized around blood pressure "are the most common black church-based health initiative," and counteracting hypertension can be a locus of ritual and spiritual practice.[24] Nevertheless, perhaps because of its status as asymptomatic, African American hypertension has been more compelling to clinicians than to broader social movements. It has been enrolled in civil rights arguments, but demands around the category have not become as associated with the movement as have those around sickle cell anemia.

In the 1970s, black physicians among others were at the forefront of trying to focus attention on the patient populations they served. African American hypertension was portrayed as both a physical fact and a result of social structures of inequality. For example, from Richard Allen Williams's *Textbook of Black-Related Diseases*:

> A typical patient is a middle-aged Black male with a history of hypertension for several years. His high blood pressure is in the moderate range, i.e. 170/110, a level which has persisted although he has been on various forms of treatment over the years. He confesses to not taking his medication faithfully because of undesirable side effects. He is "under care" at the local hospital, where he is seen every 6 months and where an intern or resident checks his blood pressure, notes that there is no change, and indifferently reorders the same medication which the patient has been taking, in the same dosages. The doctor does not bother to question the patient about new symptoms, but if he had done so, the patient might have revealed the recent

onset of dyspnea, and the need to sleep on two pillows. Had the physician taken the time to do a physical examination, he may have found engorged, distended neck veins and a very forceful cardiac apex impulse. A grade 3/6 apical pansystolic murmur radiating to the left axilla would be heard on auscultation, as well as an S_2 gallop at the lower left sternal border. . . .

If the physician is concerned and is astute enough to look for them, the changes presented in this oversimplified example should alert him to the fact that the patient has developed congestive heart failure secondary to his hypertension. Immediate action at that point such as the institution of therapy with diuretics and cardiac glycosides may forestall the rapid progression of the heart disease. However, as is frequently the case, the doctor does not investigate the patient beyond the point of recording his blood pressure, and thus the opportunity to avert further rapid advances of this morbid event is missed.[25]

In this account, Williams mixes technical medical language with an indictment of poor medical treatment for African Americans. The passage both laments the near-inevitability of poor treatment and documents the situation to advocate for change. The way that Williams describes this patient is not as an ideal case, but as a way of narrating the intersection of individual biology and long-standing poor medical care. In the process, he invokes a very different notion of "typical" than the one we saw in the previous chapter. It is like the nontechnical, mocking remark "That's typical."

African American physicians such as Williams who integrated their health research with their civil rights advocacy often claimed (and for that matter continue to claim) more than one genealogy and source of authority. On the one hand they claim mainstream medical expertise, and on the other, connection to the history and community of African Americans. Particularly in the 1970s, they sought black roots for medicine. For example, Williams often refers to Imhotep, the Egyptian god of medicine, and the first physician known by name, as an ancestor in a genealogy distinct from the Greeks, as "someone who would be recognized as Black if he walked down the street in Oakland today."[26] In the invocation of pan-African sensibility, Williams is connected to much broader cultural movements of the period. It is amid these and other black power movements that the physicians' organizing was taking place. Williams would found the Association of Black Cardiologists in 1974. The association was simultaneously a professional organization and one interested in community organizing: in the late 1970s it was through ABC that Elijah

Saunders and his colleague Waine Kong organized churches as blood pressure control centers.[27]

The focus of civil rights–oriented physicians on African American hypertension as a civil rights issue was both informed by and helped to promote larger public health initiatives in the 1970s. For example, from the inception of the National High Blood Pressure Education Program in 1972 as "a cooperative effort among professional and voluntary health agencies, state health departments, and community groups," the organization had a special focus on trying to get its message to those parts of the "general public" imagined to be most at risk.[28] The task force described those at elevated risk as falling into three categories: patients known to have hypertension, those from minority groups, and those from medically defined high-risk groups (who are pregnant, have diabetes or gout, have high cholesterol, family history of hypertension, and the like). The program's depiction of the role of minority status has a form of hedging that often characterizes such articulations: "A second large category of potential patients may be identified from certain minority groups who (not because of the minority per se) have a much higher prevalence rate of hypertension. These potential patients include blacks, Spanish-speaking groups, and American Indians."[29] The pamphlet sometimes frames African Americans as an important part of the general population, and sometimes in opposition to the "the general (Caucasian) population."[30]

Polls suggest that physicians got the message that blackness was associated with high risk of hypertension. According to the U.S. Department of Health, Education, and Welfare's 1979 survey, a strong majority (61 percent) of physicians thought that "being black" "was associated with the likelihood of a patient having hypertension." Of all the possible factors listed, only family history of hypertension received a stronger majority believing that it was related to a "definite increase in likelihood of hypertension" (69 percent).[31] Moreover, younger physicians were more convinced of this association of African Americans and hypertension risk. Among physicians under thirty-five, the belief that "being black" is something that would "definitely increase the likelihood of hypertension" was found in 73 percent of the sample, only one percentage point less than family history (74 percent).[32] These statistics suggest that the new generation of physicians gave more credence to this race-disease relationship than the generation of physicians that they were replacing. The young physicians were using an epistemology that emerged in Framingham by collapsing two kinds of risk factors—correlative and etiological—to solidify the racialization of this disease category. As risk-factor thinking was becoming characteristic of state-of-the-art medicine, a long-standing vague sense that hypertension was distinctive of African Americans was becoming durable.

As the 1970s drew to a close, professionalization around the categories of both hypertension and African American hypertension increased. The first issue of the American Heart Association's journal of its newly incorporated Council for High Blood Pressure Research came out in 1979, and included an article that would come to be widely cited: "Pathophysiology of Hypertension in Blacks and Whites: A Review and Basis of Blood Pressure Differences." It was written by Richard F. Gillum, one of the founding members of the Association of Black Cardiologists.

Two separate professional organizations were soon to come: the American Society of Hypertension in 1985 and the International Society for Hypertension in Blacks in 1986. The organizations were founded by overlapping groups of people with overlapping goals. Elijah Saunders, who was a founder of both, says he had discussed the potential of a special focus on blacks in ASH with a colleague who was then the president of that organization.[33] The then-president of ASH responded that he didn't think that the issue could be adequately addressed by ASH, and that a separate organization might better address the special needs of that community. Saunders, together with two white physicians whose practices focused on hypertension in blacks, had a meeting to write a book on the topic,[34] and out of that book project ISHIB emerged.

At its founding the International Society for Hypertension in Blacks was not only distinct from ASH, but also had two characteristics that made it distinct from two other organizations with overlapping membership, the National Medical Association (NMA) and the Association of Black Cardiologists (ABC). Where ISHIB differed from these was in its focus on patient population and its international sensibility. It was conceived of as an organization for all those involved in research on and treatment of black patients, and it aspired to lead in the treatment of black populations outside the United States.

Unlike the ABC (which began holding scientific sessions at the same time, in 1987), or the much older NMA, the defining factor of ISHIB membership was not the identity of the practitioner but the identity of the patient population that the practitioner served. This is an interesting maneuver. As we saw in previous chapters, physician professional interests and patient population needs have often been linked, and this has often led black physicians to claim particular standing to address the needs of black patients. However, even though black physicians have always overwhelmingly treated black patients, most black patients continue to be treated by nonblack doctors. To reach doctors of all backgrounds who treat black patients, ISHIB pioneered a role that minority doctors' organizations have increasingly taken on since—positioning themselves as expert resources for the care of black patients.

Also distinct from other organizations, ISHIB has had an explicitly international focus, interested from the beginning in connecting U.S.-based practitioners with those of Africa and its diaspora. After its first few meetings in Atlanta, ISHIB started to reach out geographically and had its meetings outside North America every other year from 1989 in Nairobi, Kenya, until 2003 (when concerns about security led the planned Ghana meeting to be canceled). The symposium mentioned in this chapter's introduction took place at the ASH meeting, but was in fact coorganized and cohosted by ASH and ISHIB.

The 2005 ASH Symposium emerged in a context of rearticulations of interest in health disparities that solidified in the 1990s. Much of the recent data about disparities in hypertension comes as a result of the 1993 change in National Institutes of Health policy requiring inclusion of women and minorities in studies and reporting any differences seen according to gender and race.[35] But interest in African American hypertension as a disease category exceeds interest in difference per se. Different constituencies grouped around African American hypertension have distinct interests in the disease category. From a pharmaceutical company's perspective, its status as a chronic condition might have particular draw because of its potential market of lifetime pharmaceutical consumers.[36] From a clinical researcher's perspective, its impact on the morbidity and mortality of populations served might contribute to making it a focal point. From a community organizer's perspective, the potential for interventions through health care reform and community education might make it an appealing campaign focus.

African American hypertension continues to receive attention from diverse constituencies, including mainstream medical communities, African American medical communities, mainstream media, and African American health activists. As I will now explore, explanations rooted in notions of genetic specificity have coexisted with varied explanations based on the social experiences of African Americans living in a racist society. This etiological ambiguity fosters rather than impedes the ability of diverse groups to enroll the disease category in calls for action. Those mobilized around African American hypertension as a disease category both open deep questions about the nature of race and make calls for tangible action. In risk-factor thinking and in diverse organizing against health disparities, tensions between complexity and concreteness contribute to the durable appeal of African American hypertension as a disease category.

Etiological Eclecticism Underlying African American Hypertension

In discourses of African American hypertension, there are often rhetorical moves to displace race onto some other explanatory mechanism. These include class, discrimination, segregation, and more. And yet the displacement is not successful; the disease category remains uniquely attached to race. Whenever we are told that X is "just" Y, we should be alerted to a deception. The "just" is never true. Its iteration is evidence that there is an argument, an urge to subsume. Arguments that racial differences are "just" class ones—or psychosocial stress ones, or genetic ones, or [insert causal agent]—miss the important combinatorial work that the category's very ambiguity and multivalence provides.

Cultural explanations for racial disparities are not necessarily any less reductive than are genetic ones. As the sociologist Janet Shim has pointed out, it is more common for epidemiologists to explain racial differences as "culture" than as "genetics," but these cultural explanations are also reductive.[37] The assumption that everyone who identifies as, or is identified as, black shares a common diet, lifestyle, and healthcare-seeking behavior obscures the fact that cultural practices are not precisely bounded by racial identity.

Paradoxically, at the same time that cultural reductionism paves over individual differences, it also overindividualizes. The sociologist Ruha Benjamin has noted that when health researchers characterize "African American distrust" as "a set of attitudes grounded in collective memories of past abuses and projected on to current initiatives," this fails to account for the ways in which the "sociality of distrust" is constantly reproduced in ongoing clinical practices and in larger debates about health care.[38] Cultural explanations such as "distrust" and "fatalism" hide the power that precedes the presumably neutral cultural practices. As Lundy Braun, a public health scholar, has argued, placing emphasis on "lifestyle factors or perceived cultural differences" is deeply problematic: these are "loaded with blame and direct responsibility for change to the individual rather than the society."[39]

Clinicians attentive to the ways that locating disparities in culture put undue onus on individuals do not necessarily imagine the cultural differences as fixed. Some of these clinicians have developed interesting interventions based on attention to structural impediments that make it difficult for patients to change their diet and exercise habits. Recommendations include the use of elastic fitness bands to exercise in neighborhoods where walking isn't safe, as well as urging malls to host walkers. They also address diet: efforts to modify the blood-pressure-lowering diet recommended by the National Heart, Lung, and Blood Institute to make it "soul food–friendly" coexist with critiques of the valorization of a diet with historical roots in "slave food."[40] Cultural differences—real and stereotyped—cannot be extricated from long-standing social inequality. When physicians and nurses design these kinds of interventions, it becomes even clearer that they are operating at the nexus of the biological and the social.

African American hypertension certainly has an important relationship with socioeconomic status. Class in cardiovascular etiology research is far more prominent in the United Kingdom than in the United States, but it operates as an important explanatory mechanism in the U.S. context, too, since it is widely acknowledged that access not only to basic needs of life but also to health care is difficult for those without the ability to pay. And yet, the idea that socioeconomic status should be separable from race in the experiences of any individuals, a firm assumption in epidemiology, needs to be reconsidered. A category of class that is extricated from race does not necessarily explain experience in a deeply racially stratified society. The desire to separate race from class is the desire to avoid grappling with America, and to put mathematical abstraction in its place. As Janet Shim illustrates in her ethnographic engagement with patients with cardiovascular disease, disease experiences are "lived intersections of race and class."[41] When she asked lay people with cardiovascular disease about their experiences related to class, they included in their answers experiences related to race, and vice versa. This was frustrating for epidemiologists, who wanted to eliminate the technical conundrum of confounding race and class and make them separate and independent variables. But, following Shim, we should question the desire to isolate race from class if we want to account for disease experience in America.

Experiences of socioeconomic status and of racism are deeply intertwined in the United States. In one widely cited critique of the use of race as a variable in medical research, the physician Newton Osborne and Marvin Feit, a health policy analyst, provide a guideline for the use of race in research: they disapprove of it as a variable itself, but approve of it when it is presented in a way that can allow a critical reader to identify what race is standing in for.[42] They cite a now-classic hypertension study in which the authors argue that darker-skinned African Americans suffer more from hypertension.[43] Though the first assumption might be that this would suggest a relationship between dark skin and gene prevalences, the way in which the pool of subjects was described allowed it to be explained another way. Dark skin was only predictive of hypertension when combined with lower socioeconomic status, which gave the authors an alternative explanation: namely, perhaps those of lower socioeconomic status have a harder time dealing with the stresses of discrimination based on color. In their framing, race stands in for class and the stress of discrimination in a way that promises to replace race itself as a variable. Yet because race is for them a peculiar combinatorial variable, irreducible to either of its components, their disavowal of race as a variable in hypertension does not quite undo the racialization of hypertension or the reification of African American hypertension as a disease category.

Indeed, stress is another important way of understanding the etiology of African American hypertension. Stress has long been an appealing and elusive category of risk for heart disease, and not only for African Americans. "Stress" has a far longer relationship with risks typical of ideal white masculinity, an association present in early cardiology and resilient today. Robert Aronowitz, a physician and historian of medicine, argues that the Type A personality—a notion I would mark as an elite white male risk factor—ultimately failed as a clinically tested indicator because it was not quantifiable in a way that could be compressed into risk-factor discourse.[44] It is important to qualify its failure a little. The concept of Type A has certainly lived on in the public imagination along with an image of a white male executive who dies too young of a heart attack—few in that demographic would imagine that they are *not* at risk. However, if previous attention to the stress of white men was predicated on a contrast with imagined carefree African Americans, some more recent discussions of stress have come to center on African Americans themselves. Without challenging the existence of white stress, clinical and epidemiological studies began in the 1990s to consider the stress of racism in quantifiable ways, sometimes operationalized as discrete categories such as "race-based discrimination at work,"[45] and other times in a more generalized way in the catch-all of *black stress*. The stress of racism is also a way to tell stories about connections between ways of life and experiences of disease,[46] no less now than when physicians at the beginning of the twentieth century were diagnosing their own heart disease as a "disease of modernity."[47] Stress-induced heart disease remains a compelling site to negotiate understandings of race and class, now for African Americans as well as whites. Racism has become theorized as a peculiar kind of stressor.

One of the most helpful models through which epidemiologists and physicians have analyzed African American hypertension posits that racism, rather than race, accounts for the disparity. This concept, as developed by epidemiologists including Camara Jones, includes institutional racism (e.g., lack of access to medical care), personally mediated racism (e.g., racism of medical providers), and internalized racism (e.g., accepting stereotypes as true).[48] The second two of these are deeply related to epidemiologists' understandings of stress.

For the epidemiologist Nancy Krieger, racism as risk is both intertwined with and exceeds the psychosocial stress of living in a racist society. She highlights the difference between focusing on "biological expressions of race relations" and "racialized expressions of biology": "The former draws attention to how harmful physical and psychosocial exposures due to racism adversely affect our biology, in ways that ultimately are embodied and manifested in racial/ethnic disparities in health. The latter refers to how arbitrary biological traits are erroneously construed as markers of innate 'racial' distinctions."[49] Physicians, after all, are one group that mediate the space where Krieger posits the location of the health consequences of discrimination: "The investigation of intimate connections between our social and biological existence."[50] The epidemiologist Clarence Gravlee has done some of the most helpful work on how racial categories *become* biology, by showing that hypertension is more correlated with an individual's racial category than it is with ancestry-informative genetic markers.[51]

Anne Fausto-Sterling, a biologist and STS scholar, similarly argues that the stress of racism is the underlying cause of black hypertension. She uses a thermostat metaphor to explain the problems with scientists' widespread use of homeostasis as a model for understanding the regulation of hypertension for those under chronic stress: "An increasingly accepted model of human physiology that suggests that so-called essential hypertension, the health scourge of African Americans, is in some sense a natural physiological response to the deprivations and stresses of being a person of color in America. In other words, it is not that *different* biological processes underlie disease formation in different races, but that different life experience activates physiological processes common to all, but less provoked in some."[52] Fausto-Sterling suggests that allostasis (a basal state that anticipates future demands) rather than homeostasis (a basal state that maintains a constant "normal" pressure) best helps to understand why elevated African American blood pressures do not abate. She argues: "Hypertension is an orchestrated response to a predicted need to remain vigilant to a variety of insults and danger—be they racial hostility, enraging acts of discrimination, or living in the shadow of violence. Over time, all of the components that regulate blood pressure adapt to life under stress."[53] For Fausto-Sterling, this model suggests that hypertension should be better treated with emotional and lifestyle interventions, which would address the source of the trouble, than with drugs that would treat only late manifestations. That is, according Fausto-Sterling, treating hypertension rather than decreasing stress—altering later manifestations resulting from allostasis rather than the conditions that induce the state—can exacerbate the problem by inducing the body to do even more to achieve its own norm of a heightened equilibrium. This model allows her to account for biological processes that originate not from genetic determinism but from embodied responses to stressful lived experience.

However, not all those that indict racism as the cause of African American hypertension indict pharmaceutical response as harmful. In fact, attention to drugs provides another way to understand how racism impacts biology. Even in a pharmaceutically saturated society like the United States, there are real barriers to access, and these are racially stratified. Racism also shapes biology through the deprivation of drugs. Physicians are less likely to adhere to best practices for cardiovascular disease when the patient is black.[54] African American hypertension is less likely to be aggressively medicated, in part because many physicians believe that African American hypertension is poorly controlled with drugs, and also because they often assume that African American patients will be less compliant with treatment. For disparities-focused physicians such as those at the International Society for Hypertension in Blacks, racism is also a way to label physician resistance to aggressively treating African Americans. Many of the physicians in ISHIB are investigators on huge, diverse clinical trials that have defined the gold standard for hypertension and cardiovascular disease treatment for all populations, and so it can be particularly frustrating that physicians often do not follow this gold standard when drafting their African American patients.

Amid these heated debates, it is worth considering the stakes in displacing race onto one of these alternatives, be it socioeconomics, stress, culture, or even racism. The often stated goal of epidemiology is that a more precise understanding of the cause of health disparities will lead to a more effective solution. On the one hand, epidemiologists and physicians routinely recommend nonpharmaceutical solutions—even in guidelines that focus on pharmaceuticals[55]—even though these are hard to put into practice. On the other hand, the commitment to the idea that cause and cure must be aligned—that cause and cure must be of matching pure types—is not universally shared. Etiological eclecticism is more characteristic of medical knowledge of complex diseases than is precision. Moreover, it is possible to locate the cause of disparities in social inequality, and still participate in intervening on biology.

Trying to Get Control of Race

The American Heart Association, on its website explaining hypertension to a lay audience, outlines several factors contributing to high blood pressure. Since high blood pressure is itself of interest insofar as it is a risk factor for cardiovascular disease events such as heart attack, stroke, and heart failure, these might be understood as second-order risk factors—risk factors for risk. The chart divides risk factors for hypertension into two kinds, "controllable" and "uncontrollable":

Controllable risk factors

Obesity—People with a body mass index (BMI) of 30.0 or higher are more likely to develop high blood pressure.
Eating too much salt—A high sodium intake increases blood pressure in some people.
Drinking too much alcohol—Heavy and regular use of alcohol can increase blood pressure dramatically.
Lack of physical activity—An inactive lifestyle makes it easier to become overweight and increases the chance of high blood pressure.
Stress—This is often mentioned as a risk factor, but stress levels are hard to measure, and responses to stress vary from person to person.

Uncontrollable risk factors

Race—African Americans develop high blood pressure more often than whites, and it tends to occur earlier and be more severe.
Heredity—If your parents or other close blood relatives have high blood pressure, you're more likely to develop it.
Age—In general, the older you get, the greater your chance of developing high blood pressure. It occurs most often in people over age 35. Men

seem to develop it most often between age 35 and 55. Women are more likely to develop it after menopause.[56]

On one level, the division between "controllable" and "uncontrollable" participates in the naturalization of race. It is presented in a way that makes race itself seem to explain disparities, and to exist within the bodies of racialized people. Yet it is worth noting that many of the things that we might imagine to occupy the underlying risk in the category of African American are included in the "controllable" list—high salt consumption, obesity, stress, and sedentary lifestyle—while race itself is taken out to stand on its own as well. In this sense, race appears on both sides of the un/controllable divide. Moreover, race is counted twice within the "uncontrollable," since race without those "controllable" factors presumably overlaps with "heredity."

But at the same time, the chart works to collapse controllable and uncontrollable. This is because within medical practice things on both sides of the un/controllable division are treated in the same way. The risk factors are not really imagined to be "uncontrollable" once they are incorporated into practical medical (and in particular pharmaceutical) logic. Although race is uncontrollable in this chart, its effects on the cardiovascular system can be undone by adopting the right lifestyle medications and taking the right pills. In effect, the "controllable" and "uncontrollable" risk factors are all treated the same way: principally through drugs.

For the turn toward medical and in particular pharmaceutical response, it is not necessary to argue that race is genetic. As we have seen, many factors have been enrolled in etiologically eclectic understandings of racial disparities in hypertension—including obesity, diet, and stress. These are listed on the "controllable" side of the chart, while race is conceived of as "uncontrollable." This is worth unpacking, but is at the same time beside the point for the pragmatic physician, regardless of how the physician understands race. By putting "race" under the heading "uncontrollable," this chart might at first appear to be a taxonomy of mutability and immutability, but it also plays on other medical registers of control.

The Durability of Race in Hypertension: Recordability and Calls to Action

We could question as historically contingent not just the contents but also the parameters of a whole host of things subsumed by the category "race" in discourses of hypertension. All of the alternatives to race itself that are posited to underlie African American hypertension—stress, poverty, and more—are ways of telling stories about heart disease that are racialized but not exclusive to any one race. Part of the advantage to using race as a category rather than any one of these alternatives is that it captures what antiracist epidemiologists have described as the "accumulated insults" of living in a racist society.[57] From a physician's perspective, separating out the "accumulated insults" faced by the patient before them—imagining race, class, and stress as discrete and separable phenomena—is even less tenable than it is for the epidemiologist.

Despite arguments that something besides race would better characterize disparities, race in medicine generally and African American hypertension in particular is resilient. The debate over what underlies African American hypertension does not destabilize it, but rather renders African American hypertension as a disease category that is—in Althusser's terms—overdetermined.[58] African American hypertension exists in a *contextual* relationship with genes, discrimination, socioeconomic status, and more, and need not be seen as having a definitively *causal* relationship with any of these. As Janet Shim has pointed out in her analysis of the routinized inclusion of race, socioeconomic status, and gender in epidemiological research, the multifactorial disease model itself can effectively mitigate the ambiguities of any particular factor being investigated in terms of race—whether genetic, psychological, or discrimination—and reinforce "the validity of the multifactorial model and its inclusion of race."[59]

One thing that unites all of the aspects of what race might point to is that none of them are consistently recorded—unlike race, which is routinely recorded. Telling physicians to base therapeutic decisions on whether someone is of low socioeconomic status, stressed out by racism, living a lifestyle typical of highly segregated postindustrial urban areas, or even some kind of genetic test given the expense and time that that approach still involves—all of these are less efficient than telling physicians to use a particular drug regimen for a population that is already reified and recorded, by race. If recorded race can be defined as a risk factor, this is conceivably a way to add it to other things that are also recorded that serve as indicators for prescriptions.

An evocative phrase used by Elijah Saunders, a founder of ISHIB, at a 2004 conference was that being African American can be thought of as a risk factor "like diabetes."[60] Status as African American might be "like diabetes" because it is in fact diabetes—African Americans are likely to have more conditions that compound the risks of hypertension and heart disease generally; it also may be "like diabetes" in that it is correlated with higher morbidity and mortality from heart disease. But more importantly, Saunders is suggesting that status as African American is "like diabetes" in terms of prescription guidelines. Any condition that creates the need for a lower blood pressure goal is a risk factor "like diabetes." Saunders argues that, like those with diabetes, it is particularly urgent that African Americans' blood pressure be lowered, and therefore their drug regimens should be more aggressive. In a context in which effective blood pressure control rates are going up overall, but there is a growing disparity between the effective control of blood pressure in white patients versus black patients, this operates as a demand for reaching goals.[61] In this way, he makes it as simple as possible for individual physicians to change their differential diagnosis from one that has led to less aggressive treatment for African Americans and replace it with one that leads to more aggressive treatment for African Americans.

Saunders thus seeks to intervene at the site of what John Hoberman has called "the rhetoric of exculpation,"[62] in which physicians acknowledge sociological data about the harms of physicians' racial stereotyping but refuse to take responsibility for them. As Hoberman points out, physicians use their hectic schedules as an excuse for any undertreatment of African Americans in aggregate (and deny that they themselves are guilty of such behavior). From the dais of medical conferences, as in guidelines published with his ISHIB colleagues, Saunders responds by making quick, clear, specific demands for change on the level of the individual prescribing physician.[63] As Hoberman has pointed out, "disproportionate emphasis on the *complexity* of the origins of racial disparities and how much about them remains unknown" can be a way for physicians to abdicate responsibility for them.[64] Like Saunders's move in the vignette at the start of this chapter, in which he half-joked about treating "people who look like the ones in this picture," ISHIB's advocacy of low blood-pressure goals for African Americans strives to short-circuit physicians' tendency to absolve themselves of the responsibility to use medical treatment to ameliorate disparities.

Two ideological trends are coming together to make the status of African American into a risk factor for various constituencies, including civil rights–oriented physicians' organizations and pharmaceutical companies. First, the totalization of risk-factor discourse such that everyone has at least one risk factor, which means both that ascription of a risk factor is not necessarily stigmatizing,[65] and that labeling any particular thing a "risk factor" does not suggest that someone without it is not at risk. Second, the hegemony of pharmaceutical thinking, in which drugs are almost always better than no drugs (and two drugs are better than one drug and so on . . .). In this logic, the way to get that intrinsic good of maximizing a patient's number of medications is by assigning risk factors liberally. From the perspectives both of the pharmaceutical companies and the civil rights–oriented physicians advocating the categorization of "African American" as a risk factor, there is no downside, only an upside: increased prescriptions of drugs (yielding increased profit for the one and improved patient health for the other). Even when lifestyle modifications are promoted rather than pharmaceuticals per se, these rely on the same logic: in the framework of health education, calling attention to the severity of risk is certainly not meant to lead to fatalism, but to motivate action.

Robert Aronowitz credits the allure of the concept of the risk factor to two of its characteristics: its ambiguity—it can "denote association with, cause of, predisposition to, or responsibility for disease"—and its utilitarian criteria—it can command treatment like a disease.[66] Aronowitz notes that for the designers of the Framingham Study "anything you could measure that became associated with a higher rate of heart attack or stroke later in life became a risk factor."[67] I agree with Aronowitz about ambiguity and utility contributing to the appeal of the risk-factor concept, but I would argue that the concept is in fact even more expansive than he suggests: a potential risk factor does not have to be measurable. It has only to be *recordable*.

Evelynn Hammonds argues that scientists and historians of science who have observed a shift from "gross morphological studies of racial difference" to those of "populations and gene frequencies" have misread the meaning of the shift—although the meaning ascribed to morphology has shifted, "In the US race has always been dependent on the visual."[68] And it is race as a visual category that is generally recorded on the medical record. As the sociologists Stefan Timmermans and Marc Berg have argued, the development of the paper-based individual patient record was fundamental to the standardization of medicine in the early twentieth century, and individual patient records have been central to the ongoing debates about evidence-based medicine.[69] And as Berg foregrounds elsewhere, the medical record does not merely represent the doctor-patient encounter, but is also constitutive of that encounter, because it "plays an active, constitutive role in *mediating* the relations that act and work through it."[70] In the United States, race, gender, and age are all conventionally included prominently on the patient record, together with measurements of vital statistics such as blood pressure and temperature. Distinctions between characteristics that are measured (such as weight and blood pressure) and those that are merely recorded (such as age and race) are flattened once entered on the standardized physical examination record.

In this recordability, we can see a moment of *both* labeling and action. Once the category has been recorded, no matter how messy what underlies it might be, action can be framed around it. This is true, as Karin Garrety has argued, with the most traditional of risk factors: the stabilization of cholesterol as a risk factor came not from conclusive data shifts but from the way it allowed actors in diverse social worlds ranging from activists to food companies to "do something."[71] And it is true with race as risk factor. This is the move that Saunders called for in the symposium—to let the messiness behind the category remain, while taking action to help the "people who look like those in this picture." Because of existing preoccupations with race in America, this strategy to look "for people that look like those in this picture" almost always works. Unlike alternatives like socioeconomic status for example, doctors routinely and more or less consciously look for a patient's race, and they almost always find it. One thing that Saunders is doing is trying to intervene in what they do next.

As I will explore further in the next chapter, the debate between whether the realness of race comes from the social or from the biological does nothing to stop the reification of race, or of African American hypertension and heart disease. If race is social and economic, many would argue, it is mutable, and this mutability is imagined to be negated if difference is understood as biological. But for physicians like Saunders, the biological and the social are both potential sites of intervention.

Despite the protests of those who argue for social causes of and social solutions for disease, there is no evidence that medical researchers could easily be moved away from individualistic solutions no matter where the cause of disease is located. For the turn toward medical and in particular pharmaceutical response, it is not necessary to argue that race is genetic, and social reasoning about causation does not necessarily lead to social responses for amelioration. As the anthropologist Ian Whitmarsh has argued in his work on asthma in Barbados, arguments over the origins of disease, its extent, and even the efficacy of pharmaceutical treatment do not impede the distribution and consumption of pharmaceuticals, but foster it: "Ambiguity is central to processes of pharmaceuticalization."[72] This observation is no less true in the United States. Physicians on the ground tend to be less interested in questions of disease origins than in questions of "what now?" Thus the focus of STS critiques should be not only to criticize the marking of bodies in today's medicalization, but also to grapple with the pharmaceuticalization of medical practice more broadly, in which racialized medicine plays one part.

Full participation in American society is at stake in the mobilizations for drugs into bodies, bringing African Americans more fully into the pharmaceutical grammar that Joseph Dumit has termed "drugs for life."[73] Physicians and pharmaceutical companies using the disease category "African American hypertension" to both call attention to African American distinctiveness and argue for full integration of African Americans into gold-standard treatment (i.e., hypermedication) are participating in what Omi and Winant call *racial projects*: simultaneously involved in "interpretation, representation, or explanation" *and* striving "to redistribute resources along particular racial lines."[74] To understand the terrain, we should attend to the ways that articulations of African American hypertension render race both stable and malleable. To complement attention to the ways that risk factor grammars naturalize race, we must attend to the ways that they seek to mobilize race.

Essentialist maneuvers by physician organizations, pharmaceutical companies, and epidemiologists are only part of the story of how race becomes durable. The power of the notion of racial "immutability" never lies in "immutability" itself, but rather in its tension with malleability. Stoler points out that "The notion of 'immutability' may play off deep cognitive beliefs about what constitutes human kinds, but, ironically, it only becomes a potent political principle when the attributes designated as immutable are pliable and plastic."[75] She argues that the discourse of racial immutability does "two kinds of work: it both confirms *and* calls into question the discreteness of human kinds."[76] As I will explore in the chapters that follow, something similar could be said of race and pharmaceuticals: a pharmaceutical solution both attributes biological distinctiveness to African Americans and undermines that distinctiveness. Race becomes a distinction that both can and cannot be medicated away.

CHAPTER 4

The Slavery Hypothesis
beyond Genetic Determinism

The setting was a midday colloquium at the W. E. B. Du Bois Institute for African American Studies at Harvard, featuring the rising young economist Roland Fryer.[1] The title of the talk was ambitious: "Understanding the Racial Difference in Life Expectancy."[2] Fryer's goal in his captivating presentation was to explain the persistent difference between African American and white morbidity and mortality. After controlling for such explanations as education, income, diet, geographic region, and access to health care—the explanations that come to mind most readily for economists or for that matter social scientists as a whole—Fryer turned outside these disciplines' traditional line of argument, invoking a theory known as "the slavery hypothesis."

The slavery hypothesis was described in its fullest form by Thomas Wilson and Clarence Grim in the journal *Hypertension* in 1991.[3] The theory claims that selection pressures in Atlantic slavery predispose African Americans to salt retention, leading to hypertension and thus to cardiovascular disease. The suggestion is that those Africans who were genetically predisposed to conserve salt were the ones to survive the arduous conditions and diarrheal diseases of the journey to and experience of slavery, and so as a result their descendants are salt-conserving. According to this argument, while a tendency to conserve salt might have been protective against old hazards such as cholera, it is dangerous today because it leads to hypertension and cardiovascular disease. The theory holds that the difference in salt sensitivity explains the difference in cardiovascular disease and the excessive morbidity and mortality of African Americans today.

The audience response at this particular colloquium was energetic. Here was a black scholar reactivating a racialist theory that most academics have rejected, yet the response was overwhelmingly positive.[4] When an elderly white geneticist in the audience protested, asking, "Doesn't making the cause of disparities genetic mean that there is nothing to be done, it's unchangeable?" Fryer responded, "Oh no, there's a drug for that!" "Which drug?" the audience wanted to know. Fryer drew a momentary blank, and uttered some fragments: "chloro . . . hydro . . ." A voice shot up from the front row—it was the chair of the Harvard Department of Afro-American Studies, the renowned literary theorist and public intellectual Henry Louis Gates Jr. "Hydrochlorothiazide!" he exclaimed. "I'm on that! I'm a salt-saving Negro!"

This statement was dramatic, and it was jarring, given that discussion in both African American studies and in the history and social studies of science generally operates on the consensus that race is a social construct and not a genetic one. Evelynn Hammonds, an African American historian of medicine in the audience, was at a loss to address the situation, beyond pointing out that Philip Curtin, the prominent historian of slavery, had roundly refuted the salt-saving hypothesis.[5] After a brief question about the nature of Curtin's critique, Gates and the audience returned to the thesis with enthusiasm. The historian's critique missed the emotive point at hand, which did not actually rest on the scientific and historical facts underlying the theory.

I will return to a closer reading of this encounter, but first I want to trace other debates about the hypothesis in order to show that both epistemological eclecticism underlying African American hypertension, and the availability of pharmaceutical treatment for it, are vital for understanding the appeal of this genetic explanation. This hypothesis has been critiqued vociferously, for many reasons, and it is simultaneously marginal and mainstream. On the one hand, little research has been done on it by very few people. On the other, it is widely known and referred to in venues like medical conferences and textbooks,[6] albeit with caveats of its lack of proof. Discussion of it takes place in the major journals in the field, but without earning anything close to consensus acceptance. The slavery hypothesis is appealing for history of science critique because it is a dramatic narrative combined with odd Darwinian claims brought down to a small time scale, in evolutionary terms.

In my analysis of this most sensational genetic explanation for African American hypertension, and the problems with its debunking, I argue that critics of the slavery hypothesis fail to engage with medicine as a field, one that not only arbitrates racialized bodies but also intervenes on them. Here, I will attend to several of the theory's sympathizers in order to show that critique of the theory that moves beyond a debunking mode can open up new insights into race and medicine. Attending to what is at stake for the theory's proponents and describing the failure of its opponents to grapple with those plural stakes highlights the points of consensus that underlie the arguments of both sides in these discussions.

What unites these sympathizers of the theory is not that they are genetic determinists—they are not—but something quite different that has little to do with genes per se. The hypertension clinician Clarence Grim, the humanities scholar Henry Louis Gates Jr., the psychiatrist Joel Dimsdale, and the media figure Oprah Winfrey are all in the mainstream of their respective fields and see themselves as involved in antiracist projects. As I will show, another thing that they all share is a sensibility that is amenable to myths—that is, *myths* in the sense of powerful stories about the past that matter to people in the present. They all speak of novels as a source of insight. Critique of the slavery hypothesis that rests only on scientific facts does not completely engage them, and I will attend to the critiques of these figures to show that focus on the dangers of genetic data and determinism misses important parts of why this story is compelling for actors such as these. I suggest that opponents of the thesis also participate in the reification of African American hypertension, and that it is more productive to track the simultaneously social and biological discourses of race that pervade the debate than to argue about the racism of the theory's proponents.

Origin Stories of the Hypothesis

To understand how the slavery hypothesis participates in medicating race, it must be seen not only as a natural science theory that arbitrates race but also as a story that can be enrolled in clinical practice that intervenes upon race. Consider two conflicting origin stories of the slavery hypothesis—only one of which has a role for medical intervention.

The most extensive review and critique of the slavery hypothesis was written by Jay Kaufman and Susan Hall and appeared in *Epidemiology* in 2003.[7] They provide a compelling debunking, drawing on arguments from history, population genetics, and evolutionary biology. Yet their explanation for the wide acceptance of the theory—the pervasiveness of genetic essentialism in medicine—is less convincing. Here is the origin story of the hypothesis that they provide. Kaufman and Hall suggest that the hypothesis emerged in dialectical response to earlier medical literature that posited that high rates of African American hypertension were the result of high rates of hypertension in Africans. However, Africans were shown to in fact have low rates of hypertension.

And so, according to Kaufman and Hall, the slavery hypothesis was a way for physicians who were committed to genetic explanations for racial disparities to continue to understand African American hypertension as genetic, and yet account for genetic difference between Africans and African Americans. The language that Kaufman and Hall use is highly deterministic. They describe the researchers as "locked in a paradigm that favored genetic explanations for the black-white disparity."[8]

Here is the origin story of the hypothesis provided by the hypertension clinician, Clarence Grim, as he described it to me in 2005.[9] He explained his interest as coming from two simultaneous sources: clinical experience, and the science of salt in physiology and history.

On the one hand, Grim has had formative and long-standing clinical experiences with successfully treating severely hypertensive black patients. This included a case of an extreme form of treatable hypertension (now called Conn's Syndrome) that he saw in a black woman when he was a medical student in Missouri in the early 1960s, in addition to the many black patients with renal failure he saw during his residency at Duke, his work on the Evans County Study in Georgia,[10] a fellowship at the Martin Luther King Hospital in Los Angeles in the 1980s—where he started reading black history at the urging of fellow clinicians there—and his long-standing practice in Milwaukee.

On the other hand, Grim became convinced of the importance of salt metabolism in his training by two key advisors: Walter Kempner and Derek Denton. The two had very different emphases. Dr. Kempner, with whom Grim worked at Duke, became famous for his "rice diet," which was designed to treat kidney disease but which also dramatically decreased blood pressure—in the rich white patients who could afford to stay in his care for six months.[11] In the early 1980s, Grim spent a year with Dr. Denton, an Australian who put appetite for and endocrine response to salt at the center of anthropological, physiological, and medical analysis in a virtuosic 1982 tome called The Hunger for Salt.[12]

Grim described these two aspects of his training and experience as starting to come together when he read descriptions of the stench of slave ships in James Michener's historical novel Hawaii.[13] The more he read about the nature of black mortality in the Atlantic slave trade, the more he became convinced of the connections between salt, black history, and the hypertension he treated in his patients. Grim attributes his skepticism of the alternative explanation for black hypertension—psychosocial stress of living in a racist society—to the fact that blacks in the Caribbean have high rates of hypertension even though, according to Grim, they do not deal with racism on a day-to-day basis. Grim characterizes his argument as a minority one, one that has always led people to attack him for being racist, but one that he perseveres with because of his dedication to the validity of the theory. He has done research in the basic science: twin studies in Barbados to show that salt sensitivity is genetic,[14] for example, and there are many more studies he would like to do. He described with disdain the previous hypothesis for black hypertension—that African Americans hadn't evolved enough for the modern world—and sees his theory as a nonracist alternative that fits well with clinical practice.

What is at stake in these differing origin stories of the slavery hypothesis? For Kaufman and Hall, what is important about the slavery hypothesis is that clinicians refer to it at all, in spite of its poor evidentiary basis. They are particularly critical of its proponents' scant explication in peer-reviewed journals and their failure to respond to critiques of the theory. For Kaufman and Hall, the fact that the theory nevertheless has widespread knowledge in the community of hypertension researchers demonstrates the continuation of a pernicious racialization that has long characterized unequal medicine. What they are not attentive to, however, is where these conversations are taking place, and what precisely underlies them. In most of the citations of the theory, reference to the theory is markedly agnostic. The textbooks are not "locked" into genetic ideas alone, but rather intrigued by genetics as they tell a story of race that draws on a messy complex of nature and nurture.

For Grim, what is important in this hypothesis is that it brings together biology and history with practical medical interventions. Throughout his scientific research, Grim has used the model that "all humans are salt-sensitive, the question is the level," and that responsiveness to thiazide diuretics is a measure of salt sensitivity.[15] All the while, he has been a practitioner advocating careful measurement of blood pressure, and salt restriction and diuretics as preferred treatments for everyone with hypertension, especially for blacks. I asked Grim whether it was scientific interest or clinical interest that primarily drove him, and he said, "It's all together. The ultimate experimental animal is humans. I don't care about those rats. I don't treat any rats. So everything that drives my interest [is] in trying to control high blood pressure and find out the causes of high blood pressure."[16]

If I sound like something of an apologist for Grim, this is not to discount the speciousness of his theory. Rather, I want to highlight that his epidemiologist critics and Grim both participate in racial discourses, and it is more productive to track those than to hunt for racists. I am guided here by Ann Laura

Stoler, who has pointed out that "a common historiographic assumption is that racial discourse is a discourse of those with power (or those trying to maintain their hold) rather than a 'dense transfer point' of it."[17] By assuming that the fundamental thing done by Grim's theory is to prop up racism in natural science, Kaufman and Hall miss the clinical and other arenas at stake. For Kaufman and Hall, science precedes practice, but attending to clinical practice helps us to see that—whatever his other failings—Grim is right that, in medicine, science and practice are immanent.

When Kaufman and Hall describe the implications of the theory, they write as if Grim and others sympathetic to the theory were merely basic scientists observing natural states, not also clinicians intervening in them:

> Finally, the seemingly irresistible siren song of the Slavery Hypothesis may derive in part from its implications for scientific conceptions of race and identity. Once Grim had devised the evolutionary hypothesis of rapid genetic selection during the period of slavery, it provided a basis for exceptionalism in discussion of African American hypertension, a basis for treating American blacks as a group that had been uniquely and intractably transformed, genetically mutilated. The essential "defect" or "abnormality" in this group therefore achieved not only rational basis, but became something innately pathologic, thereby reinforcing blacks' essential physical inferiority in the modern world. Given the common African origins of all humanity, therefore, the Slavery Hypothesis may serve not merely to provide an explanation for the biological distinction between racial/ethnic groups, but to judge that distinction as a deformity rather than a mere divergence.[18]

In this critique, there is a failure to engage with Grim as a subject rather than as a caricature. For Grim, who was trained by a physician renowned for the belief in radical dietary change, and who is a proponent of low-salt diets and aggressive diuretic treatment for hypertension, difference in blood pressure is far from "intractable." Indeed, responsiveness to salt restriction and treatment through diuretics is part of how black hypertension is characterized. The language of "inferiority" that Kaufman and Hall use would be abhorrent to Grim himself (and indeed his response published in the same issue of *Epidemiology* took issue with that characterization).[19] Moreover, for Grim, the salt aspect of both the cause and intervention for hypertension is as important as the genetics aspect. And, as Kaufman and Hall themselves note, medical beliefs in African American inferiority, including ones that used hypertension as evidence, preceded Grim by a good deal. Those beliefs do not rise or fall on the truth value of the theory. To frame a debunking as an antiracist project is a common error that Stoler documents in antiracist historiography: the fantasy "that if we can disprove the credibility of race as a scientific concept, we can dismantle the power of racism itself—that racisms rise and fall on the scientific credibility of the concept of race."[20]

In their critique of the slavery hypothesis, Kaufman and Hall acknowledge the identity practices around seeing black hypertension in terms of the legacy of slavery, but they reject the value of that because of the danger of discrimination that would result from calling black hypertension genetic. They make references to the problems of discrimination based on sickle cell anemia to argue: "As in the case of sickle cell anemia, the presence of a biological trait that is understood to derive directly from Africa or from the initial passage from Africa may . . . become an authenticating characteristic. The myth of genetic determinism cuts both ways, however, for although it absolves the individual of responsibility, it also absolves society at large."[21] They cite Dorothy Nelkin to suggest: "Deterministic biological explanations ('it's in my genes')—much like theological explanations ('the devil made me do it')—locate problems (and, therefore solutions) within individuals."[22] However, in its context of cheap and effective treatment, "black hypertension" is radically different from "black sickle cell," much less demonic possession. Kaufman and Hall's suggestion that genetic determinism absolves both the individual and society of responsibility is in brazen disregard for how Grim actually uses the theory in practice. On the contrary, when the theory is combined with interventionist medicine, it becomes a way to locate blame in the social processes of a horrific history *without* abdicating responsibility for changing an unacceptable present. Grim conceptualizes change as possible through diet, clinical care, and the social distribution of drugs. When disease definition and therapeutic promises are immanent, the stakes of biological arguments change, and critiquing genetic determinism is not up to the task.

Kaufman's critique of the genetic framing of African American hypertension extends that of his advisor, Richard Cooper, who gave a presentation on African American hypertension at the ASH symposium described in the previous chapter, a talk that continued his decades-long work arguing for social and environmental causes of hypertension and disease disparities.[23] However, in Cooper's critique, as in Kaufman and Hall's, there is a remarkable failure to engage with what is at stake for his opponents in the debate. For example, writing in 1986 in the *Journal of Health Politics, Policy and Law*, Cooper and his colleague Richard David suggest that the danger of assuming that genetic factors are more important than social ones, and that a sophisticated analysis of class is unnecessary, is that important public health interventions are ignored and the high rates of black hypertension are imagined to be immutable. They connect conceptualizations of black hypertension as genetic to the histories of "drapetomania" and syphilis and more, cases in public health in which "the theory of race serves to justify racial inequality."[24] Yet Cooper does not challenge the existence of the disparity itself, and opens a 1997 article coauthored with Charles Rotimi with the unequivocal claim that: "The excess of hypertension among blacks has been recognized since early in this century and explains a substantial portion of the black health disadvantage."[25]

Kaufman's and Cooper's "race is not genetic" mantra, while true, does not counter racial reification in medicine. Clinicians are perfectly capable of using a wide variety of modes of understanding race that do not rely on genetics alone. Moreover, for both sides in each of the debates over the etiology of black hypertension, there is consensus that action can be taken. Neither side of any of these thinks that disparities, whether genetic or psychosocial, are inevitable and should be accepted.

More unites the two sides than Kaufman and Hall let on, in particular, the belief that African American hypertension is a legitimate topic of research and intervention. Kaufman and Hall suggest that a genetic theory precludes intervention, but Grim actually participates in both medical and social change. Grim is a white physician participating in white-dominated discussions of basic science–oriented arguments about racial difference, and this is the aspect that Kaufman and Hall address. Yet Grim is also a clinician treating hypertension in blacks. He is intervening, not just observing, and changing the biology that Kaufman and Hall assume is fixed.

If we take seriously Peter Wade's call to historicize racialized natures, rather than assume that every naturalizing discourse across time and space is a deterministic one,[26] Grim's historical position in this period of pharmaceuticalized medicine matters. In this sense, we might read Grim as less a practitioner of genetic determinism of an old school than as part of what David Skinner has characterized as a new biologism. Skinner argues: "Dystopian critics associate biological arguments with determinism, essentialism and the naturalization of difference, but new biological knowledge can and does take contrary forms that challenge conformist assumptions and existing divisions with an account of material heterogeneity and contingency."[27] Grim is not a passive natural scientist; he participates in organizing with diverse health care providers committed to improving the health of African Americans. Context matters, and

Grim's contexts are plural. As important as the scientific argument between him and his nemesis the genetic epidemiologist Richard Cooper is, it is also important that they are both members of the International Society for Hypertension in Blacks and that both participate in practical efforts to ameliorate disparities. Thus, neither the theory's proponents nor its opponents really think that no action can be taken. When Cooper and Grim debate the hypothesis in venues such as the International Society for Hypertension in Blacks, neither argues that disparities are inevitable and should be accepted. Kaufman and Cooper are far less clinically oriented than Grim, so it is not surprising that they see the social as malleable and the biological as fixed. However, it is important not to take this dichotomy for granted. Grim has made his career not only by describing but also by altering patients' biologies.

The Hypothesis amid Epistemological Eclecticism

Each time that the debate over the slavery hypothesis is reenacted, it does not challenge but rather takes for granted the existence of African American hypertension as an entity. To illustrate how this works, consider a debate about the slavery hypothesis that took place in the journal *Psychosomatic Medicine* in 2000. A leader of the journal, the psychiatrist Joel Dimsdale, wrote of the theory sympathetically in the context of a larger piece that described diverse etiologies for persistent ethnic disparities in health, in which hypertension was a major focus.[28] He used the theory as an additive explanation to psychosocial stress (which is his area of specialization) rather than an alternative to it. After defining phenotype as "a composite of culture, genotype, and the physical environment"[29] in which all elements come into play, considering the shaky definitions involved in self-reported ethnicity, and remarking at the nonetheless powerful influence ethnicity has on health, Dimsdale wrote about relationships between ethnicity and memory in an epistemologically eclectic way: "At its heart, ethnicity involves the legacy of the past, and that legacy comes from many sources of memory. There is memory in our genes. William Least Heat-Moon recognizes this legacy by speaking 'of genetic inclinations whereby ancestors seem to stalk our blood.' Memory also comes, of course, from our personal life experiences and our families' experiences. As Faulkner points out 'the past is not dead; the past is not even past.' Thus, there are reverberating levels of history and ethnicity that influence health on multiple levels."[30] Dimsdale devoted roughly equal space to consideration of the possible roles of "salt and slavery" and "stress and physiology," and smaller sections on "emotional expression" and "letting go." He concluded with his quirky ideas about memory as well: "I have tried to summarize many of the approaches my colleagues and I have used in our studies of ethnicity and health. Low social class, invidious life treatment, and differences in physiological vulnerability all determine risk trajectories across ethnic groups. Every one of us carries legacies (bequests and burdens), which are encoded in our genes, immune system, our group's experience, and our own individual life experiences. These 'memories' must be considered in understanding different susceptibilities to illness."[31] This is a rich way of reading history, with a literary and mythic sensibility in which both ancestors and individuals matter.

The epidemiologist Jay Kaufman wrote a letter in response to Dimsdale's piece.[32] In it, he suggested that the rest of the article was "thoughtful and illuminating," but focused his response singularly on refuting what he called "Dr. Grim's fairytale." He warned that "the essay in *Psychosomatic Medicine* has unwittingly perpetuated this old pseudoscientific canard, which plays into the hands of racial essentialists and biological determinists." This rhetorical construction is common in critique of the hypothesis: Kaufman suggested not that this particular sympathizer of the theory was malicious, but that he was an "unwitting" proponent of the racist and incorrect theory, and thus a potential danger abetting unnamed others.[33] Kaufman did not suggest that Dimsdale himself was a reductionist biological determinist (and such a claim would be an odd one since Dimsdale is an elite psychiatrist who is a leader in the field of the relationships between stress and physiology and cultural factors in illness). Instead, Kaufman suggested that Dimsdale's article would aid and abet the elusive and dangerous biological determinists out there.

Kaufman concluded his critique with a statement of bafflement, "We may wonder why, despite an absolute lack of supporting evidence, in fact a great weight of contradictory evidence, otherwise smart and reasonable people continue to rehash this fantasy as though it were sensible and respectable science."[34] But the fact that "smart people" *are* sympathetic to the theory could actually be a starting point for further analysis of the productivity of the theory, opening the question of whether the only thing it can do is promote pernicious racism. It is Kaufman's drive to purge genetics from other racial arguments that leads Kaufman to wonder at the invocation of the theory, nonplussed about the role it is playing for his interlocutors, including the epistemologically eclectic Dimsdale. Dimsdale is a leader in psychosomatic medicine, and particularly invested in the immanence of the psyche and the soma, but Kaufman's response seeks to purify psyche from soma.

Kaufman's singular focus on the debunking of genetics leaves uninterrogated more fundamental ontological questions of racial difference in hypertension. For example, Dimsdale's piece acknowledged debate on the slavery hypothesis itself but stated a point of consensus: "Most readers of this literature would agree that black individuals hyper-respond to stressors."[35] Kaufman's response ignores this point, which is not surprising given that there does indeed seem to be consensus on this in the literature. But the noncontroversial claim—that African Americans "hyper-respond" to stressors—is itself worth unpacking. Kaufman only sees racism's return in the genetic aspect because he has not seen its continual persistence in the other aspects. As Dunklee, Reardon, and Wentworth have argued, "Sociologists and humanists can only encounter race's return when they fail to see it all along."[36] It is striking that Dimsdale's statement of consensus conforms to stereotypes of black personalities. That is, if stressors in the world are imagined to be constant, white people respond to them in a standard way while black people respond to them with overreaction. That overreaction, in turn, is purported to be (at least in part) the cause of the increased harm experienced by black people. If this narrative is oversimplified, it does resonate with mainstream racism. As Angela Jenks has pointed out in her analysis of cultural competency, locating disparities in a concept of culture that is understood as individual personality traits that harm health or impede access to care is not necessarily better than locating them in biology.[37] Dimsdale's arguments about the "withheld anger" of African Americans and their "hyper-response" to stressors are not any less enrolled in racial discourse than his points about the slavery hypothesis, and yet exclusive focus on genetics leaves them unaddressed in the only critique published.

It is simply not the case that the category of African American hypertension, whether enrolling genetics or not, is proposed by racists and critiqued by antiracists. That it is a racial discourse does not by itself determine precisely how it will be mobilized. Suggesting that blood pressure elevation comes from the social rather than the genetic does not take it out of the bodies of African Americans.[38] Critique of explanations of African American hypertension must not lean too heavily on critiques of genes and medicine, because the category does not rest on genes alone.

Seeing stress as an explanation *opposed* to genetics is something that makes Kaufman's perspective distinct from Dimsdale's. Even though Kaufman is right that there is scant evidence for the slavery hypothesis, Dimsdale is onto something epistemologically important: if racism is posited to lead to disparity, we need not decide in advance that racism exists on only one level, that current stressors need to be understood to be completely separate from historical experiences of slavery on plural biological, psychological, and social registers.

Debate about whether African American hypertension is social or biological does not undo the durability of the racialized disease category. Debate over whether African American hypertension is caused by genes or by environment does not throw into any question the reification of black hypertension itself. There can be eclecticism in etiology that helps interest in it to proliferate. As Ann Laura Stoler has argued, "The ambiguity of those sets of relationships between the somatic and the inner self, the phenotype and the genotype, pigment shade and psychological sensibility are not slips in, or obstacles to, racial thinking but rather conditions for its proliferation and possibility."[39]

At stake, then, on all sides of this debate is not whether "race is real" generally or whether African American hypertension is "real." Both explanations of African American hypertension—social and genetic—are racial discourses, and clinicians like Dimsdale are perfectly capable of being epistemologically eclectic. Both sides of the debate contribute to the durability of the category of African American hypertension, because both the claim that "African American hypertension is genetic" and the counterclaim that "African American hypertension is psychosocial"—as well as theories that embrace both—presuppose that "African American hypertension *is*."

Beyond Whacking Moles

The appeal of the slavery hypothesis extends far beyond medicine and epidemiology. A recent debate about the slavery hypothesis outside of the academic realm also helps to illustrate the failure of the theory's critics to engage with what is actually at stake for its sympathizers. On a show about health questions in April 2007, Oprah Winfrey invoked the theory uncritically as a way to describe why African Americans have high rates of hypertension.[40] The show's theme was "Ask Dr. Oz II," a chance to ask Winfrey's doctor questions that are too embarrassing to ask one's own doctor. After a series of questions ranging from whether it is dangerous to hold in flatulence or talk too much on a cell phone to what to do about a smelly navel or feet, an African American woman in the audience asked the tenth and final question: what could be causing her excessive sweat? After talking about the possibility of thyroid problems or toxins, Dr. Oz raised the possibility of hypertension and emphasized that hypertension is dangerous and should be aggressively treated not just to the average level but to the optimal level. He chattily asked Winfrey why it is that African Americans have hypertension. She answered by saying: "The reason why African-Americans have higher blood pressure, Dr. Oz, is because during the Middle Passage, the African-Americans who survived were those who could hold more salt into their body. And those who didn't survive were the ones who couldn't hold more salt into their body."[41] Pleased, Dr. Oz said that his work there was done, and the show was over.

It was a passing mention, but one that spurred critique from academic and nonprofit commentators concerned with race and science. Osagie Obasogie, who directs the project on bioethics, law, and society at the Center for Genetics and Society in Oakland, California, wrote an op-ed in the *Los Angeles Times* in which he described the poor evidence for the theory, and warned of the danger that it would suggest that racial disparities should be seen as genetic and unchangeable rather than social and demanding change.[42] Obasogie's piece was titled "What Oprah Doesn't Know," an implication similar to Kaufman's characterization of Dimsdale as "unwitting." Obasogie's piece seemed to assume that if a smart and well-intentioned person like Winfrey *did* know, it would be different, and lamented that her good intentions were subverted by her ignorance: "Though well-intentioned, Winfrey's answer last month effectively lent her credibility, star power and billion-dollar brand to a dubious theory known as the 'slavery hypothesis.'"

Like Kaufman in his critique of Dimsdale, Obasogie did not suggest that Winfrey herself is a pernicious racist, but that pernicious racism follows from the theory that she naively propagated. The critique rests not on the suggestion of racism on the part of Winfrey, the actual proponent of the theory in this instance, but on concern over the hypothetical support for racism that the theory could provide to members of her audience who might be naive or malicious. In this way, Obasogie is like Kaufman. Obasogie prefers to critique those he thinks should be the logical constituents for the hypothesis, people with unexamined racist ideologies. In the process, he disregards the actual ideologies and political practices of those sympathetic to it, who include people who have given extensive thought to race and see themselves as engaged in antiracist projects, such as Oprah Winfrey.

Also like Kaufman, but unlike Dimsdale and Winfrey, Obasogie implied that stress could only be an alternative explanation to genetics, rather than an additive one: "Countless studies show that stressful environments and situations raise blood pressure. And few things are as consistently stressful as being black. By almost every measurable social category—such as income, infant mortality, education, incarceration rates and employment—blacks fare poorly, making everyday life a constant struggle. Only a buried-head ostrich would say that racial discrimination does not play a role in many African Americans' poor health."[43] There is something peculiar in the suggestion that Winfrey "doesn't know" that racism is a cause of disparities. Winfrey would presumably agree with everything Obasogie said about racism being stressful, and has after all put vastly more of her copious airtime and money into promoting stress relief and social change against racial inequality (and fiction reading and dieting and so much more) than into publicizing this theory. What sense does it make to suggest that she is a "buried-head ostrich"? Obasogie wrote: "What's so pernicious about this 'bad gene' theory is that it attributes current health disparities to actions taken nearly four centuries ago, when the more relevant issue may very well be what is happening today. Reducing health disparities to genes obscures more sensible conversations about the contemporary nature of discrimination, how it affects minority health and how best to improve health outcomes."[44] However, Winfrey's embrace of the theory should make us question whether propping up racism in natural science and rendering poor black health immutable are the exclusive and inevitable results of the theory. Neither of those things seems to be part of Winfrey's project. If there is anything that we know about Winfrey's worldview, it is that she thinks that change can happen, on both individual and social levels. In this sense, we should read her invocation of the theory as of a piece with references to it in womanist and African American self-help writing.[45] In the context of this particular show, her performative repetition of the theory seemed to express a fondness for fun health factoids, rather than intellectual or political commitment to one or another etiological model. It may also be part of her affinity with the efforts to build a "liberal anti-racist genomics," a term Jenny Reardon has articulated through engagement with Winfrey's participation in genetic ancestry testing.[46]

Winfrey's embrace of this incorrect theory should not be dismissed as ignorance or wholesale seduction by pseudoscience. We can read Winfrey's invocation of the theory as part of her overall interest in articulating African American experience as simultaneously: connected to the historical experience of slavery, *and* an urgent site for social change, *and* a site of individual self-help. Indeed, if we read the theory within her show's narrative tropes, the slavery hypothesis fits into a familiar narrative structure: a family has survived tremendous violence and found the resources within themselves to persevere; the family bears the scars of violence, but they display resilience and tenacity as they take initiative to move forward with their lives. To operate as if Winfrey's most fundamental stakes are the truth or falsity of this theory, or to suggest that the theory can only be used by those ignorant of the health effects of racism, is to isolate this theory from its plural contexts.

The analogy that Obasogie made to understand the invocations of the theory is an evocative one that I will use to set up an analytical point about the durability of race in medicine: the game of whack-a-mole. Obasogie wrote: "Like a game of whack-a-mole, the slavery hypothesis keeps popping up in the media, popular culture and even medical texts no matter how many times it is slammed down. It has come to symbolize the incessant way in which unfounded biological theories of racial difference continue to thrive despite significant evidence to the contrary."[47] Taking Obasogie's metaphor seriously gives us an opportunity to think through how we could actually address racism in medicine. Obasogie described the problem of the perniciousness of the theory in terms of the game of whack-a-mole, but did not follow that metaphor to a conclusion about strategy. But following the metaphor a little further might be fruitful. Consider: whacking moles feels like defeating moles, but that is an illusion. The game is designed such that the moles will return to their holes whether or not they are whacked, though points are only scored if the player whacks the mole while its head is sticking out. The moles are built to be able to endure repeated whacks, and will keep popping up as long as there is power behind them. Even if any one given mole were to get broken, it could easily be replaced, and there are plenty more to whack in the meantime. Whacking the same moles over and over again is a fine way to spend time if it seems enjoyable. But any sense that this action decreases the total number of moles in the world is an illusion. If what is really desired is no more moles, whacking them is irrelevant to that goal. It is necessary to find a way to unplug the game.

The game of whack-a-mole comes with a mallet tethered to its front, and the slavery hypothesis analogously comes with ready-at-hand modes of rebuttal. Less accessible is the power source of this whack-a-mole machine: racial inequality in health. As long as these disparities exist and provide fodder for broader preoccupations, this slavery hypothesis mole or one like it will keep popping up. But the cord powering this game is a lot harder to get our hands around than the mallet that came tethered to its front, and no one knows how to reach it. In the absence of that plug pull, mole-whacking is a morally neutral way to pass the time rather than a righteous way to attack racism itself. Moreover, if we come away from a critique of race and medicine feeling satisfied that we have won anything, that's a clue that we may have mistaken a mole for the game, a whack for a kill. So long as inequality endures, we should feel unsatisfied.

I would suggest that it is an open question whether whacking this theory every time it pops up does anything more productive than whacking the mole in the game. It passes the time, scores points of a kind, and gives the satisfaction of the whack, but does it effectively further goals like increasing truth or justice with regard to race in medicine? The expressed antiracist political commitments of many of its sympathizers and the persistence of the theory after so many whacks present doubts.

"There's a Pill for That!"

Since the allure of genetic determinism does not explain the appeal of the slavery hypothesis for these diverse antiracist actors, it is important to pay attention to other elements that help the story to resonate. So far, we have seen its appeal not only in scientific terms, but also in mythic ones. For the hypertension clinician-researcher Clarence Grim, another key element was the alignment of the theory with ready-at-hand intervention. To see how these elements come together, it is worthwhile to pay attention to *how* intervention on biology takes place. Pharmaceutical treatment for salt-sensitive hypertension comes in the form of a particular class of drug, a cheap old generic pill called a thiazide diuretic. That brings us back to the opening exchange, between Henry Louis Gates Jr. and Roland Fryer, where the appeal of the slavery hypothesis for the audience of that colloquium was bolstered by the availability of pharmaceutical treatment: "There's a pill for that!" How does the slavery hypothesis become enrolled in this pill, and why does this intersection become compelling for a scholar and public intellectual such as Gates?

I have left this encounter for last because I want to use it to shift to more complex theoretical questions, while at the same time bringing into focus how it matters that the slavery hypothesis is enrolled and embedded in a commodity, a pharmaceutical. This requires stepping back from the slavery hypothesis itself to introduce the concept of commodity fetishism, before returning to a close reading of the Fryer-Gates exchange. My analysis of this encounter is more theoretically dense than the ones so far, reading Gates's statement—"I'm a salt-saving Negro!"—in terms of his own literary theory as well as through a series of other theoretical frames. This provides an opportunity to use this encounter to engage with critical theory in spheres beyond race and medicine per se, while highlighting the relevance of the immanence of the slavery hypothesis and its generic drug for pharmaceutical meaning-making more generally, as well as race and medicine.

In the science studies of pharmaceuticals, there has been rich analysis of the ways in which doctors, patients, and society as a whole can both incorporate and contest the language of drugs' marketing into their descriptions of disease experience and identity.[48] But if we want to understand the allure of pharmaceuticals, we need to look beyond both medical efficacy and profit motives. The success (or failure) of a drug depends not only on these, but also on how it mobilizes prior conceptions of identity. The extent to which a drug is taken—or talked about—is related to commodity properties that exceed the physiological and the economic.

That Gates invokes his consumption of a generic drug to make an identity claim shows that the meaning-making capacity of pharmaceuticals does not necessarily have marketing at its base. Marketing is rather drawing on something prior, which I argue has to do with pharmaceuticals' nature as objects, as commodities, whether or not they have high-budget advertising campaigns. This is a theme that I will return to in the next chapter, which focuses on debates about thiazides within medicine, where both the same and distinct aspects of commodity fetishism come into play. Analyzing the commodity fetishism of generics is an opportunity to get conceptually closer to the processes of fetishization of pharmaceuticals generally. And so I will review the concept of the commodity in terms of medicine, and then examine a variety of lenses through which to read this Fryer-Gates exchange, each of which will provide partial perspectives on it. My goal is to leave the terrain unsettled, to show that the reification of race in contestation over this theory and its drug is always incomplete even as it is always being done.

The pharmaceutical as an object can be understood as a commodity. According to Karl Marx, a commodity is an external object that satisfies human needs of whatever kind and has a dual nature: it has use value and it is a bearer of value.[49] Though all commodities are expressions of human labor, and so are purely social, they come to be understood outside of social relations and to take on a magical quality. The commodity reflects the social characteristics of human labor in objective form, and through this substitution human labor becomes a sensuous thing that is simultaneously suprasensible. Marx makes an analogy with religion to explore the peculiar agency that commodities come to take on. Like gods, commodities are "products of the human brain [that] appear as autonomous figures endowed with a life of their own, which enter into relations both with each other and with the human race."[50]

As soon as objects become commodities, they become amenable to this fetishism, in which it is possible to fantasize that the objects of our own creation have mastery over us. This fantasy is itself structural, and cannot be punctured by simply naming it as such. As objects that can be understood to have an embodied as well as ideological mastery over us, pharmaceuticals are peculiar commodities. Yet like all commodities, pharmaceuticals come to have a life of their own that exceeds their design and distribution.

In this moment of the colloquium, the economist Fryer and the literary theorist Gates are participating in the meaning making of thiazide diuretics. For each of them, in different ways, the thiazide becomes a thing to think with as they invoke it to talk about their own economic research and racial identities respectively. Hydrochlorothiazide becomes an *evocative object*, in Sherry Turkle's terms,[51] one that can be encountered on many levels: one-on-one as a physical object (the pill itself); as a gateway to health (its promise of protection from sickness and death); and as an artifact with which we can relate to define our own sense of self (something "extra"). The thiazide offers something physiologically: to lower blood pressure by 10 millimeters of mercury. It also makes a larger promise of health: to provide protection from cardiovascular disease economically and effectively. These two aspects may seem to be the same thing, but in fact only after medical knowledge on an individual level becomes biomedical knowledge on a large scale can the intervention into asymptomatic states of risk be understood to have an impact on something we can understand as "health."[52]

It was on these relatively narrow promises that Gates originally took the drug. But for Gates and Fryer, invoking this commodity also invokes something "extra," which reaches a scale that exceeds the mundane or the individual and touches on the projects that frame not only their lifetimes but also their respective life's work. The thiazide makes two new promises after it has already been consumed: it promises to connect Gates to his kin, and for Fryer it promises to solve one part of racial inequality in America. The magical potential of this commodity is underscored when it is revealed to be doing more work than it had been advertised to do.

Indeed, the notion of what a drug is advertised to do is important here, and connects to the well-developed STS critique of processes of interpellation in the pharmaceutical advertisement.[53] For Louis Althusser, the subject is interpellated in an encounter with the police who yell, "Hey, you!"[54] The subject is the one who responds with "It's me!" Donna Haraway has noted that the process of interpellation extends to technoscience, through which we all—not just scientists and engineers—are interpellated with its "Hey, you!"[55] Joseph Dumit has extended this to explore the ways in which the pharmaceutical advertisement interpellates particular kinds of subjects, in a way that is simultaneously partial and effective: provided with diffuse symptoms that had been obscured in everyday experience, we respond, "Oh! so that's who I am."[56]

Now, in this exchange between Fryer and Gates before an audience, we can see something similar happening, but without the intervention of physician-scientists or pharmaceutical marketers. We can see Gates's subjectivity interpellated by invocations of a disease category and a drug outside of its explicit marketing or a medical encounter. This suggests that the interpellation of the subject by a pharmaceutical is not, at base, marketing, but rather that marketers are using the pharmaceuticals' prior interpellative potential. But in this case as in Dumit's, if the interpellation is successful and the drug is taken, it makes the patient him- or herself into a particular kind of subject, one who is the object of scientific knowledge, in this case, a "salt-saving Negro."

We can tell from his entire oeuvre that Henry Louis Gates Jr. is not naive about the volatile power of inscribing the body with race. He is one to put the word "race" in quotes in many a title, and is always careful to connect it to a mode of historical experience and not a biologically deterministic given.[57] When Gates appeals to his use of the drug to describe a kinship with his ancestors, he is not doing so in a simply naive way. Reification is something that Gates knows is a dangerous path, and he does it in the form of a half-joke with the odd logism "salt-saving Negro." But to point out that reification is potentially perilous does not refute the work that it is doing.

Indeed, the locution "salt-saving Negro" may be read as part of Gates's African American literary criticism, as being in the voice of the trickster, and meant to be figurative and ambiguous.[58] In this locution, Gates performs the process of signifying that he theorizes. When Gates makes this interjection, he is not only making a claim, but also playing a prank. He is disobeying normal rules of behavior for the academic setting of a colloquium in which ideas and not individuals are the subject of discourse, and there are no Negroes, only African Americans. In doing this, he is displaying many of the characteristics that he ascribes to the trope of the trickster in African and African American literature, including indeterminacy and disruption and reconciliation. And he is not only making a polemical claim based on either a scientific theory or the literal ingestion of a drug, but making the kind of double-voiced statement he characterizes as fundamental to African American vernacular tradition: inciting action and debate through playing on rhetorical principles.

So what is at stake is not whether Gates—or the audience of the colloquium, or the reader of this account—"really believes" in either the risk category of the salt-saving Negro or in the efficacy of a thiazide diuretic as the solution. If we limit our critique of the ideology of racial theories or of pharmaceuticals to the authority of medical experts and gullibility of patients, or of the machinations of pharmaceuticals' sellers and the naiveté of their consumers, we only understand the most straightforward of situations. But there is more than one way to "buy in." Some patient-consumers may indeed be ignorant, but many are perfectly capable of simultaneously being skeptical of and participating in what Joseph Dumit has called "pharmaceutical grammars,"[59] even trying to shape them a bit along the way.

And so, I would suggest, it is possible for the subject interpellated by this concept of the salt-saving Negro on hydrochlorothiazide to be read not necessarily as a naive believer in specious science. The salt-saving Negro is a postmodern subject, already a locution of "ironic distantiation" as described by Slavoj Žižek.[60] Like Marx, Žižek frames his argument about ideology and commodities with a comparison to religious thinking. Žižek argues that since a mark of modernity is that religion becomes something separate from a way of life, contemporary subjects assume one of two roles: either the Christian who says, *I really believe!* or the skeptic who relies on the figure of the "other" who *really believes*. Žižek argues that cynical subjects cannot understand what (or even that) we really believe, because we always insert this distance.[61] Disease categories and pharmaceuticals can be successful in interpellating both kinds of contemporary subjects, both the Christian and the skeptic. Real belief is not necessarily more compelling as a motive for identifying with a disease category or consuming pharmaceuticals than is provisional consideration, unreflective compliance, or self-aware doubt. If we critique the ideology of pharmaceuticals on the basis of false consciousness of their pushers or their consumers— they know not what they do, so they do X—we miss the insight from Žižek that the cynical subject is perfectly capable of knowing what they are doing and doing it anyway.[62]

Not every claim we make that invokes racialized genetics or pharmaceuticals is literal, and so the claims cannot necessarily be refuted on the basis of scientific evidence. If we understand the connections we see between our identities and disease categories or pharmaceuticals as commodity fetishes, we can understand both the identity and the distance invoked. In Donna Haraway's work on gene fetishism, she has unpacked the fetish in this way: "The fetishist is not psychotic, he 'knows' that the surrogate is just that. Yet he is uniquely invested in this power-object. The fetishist, aware that he has a substitute, still believes in—and experiences—its potency, he is captivated by the reality effect produced by the image."[63] The "reality effect" she refers to, and which is also provoked in this Fryer-Gates encounter, is that of the Barthesian realistic novel in which the story is infused with verisimilitude by attending to details that appear to have no reason to be there besides their correspondence with historical reality.[64] In this encounter, the presence of a cheap generic drug in Gates's medicine cabinet provokes a reality effect. It had seemed irrelevant, but it was now part of the evidence for Fryer's story of uniquely black hypertension. It is convincing in the same way that a novel is, not in the way of a scientific argument. That is why refutation based on citing a prominent historian did not undo the audience's captivation with this theory. The exchange produced the reality effect not only in spite of, but also because of, the contingency and coincidence of Gates's own case.

The resilience of this reality effect in the face of contestation based on the limitations of the scientific data is also captured in the work of Alondra Nelson, who describes the complicated ways that African Americans who have used genetic ancestry testing as part of their genealogical research enroll that data in the construction of their life stories.[65] Drawing on rich ethnographic material, she demonstrates how the genetic tests are part of an active process of fashioning identity—"affiliative self-fashioning"—not its conclusion.[66] Narratives of connection preceded the procurement of the tests, and have power that does not rise or fall on their results. As she demonstrates, the limits of the science on which the tests are based do not diminish their productive enrollment in life stories that seek to align biography and biology, but make that productivity open-ended.

In an important sense, when Gates points to his consumption of this particular drug as a way to narrate a connection with the history of slavery, he becomes what Nikolas Rose describes as a "somatic individual."[67] Rose argues that we should not see every instance of the invocation of biology in race—whether genetic ancestry testing or epidemiological research—"on a trajectory of 'racial science' or see them as the most recent incarnation of the biological legitimation of social inequality or discrimination." Instead, Rose argues:

They should be located within an emerging form of life, in which human beings are coming to understand and act upon themselves and others as "somatic individuals," to construe their identities partly in biomedical terms, to
believe that medicine can and should help identify and combat susceptibilities to disease, and to enact their own relation to their biomedical future in
the light of this knowledge. These new forms of biomedical and genetic
prudence are attentive to biological differences, but they are not elements in
a new science of race, but part of a different politics, of new forms of
individual and collective subjectification in which our "biology"—not just
our genome—has become highly salient to practices of identity formation.[68]

It is precisely the malleability of the biology of the "salt-saving Negro" that
makes it a particularly rich site for this new form of articulating racial identity
in biological terms.

In the media response to Fryer, much was made of the fact that he is black
and pushing this theory of biological race that can be medicated. There was
tut-tutting about his naiveté.[69] If he were touting a branded pharmaceutical, it
would be easy to let the explanation rest with an argument about economic
motivations. But instead, Fryer was touting a generic drug. His lack of financial stakes in the drug illustrates an important way in which the commodity
fetishism of a pharmaceutical exceeds that of its marketing and moves in
unpredictable ways.

We might turn again to Roland Barthes for another mode of reading this
encounter: mythologies and identification. We can read the images of Fryer as
a proponent for pharmaceuticalized race the same way that Barthes reads the
image of the Negro soldier before the French tricolor.[70] Barthes reads that
image in three ways: as an *example* of French coloniality, and as an *alibi* for it,
and as simply the *presence* of it.[71] The analogy between French coloniality and
American pharmaceutical hegemony is dramatically imperfect and yet evocative: Fryer as example of, alibi for, and demonstration of the presence of a
particular model of racial disparity that is simultaneously biologically real and
capable of being medicated away.

In this sense, we can see that the modes of biological citizenship that become possible when the slavery hypothesis meets thiazides are plural. Like the
biological citizens after Chernobyl described by Adriana Petryna, in which "the
damaged biology of a population has become the grounds for social membership and the basis for staking citizenship claims,"[72] there are powerful ways in
which the invocation of the slavery hypothesis by such actors as Fryer and

Gates becomes both a way to locate the harm and to articulate entitlement to treatment.

However, as the next chapter will explore, the invocations of thiazides in biological citizenship demands are more than claims to damaged biology in Petryna's terms, or, in Rose's framework, "the constitution of active subjects."[73] Any hope that thiazide diuretics offer in changing the situation of racial disparities is, depending on one's point of view, either insufficient or tantalizingly (if frustratingly) right here right now.

It is worth highlighting that Fryer's model of what kind of problem race presents here is not exactly the same as Gates's. Fryer responds to the concern raised by the geneticist in the audience about "fixing race" in the sense of making it unchangeable with an answer that promises to "fix race" in the sense of easy repair: "There's a pill for that!" He uses a racialized invocation of that pill to hold out the promise of putting an end to the only racial difference that he is paying attention to: mortality disparity. Gates, on the other hand, is invoking his use of the pill to connect him to the racial differences that he is most interested in: the role of the common history of slavery in shaping the African American experience, his own place in that history, and as a mode of narration. Fryer has a model of racial disparity that is simultaneously biologically real and capable of being medicated away, but Gates has a model of race that is socially real yet capable of being medicated in. For each of them, the drug's capacity to traffic between the material and the semiotic helps to move race across that boundary, and yet the traffic is in differing directions. And so we can see the limits of an analogy to Barthes, who promised to reveal the cultural logic of the Negro before the tricolor. These identifications and mythologies are unstable, diverse, ambiguous, even among African American Harvard professors, let alone as they move across other venues.

The Stakes in the Simultaneity of the Slavery Hypothesis and Thiazide Diuretics

In these multiple meanings of what it might mean to "fix race," we can see a gap between race as an object of bioscientific inquiry into states presumed to be natural, and race as a medical taxonomy that drives intervention into those states. I argue that in order to understand the productivity of race in medicine, it needs to be understood as a category that is simultaneously a subject of identity practices, bioscientific inquiry, and practical clinical taxonomy. The task for critical scholars should not be to call for a true or innocent science that seeks to purge the material-semiotic category of race from biology, but to track plural noninnocent discourses that are simultaneously biological and social. I argue that critique that rests only on scientific reification without attending to clinical intervention is both a failure to engage, and contributes to the durability of the categories that it ostensibly critiques.

The slavery hypothesis is an excellent site at which to interrogate race at the intersection of the social and the biological because it is enrolled in articulations of medical research and practice at precisely this intersection. The slavery hypothesis is a theory located not just in epidemiology but also in clinical medicine. Clinical medicine's emphasis on *intervention* on the social and the biological makes the theory a distinct site for analysis of race and genetics, with slightly different implications from the sites usually explored by scholars of science and technology studies, such as genetic databanks and genetic ancestry tests. If the Human Genome Diversity Project, for example, fixes (reifies) race in order to put it into the corpus of scientific knowledge,[74] a conceptually different process is at work as practitioners fix (reify) race in order to act on it. By turning from debates centered around the slavery hypothesis to broader debates centered around thiazide diuretics, we will see how this cheap, reliable, old drug class is remarkably polyvalent with regard to race.

CHAPTER 5

Thiazide Diuretics
at a Nexus of Associations:
Racialized, Proven, Old, Cheap

I n the previous chapter, we saw one volatile intersection between thiazide diuretics and race: the slavery hypothesis for African American hypertension. Henry Louis Gates Jr., the African American studies scholar and public intellectual, invoked his consumption of hydrochlorothiazide to identify himself with the slavery hypothesis—"I'm on that! I'm a salt-saving Negro!" The immanence of the drug class and that disease category was important also for the principal medical proponent of the slavery hypothesis, Clarence Grim. But there are many more intersections of thiazide diuretics and race worth mining. Thiazide's durable appeal does not rest on genetics alone. When the drug class becomes enrolled in intertwining debates about access to medicine and racial difference in drug response, it rearticulates racialized American identity in consumer capitalism as simultaneously biological and economic.

By attending closely to debates within medicine that enroll this drug in questions about race and therapeutics and about expansion of access to pharmaceuticals, I will show that although the appeal of pharmaceuticals draws on scientific data and marketing, these commodities are in fact also subject to claims on many more registers that cannot quite subsume or refute each other. Gates and Grim are not alone in using the drug class to articulate narratives of difference—or narratives of hope. As we will see, two more commodity aspects of thiazide diuretics become key: use value (efficacy) and exchange value (price). Thiazides exist at a nexus of associations—racialized, proven, old, cheap—and attention to the drug class provides a site for unpacking some of the plural productions of coherence and incoherence at the intersections of race and pharmaceuticals.

Thiazide diuretics—also called thiazide-type diuretics, thiazides, or simply diuretics—are a class of drugs introduced in the 1950s and, as the first class of antihypertensives to be developed, they have long been available in generic form. Thiazide diuretics treat hypertension by reducing the amount of fluid in the body.[1] Decreasing the volume of fluid decreases blood pressure, and hence the work that the heart has to do. Thiazides' impact on morbidity and mortality seems to exceed this effect as well. Thiazide diuretics are often combined with other antihypertensives to increase their antihypertensive effect while mitigating side effects such as increased blood sugar and lowered potassium. Thiazide diuretics also (relatedly) decrease the sodium level in the body. When debates about thiazides intersect with debates about race, this relationship with salt is important. African American hypertension as a disease category is generally characterized as "salt-sensitive," and this characterization extends far beyond the slavery hypothesis. There is a gap between genetics and physiology, and to posit physiological difference is not necessarily to posit genetic difference. Differential salt sensitivity has been explained in epistemologically eclectic ways, ranging from genetic frequencies, to diet, to psychosocial stress.[2] Etiological ambiguity bolsters rather than hinders the widespread claim that African American hypertension is distinctly salt sensitive. And receptivity to diuretics has been part of defining African American hypertension as a disease category.

Racial Prescriptions

Well before BiDil became the first drug approved with a racial indication, debates festered about racial differences across classes of antihypertensive medications. These debates are ongoing, and both include and exceed arguments about genetics. Thiazide diuretics can be mobilized by those with genetics-oriented understandings of racial difference, whether or not they articulate them in terms of the slavery hypothesis per se. For example, Jared Diamond (author of the best-selling *Guns, Germs, and Steel*) and his coauthor Jerome Rotter write in their contribution to the volume *The Genetic Basis of Common Diseases*:

> Hypertensive blacks are not merely similar to and proportionately more frequent than severely hypertensive whites. Instead, physiological differences seem to contribute as well. On consuming salt, blacks on average retain it much longer before excreting it into the urine, and they experience a

greater rise in blood pressure on a high-salt diet. Hypertension is more likely to be salt-sensitive in blacks than in whites. By the same token, black hypertension is more likely to be treated successfully by drugs that cause the kidneys to excrete salt (thiazide diuretics) and is less likely to respond to drugs that reduce heart rate and cardiac output (beta blockers, such as propranolol). These facts suggest qualitative and not just quantitative differences between the causes of black and white hypertension, with black hypertension more likely to involve renal salt handling.[3]

On one level, this is just another simplistic genetic argument, and could be debunked just as the historian of medicine David Jones has incisively debunked the "virgin soil" theory of Native American epidemics that Diamond has participated in promoting.[4] Moreover, since we know that there is more genetic difference within racial groups than between them,[5] and since we know that African Americans have considerable shared ancestry with white Americans, we should therefore be particularly skeptical of claims that genetics can sort these populations into two kinds.

But what I am most interested in here is that even in this very simplistic framing of racial genetics' contribution to disease, before even introducing the slavery hypothesis, it is the variance in drug response that helps to make the claim of racial difference particularly durable. Diamond and Rotter's argument mediates race in the sense of both arbitrating and intervening: it arbitrates difference by sorting populations into two types, at the same time that it advocates intervention with the appropriate pharmaceuticals. The intervention becomes evidence for the arbitration, as much as the other way around, validating specious racial group sorting according to which drug class is believed to be appropriate for each group. The pharmaceuticals allow traffic between race as an object of bioscientific inquiry and race as a category of practical clinical taxonomy. In an important sense, the practical is primary: many debates about the distinct appropriateness of thiazide diuretics for African Americans make no particular claim about the etiology of the differential in drug response.

Debates about the differential effects of various classes of antihypertensives have been central in the arguments about whether there are racial differences in the efficacy of drugs more generally: Jonathan Kahn has pointed out that contested claims about antihypertensives have been the grounds of the overwhelming share of racialized physiological claims.[6] As researcher-clinicians focused on the treatment of African American hypertension have compellingly shown, race is in fact a very poor predictor of any individual patient's drug response, since intraracial variation in drug response is much larger than interracial variation.[7] Clinical guidelines produced by the major organization for blood-pressure treatment guidelines, the Joint National Committee, and separate guidelines produced by the International Society for Hypertension in Blacks,[8] both discuss aggregate differences in response by race, and emphasize that combining lifestyle modification with multidrug therapy is effective for blacks.

However, even tiny differences in mean response by race are reported and read in the context of larger racial preoccupations. Thus, debate remains unsettled about how to grapple with this data at the level of clinical practice: even though racial difference is tiny and only visible in aggregates, racial profiling in prescription selection exerts a strong appeal.[9] The debates about drug response have a volatility of their own, whether or not their arguments about physiological processes, such as salt sensitivity, are based on genetic claims.

Thiazides have been of renewed interest in clinical practice because of a landmark drug trial known as the Antihypertensive and Lipid Lowering Treatment to Prevent Heart Attack Trial, or ALLHAT.[10] This trial, which ended in 2002, is the largest antihypertensive trial ever conducted, with over forty-two thousand participants—a third of whom were African American.[11] It was conducted by the National Institutes of Health to compare four classes of antihypertensive drugs head to head. According to this landmark study, the newer antihypertensives—which were at the time still under patent and thus much more expensive—didn't work any better than the older, cheaper generic diuretics, and that this was particularly true in African Americans.[12] One of its first press releases announcing results, in 2005, included attention to race in its opening sentences: "Diuretics work better than newer therapies in treating high blood pressure and reducing risk of heart disease in both black and nonblack patients, according to a long-term, multi-center trial of antihypertensive therapies funded by the National Heart, Lung, and Blood Institute of the National Institutes of Health. This analysis by race confirms earlier findings on the effectiveness of diuretics and emphasizes that diuretics should be preferred as a first therapy for most patients with high blood pressure."[13] A slide from the trial's publicly available slide deck summarizes its implications, both general and racially specific (figure 3).

In the reports about ALLHAT, there has been a repetitive promotion of diuretics, especially for African American patients: "While the improved outcomes with [the thiazide] chlorthalidone were more pronounced for some outcomes in blacks than in nonblacks, thiazide-type diuretics remain the

ALLHAT **Antihypertensive Trial: Implications**

- Diuretics should be the drug of choice for initial therapy of hypertension. The evidence for this recommendation is even stronger for Black hypertensive patients..

- For the patient who cannot take a diuretic (which should be an unusual circumstance), CCB's and ACEI's may be considered. However, in Black hypertensive patients, ACEI's should be considered second-line therapy.

- Most hypertensive patients require more than one drug. Diuretics should generally be part of the antihypertensive regimen. Lifestyle advice should also be provided.

7/27/2006

3. "Antihypertensive Trial: Implications." From "Outcomes in Hypertensive Black and Nonblack Patients Treated with Chlorthalidone, Amlodipine, and Lisinopril," ALLHAT Slide Deck.
At http://allhat.uth.tmc.edu/Slides/RaceSexAge.ppt.

drugs of choice for initial therapy of hypertension in both black and nonblack hypertensive patients."[14] These kinds of claims about ALLHAT's application to "black and nonblack" patients appeared in the context of broader arguments about racial differences in drug response.

We should not be surprised that the ALLHAT data has been broken down to draw contrasts between racial groups. The ALLHAT study was remarkably inclusive of African Americans, and as Steven Epstein demonstrates, attention to inclusion and to difference are often linked.[15] When Jason van Steenburgh wrote about the implications of ALLHAT in the *American College of Physicians Observer*, he mentioned that African Americans' salt sensitivity makes them particularly good candidates for diuretics: "There is one group that researchers say you should definitely consider switching from ACE inhibitors to diuretics: black Americans. ALLHAT found diuretics lowered systolic blood pressure 4 mm Hg more than ACE inhibitors, probably because black Americans' salt sensitivity makes them especially responsive to diuretics."[16] Van Steenburgh went further, suggesting that such a high rate of inclusion of blacks may have thrown off ALLHAT's statistics: "Even more significantly, the study found that black Americans taking ACE inhibitors experienced a stroke 40%

more often than their counterparts taking diuretics. (Black Americans typically require high levels of ACE inhibitors to control their blood pressure.) Black Americans responded so well to diuretics in the ALLHAT study that some physicians questioned whether the high percentage of blacks in the study (35%) skewed the overall results against ACE inhibitors."[17] The idea that high inclusion of African Americans "skews" otherwise normal results rests on a noninclusive definition of the population. This resonates with enduring questions, ones that earlier chapters have highlighted in terms of longitudinal research at Framingham and Jackson, about who can stand in as normal Americans from whom to extrapolate.

But elaboration in the *Observer* article acknowledges that there is something unsettling about the implication that expensive drugs are inappropriate for black people. Part of the skepticism of the cheap drug is related to its quality as a commodity, and the piece noted that the price of diuretics was just 5 to 10 percent of that of the newer drugs.[18] The piece suggested that "because diuretics cost less and are much older than ACE inhibitors and calcium channel blockers, patients switched to diuretics from more high-profile drugs may think they are getting substandard care." Seeking to "dispel that notion," a Yale clinical professor of medicine was quoted saying: "We aren't advocating good medicine for people who can afford it and bad medicine for people who can't. . . . The data are clear: The less expensive medication is at least as good."[19] This statement illustrates even as it contests slippage between exchange value and use value of the drug. By attending to ways that physicians talk about the relative value of different classes of antihypertensive drugs for racially and economically stratified populations, we will see that clinical discussions—like those in nonmedical settings described in the previous chapter —are working through aspects of the inextricability of use value, exchange value, and magical thinking that are part of commodity fetishism. There are two things that complicate the simple assessment of drugs' relative natural properties: the role of price in a commodity's fetish, and the difficulty of assessing the use value of drugs—especially for asymptomatic conditions.

Debating Diuretics

At the 2006 meeting of the International Society for Hypertension in Blacks, there was a debate between two physician-researchers on the topic "Diuretics are over-emphasized as antihypertensive therapy."[20] The doctor arguing for that case was a University of Michigan professor, Kenneth Jamerson, and the

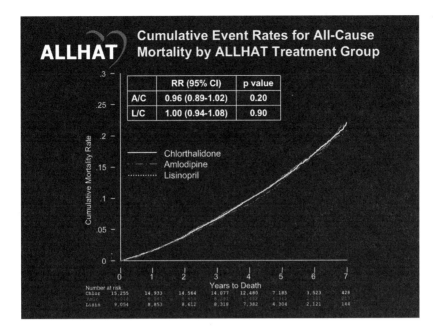

	RR (95% CI)	p value
A/C	0.96 (0.89-1.02)	0.20
L/C	1.00 (0.94-1.08)	0.90

4. "Cumulative Event Rates for All-Cause Mortality by ALLHAT Treatment Group." From "Major Outcomes in High Risk Hypertensive Patients Randomized to Angiotensin-Converting Enzyme Inhibitor or Calcium Channel Blocker vs Diuretic," ALLHAT Slide Deck. At http://allhat.uth.tmc.edu/Slides/Results.ppt.

one arguing against it was a Case Western professor and ALLHAT researcher, Jackson Wright. Both showed the same slides from ALLHAT, and both agreed that multidrug therapy was ideal. However, they disagreed about whether the data suggested that the thiazide was "best."

Jamerson started out his presentation by emphasizing first that ALLHAT did not show that diuretics were "best." Showing a PowerPoint slide from ALLHAT with the lines on a chart comparing "All-Cause Mortality" over time for three drug classes tested head to head—in which the lines representing each drug almost completely overlap (figure 4)—he said, sarcastically, that "clearly" diuretics are best.

Since these lines were too similar to settle anything, Jamerson suggested that another consideration be taken into account, one that was missing from the slide: metabolic effects. Diuretics have low side-effect profiles, but that is not the same thing as having no side-effect profile at all. From the perspective of physicians focused on heart disease risk, diuretics' most significant side effect is increased blood sugar levels.[21] Averting the risk of inducing diabetes,

Jamerson suggested, was a reason to choose newer drugs even if they didn't lower blood pressure any more than diuretics or improve morbidity and mortality within the time frame of the trial.

The con argument—that diuretics are not overemphasized in the treatment of hypertension—was made by the ALLHAT investigator, Jackson Wright. He suggested that Jamerson's concern was merely speculative while the data were definitive. He presented data that showed that although there was an increase in the blood sugar levels of those on diuretics (as expected), there was not an increase in adverse events. At stake here is which kind of counting is more compelling: that of blood sugar levels or that of strokes, heart failures, heart attacks. It seemed clear to Wright that the latter are obviously more compelling, but their conclusiveness is diminished by the limited eight-year time span of the trial. Wright had no answer for Jamerson's central point: what metabolic dangers lurk in the timeframe beyond the trial's scope? For his part, Jamerson could not quantify those, either.

Wright blamed physicians' lack of enthusiasm for diuretics—despite what he saw as ALLHAT's conclusive evidence—on diuretics' lack of marketing: no pharmaceutical representative had ever taken him out to dinner to promote these old, cheap generics. He was frustrated that although ALLHAT was conclusive on the safety and efficacy of diuretics, its results had not been widely followed. Far from overemphasizing diuretics, Wright said, physicians have continued their prescription practice of focusing on the new, expensive drugs. He made numerous references to his lack of reliance on pharmaceutical industry funding.

In terms of the science, we can understand Wright and Jamerson as differing on perfectly legitimate grounds. Whereas Wright could base his argument on observed cardiovascular events, Jamerson could appeal to convincing physiological mechanisms. Balancing the competing abstractions of statistics and physiology with the idiosyncrasies of each presenting patient is precisely the challenge of what the theorist of science Ludwik Fleck called the "specific intuition" of medical thinking.[22] Weighing clinical trial evidence against knowledge about physiological mechanisms is a typical grounds for debate. The tenor of the debate at the ISHIB conference, however, merits further consideration.

In this debate, narrow economic interests were invoked, as they rarely are on the podiums of these medical conferences. Pharmaceutical companies' support is always recognized by name before presenting data, yet there are rarely the sort of accusations of bias that attended government support of

ALLHAT. When dinners are provided by pharmaceutical companies at conferences or outside them, there is of course a sense that the companies are doing this in the hope of persuading physicians to prescribe their wares. Although casting doubt on the independence of "continuing medical education" from the commercial interests that fund it has been a prominent feature of recent arguments for reform of the links between the pharmaceutical industry and the medical profession,[23] there is also some understanding that the speakers are not merely representing the pharmaceutical companies. The system of continuing medical education of which this ISHIB conference was part operates on the assumption that sponsorship and science are separable. The knowledge being presented, while it is paid for, is not simply bought. When ALLHAT's investigator Jackson Wright suggested base economic motives in his opponents, he rankled the sensibilities of the many physicians who accept gifts from the pharmaceutical companies without thinking that it affects their own professional judgment. But neither the government nor pharmaceutical companies are disinterested parties in this debate. There is no innocent place from which to judge.

Clinicians grappling with the implications of clinical trials for their own practices are facing a situation of information overload, and many clinicians, including those who focus on the treatment of African American populations as those in ISHIB do, have come to embrace the aspect of ALLHAT that has generated consensus among industry, professional, and to a lesser extent governmental sources: the importance of combining a diuretic with a new expensive drug in a multidrug "gold standard" treatment regimen. The difficult situation that the physician is put in is one that Jeremy Greene and Scott Podolsky have argued has been in place since the middle of the twentieth century: "Physicians came to use both commercial and professional sources in an attempt to 'keep modern' by incorporating emerging therapeutics into their practices."[24] Professional sources have had a hard time competing with commercial ones, and so has the government. Moreover, because of the government's involvement in the healthcare system as a payer, it is hardly a disinterested player in the treatments given to patients.

When international hypertension researchers collaborated on the book *A Century of Arterial Hypertension: 1896–1996*, their discussion of treatment options was illuminating. Complaining about the fifth Joint National Committee recommendation that cheaper agents be used before new, expensive ones unless the latter can be shown to be advantageous, they characterize the quandary this way:

In the midst of this debate, how can general practitioners, the main pre-scribers of antihypertensive drugs, find their way? They are trapped between the pressure of pharmaceutical advertising which constantly reminds them that increasingly effective drugs are available, and official bodies which encourage them to be more economical in their prescribing. Both parties refer to the conclusions of their "experts" which overwhelm the modest practitioners trying to do their best for their patients. The confusion of doctors faced with these recent developments is a totally new facet of the impact of contemporary society on hypertension and its treatment.[25]

In this account, pharmaceutical companies are read as telling the truth about the newest things being best, but alas the government steps in and pressures doctors to consider price as well. In a context otherwise saturated with pri-vately funded drug research, the doctors' skepticism of ALLHAT, and govern-ment advocacy of generic drugs broadly, was conspicuous.

Even if we accept ALLHAT's basic assessment that cheap, old thiazide was as effective as the new, expensive drugs, commodity arguments don't rest there —even if then and in this one case, the NIH was correct in recommending the cheap, old drug first. In consumer capitalism, citizenship can be staked out in terms of who can indulge in consumption of the brand name, and when race becomes part of arguments about entitlement to brand-name drugs these be-come inextricable from broader racialized citizenship claims.

The Commodity Fetishism of Generic Drugs

Given many physicians' (and consumers') general preference for the new, it is worth considering why an array of actors have found championing diuretics appealing. Such ALLHAT investigators as Jackson Wright, and their govern-ment supporters, have no monopoly on self-righteous embrace of the cheap generic. Before returning to thiazides' other champions, I will attend to the ways that the category of the generic can draw its own commodity fetish, and thiazides in particular can be a way to articulate particular kinds of publicly oriented medicine.

Commodity fetishism of pharmaceuticals precedes their branding, histor-ically as well as conceptually. The historian of medicine Robert Bud has com-pellingly argued that penicillin can be fruitfully analyzed as a "brand"—one that became enrolled in propaganda for the prowess of big medicine in the Second World War, and later became a problematic locus of patients' hunger for "wonder drugs."[26] Thiazides can also be fruitfully analyzed as an untrademarked brand—one that in the 1980s, 1990s, and especially the first decade of the 2000s, became enrolled in arguments for evidence-based medicine and against ever-escalating drug costs.

As economic sociologists have pointed out, a prerequisite of consumerism is the fact that commodities do not just meet consumer needs but "allow consumers to express their values and make public statements about self-image, social status, and personal identity."[27] This is true whether or not the commodity in question is branded. In an era rife with conspicuous consumption, thiazides' advocates could use the drug to construct an alternative framing of participation in American ways of life. In the context of the early twenty-first-century social movements against corporate brands—epitomized on the left by the journalist Naomi Klein's No Logo: Taking Aim at the Brand Bullies, an international bestseller decrying corporate globalization—advocacy of a generic class of drug could become a way to articulate a vision of escape from the hegemony of private interests. But there is no escape here.

Getting at the pure biomedical knowledge amid competing biases of government and pharmaceutical companies turns out to be a goal of considerable difficulty, for reasons related to the commodity fetish. As discussed in the previous chapter, like all commodities, drugs are subject to commodity fetishism. According to Marx, one aspect of this fetishism is that commodities' different equivalent values are imagined to be inherent to them.[28] We might imagine that because drugs have scientifically demonstrated "natural properties," they could be—and in an ideal case would be—exempt from the fetishism that attends all commodities. Yet we should remember that Marx's key example of commodity fetishism, a coat, has physical aspects too, and its value as something useful and its value for monetary trade are often easy to conflate.[29] But if we do so, Marx argues that we are making an error: its ability to keep us warm is physical, but its price is purely social. When we say that randomly controlled trials show that generic drugs have "the same" efficacy as brand-name new ones, we ignore the real and continuing power of the magical thinking of the commodity's fetish that can never quite divide exchange value from use value.

Second, the clarity of the data turns out to be tricky to establish. Unlike exchange value, use value is hard to pin down. Even determining what utility means is complicated for a drug used for an asymptomatic condition such as hypertension. When choosing a commodity like Marx's coat, we know that we choose not only on the basis of its temperature control. We might choose one that is class-marked, regionally marked, racially marked, or associated with any combination of characteristics that transcend simple functional utility maximization. In an age of market-driven pharmaceuticals, we should attend to these diverse identity forms with regard to pharmaceuticals as well.

Moreover, our choice of a coat or a drug is based not only on maximizing utilities but also, perhaps predominantly, on minimizing disutilities. Consider the coat-drug analogy a little further, to consider utility versus disutility. For example, one problem with coats is that they can cause sweating. We could consider as analogous to a side effect of a drug the problem of sweating being caused by something that is designed to protect from cold. We might choose a coat then not only for its ability to keep us warm, but also for its ability to ventilate and prevent sweat: these effects need to be weighed against each other. Weighing utilities and disutilities of drugs that do not treat symptoms is analogous to, but much more challenging than, the choices involved in coat selection. Unlike drugs that have a transparent utility to the patient because they cure disease or treat symptoms—or the purchase of a coat to provide warmth—selection among antihypertensive drugs is, from the patients' perspective, mostly about minimizing disutilities.

The utility of something as far-off and abstract as a "statistically significant reduction in cardiovascular events" must be weighed against short- and long-term disutilities. While the disutilities of thiazides are generally mild, they can be important to patients' experiences: the hassle of taking a drug, the cost, and side effects such as increased urination (which should subside after the first few days but often is experienced as continuing). More rare side effects include gout and impotence (an iatrogenic erectile dysfunction that sociologists Laura Mamo and Jennifer Fishman have insightfully analyzed as part of the context of Viagra[30]). At the same time, the fact that both hypertension and its treatment often have no effect that is immediately perceptible to the patient can itself inhibit adherence to a treatment regimen, with a thiazide or otherwise.[31] Thiazides' long-term side effects are the subject of much debate about the differential value of thiazides compared with other drugs. As we saw in the debate at ISHIB, establishing that the efficacy of thiazides is "the same as" or "better than" other drugs turns out to be a very complicated task, and has been widely challenged.

Indeed, there has been ample criticism of the governmental endorsement of the old, cheap drugs, and it is continuous with medical criticism of federal efforts to encourage physicians to use generic equivalents, an issue that has emerged periodically since the 1960s.[32] Although the earlier efforts were distinct from this case because they were examples of encouraging the prescription of generic equivalents rather than prescription of drugs of a class different from the branded drug, the suspicion of governmental motives and righteous indignation of professional prerogative around ALLHAT are continuous with this long-standing embrace of brands. In his scathing indictment of the design of ALLHAT, its application beyond its primary endpoints, and the hastiness of its peer review, Jay Meltzer argued in the *American Journal of Hypertension* that contrary to what it deserves "ALLHAT has had widespread acclaim in part due to a massive government sponsored public relations campaign."[33] Part of the disconnect between Meltzer and diuretics' proponents is the uncharted space that Meltzer identifies as "public relations." It is something that we might situate between "marketing" and "publicity."[34] Publicity becomes like punditry in this framework: in a sleight of hand like that of television news, the construction of a narrative around "two sides," public and private, conceals considerable differences between the scale, scope, and interests of the sides.

At stake is the integrity of the science and art of medicine. In the words of one poetically minded physician: "*The recommendation to prescribe the cheapest drug is a denial of both scientific progress and medical art.*"[35] Nostalgia for the artistry of medicine is resonant with that for premodern modes of production. Theories of visual media can help to think this through. In his essay "The Work of Art in the Age of Mechanical Reproduction," Walter Benjamin celebrates the diminishment of the aura of the artist in an era in which the necessarily original painting ceded ground to the reproducible photograph or film. Benjamin differentiates the painter and the cameraman by making an analogy to medicine, distinguishing the medical practitioner as the painter-like magician, who lays on hands, from the photographer-like surgeon, who radically decreases the space between practitioner and patient.[36] Both magicians and surgeons create pictures of the patient, but of very different kinds: whole versus fragmentary, obscuring the technique versus foregrounding it, and Benjamin privileges the surgeon-cameraman in each of these binaries. It remains an open question what role mass production has in medicine as art.

Even the brand-name blockbuster drug has a problematic relationship with art, of both the same kind as the blockbuster film (the blockbuster's consumer is unsophisticated and unoriginal, susceptible to marketing), and of its own kind (its provision is driven by guidelines that draw on scientific evidence rather than clinical intuition). Once mass production of branded drugs cedes to mass production of generics, this in turn raises a question about whether generic drugs, stripped as they are of authorship and innovation, can play any role in medical art. But there is something even more peculiar about the ways in which art versus lowest-common-denominator science are played off against each other here. At the intersection of generic drugs with a racially stratified society, it becomes particularly clear that to embrace or to disavow the generic is a complicated and meaning-laden maneuver. To bring the commodity fetishism of generic drugs to bear on the larger arguments of this book, I will now turn to their role in biological citizenship.

American Biological Citizenship

Throughout this book, I have made references to notions of *biological citizenship* to understand diverse mobilizations around African American disease and health. Now I will elaborate this concept. The appeal and aversion provoked by a cheap racialized drug can illuminate the contours of a distinctly American biological citizenship in which consumer capitalism and racialized deprivation coexist.

The term "biological citizenship" emerges from two related literatures: one developed for analysis of resource-poor settings and the other for the Global North. Both strands help to understand how it is that medical treatment should be seen as a site of, rather than an alternative to, social and political contestations. Attention to debates about generic pharmaceuticals shows how mobilizations around African American health can be betwixt and between, enrolled in both kinds of biological citizenship projects.

One origin of the term "biological citizenship" is in the anthropology of resource-poor settings. It comes from Adriana Petryna, who has given a rich anthropological account of post-Chernobyl Ukraine where "the damaged biology of a population has become the grounds for social membership and the basis for staking citizenship claims."[37] She shows that bureaucratic practices that mediate illness also mediate claims to biological citizenship, defined as "a massive demand for but selective access to a form of social welfare based on medical, scientific, and legal criteria that both acknowledge biological injury and compensate for it."[38] In Ukraine, the struggle for scarce medical resources is happening in a postsocialist terrain. In the invocations of African American health emergencies—whether high rates of infectious disease in the early twentieth century, or premature heart disease mortality in the twenty-first—efforts to mobilize state resources to address "the damaged biology" of African Americans are part of social membership and citizenship claims. Demands for access to pharmaceuticals are biological citizenship demands, whether the drugs in question are generic or branded, but the modesty of the citizenship demanded is clearer when the drugs are cheap.

At the same time, the more consumerist model of biological citizenship posited by the sociologist Nikolas Rose and his colleagues is also at play here. Rose and his coauthor Carlos Novas write about a new kind of biopolitics that has emerged in North America, Europe, and Australia, and use the term "biological citizenship" to describe "all those citizenship projects that have linked their conceptions of citizens to beliefs about the biological existence of human beings, as individuals, as families and lineages, as communities, as population and races, and as a species."[39]

Rose and Novas compellingly argue that contemporary biological citizenship projects such as personalized genetic testing are distinct from earlier racialized national projects, such as eugenics and hygiene. Biology becomes the grounds for hope and creative identity practices, rather than pathology and determinism: "As aspects of life once placed on the side of fate become subjects of deliberation and decision, a new space of hope and fear is being established around genetic and somatic individuality. In Western nations—Europe, Australia, and the United States—this is not taking the form of fatalism and passivity, and nor are we seeing a revival of genetic or biological determinism."[40] This framework captures something important about thiazides' appeal for Henry Louis Gates Jr. in his identity claim "I'm on that! I'm a salt-saving Negro!" Rose and Novas characterize this form of biological citizenship as distinctive of contemporary liberal democracies, and posit that the forms of biosociality that they find most novel are available in Paris, San Francisco, or London, but not sub-Saharan Africa.[41]

There are two problems with this temporal and geographical cartography of the new biological citizenship. First, Rose and Novas's framework paves over heterogeneity both within the Global North and within the United States. Eliding distinctions between and within rich countries evacuates their particular racial histories; the United States was founded on racial genocide and racial slavery as fundamentally as it was founded on notions of liberal democracy. Second, the new biological citizenship does not simply replace the old. As the legal scholar Dorothy Roberts has pointed out, race is as fundamental to the new biocitizen as it was to the old, and Nikolas Rose's optimism about the freedom that citizens can exercise in private domains of family and market reflects a neoliberal moment.[42] It does not capture the radically unequal access to consumption in America.

Thus, the Petryna model is helpful for understanding situations of scarcity and deprivation, and the Rose model is helpful for understanding situations of consumerist excess. I argue that both models must be combined in order to understand mobilizations around African American health. Indeed, the tension between racialized exclusions and the promise of consumerist freedom is foundational to a distinctly American biological citizenship. In a context in which American society is widely characterized as saturated with pharmaceuticals, pharmaceutical consumption is central to biological citizenship, and access to pharmaceuticals and especially to brand-name ones becomes part of articulating inclusion in American ways of life.

Generic Drugs and the Scope of Inclusion

To grapple with this distinctly American biological citizenship, I will attend to how advocacy around this generic drug has resonances with both Global South critique and consumerist models of medicine. I will start by discussing the ways in which access to drugs in resource-poor settings—often generic drugs —is a simultaneously compelling and inadequate means to accomplish access to health and demarginalization in society. I then attend to American articulations that situate generic drugs in contrast to expensive, especially pharmacogenomic, drugs. In these contrasts, generics are sometimes portrayed as preferable, and sometimes as second-rate. Either way, the nature of a consumerist model of health is at stake. The volatility of the coincidence of the generic drug and the drug for blacks illustrates the foundational tension in a society that straddles freedom and inequality.

The democratic ways of life staked around generic drugs and African American health have resonances with pharmaceutical grammars emerging in the developing world, and bear some of the same promises and perils. As anthropologists working in the Global South have shown, even as generic drugs can be a powerful focus of advocacy for more inclusive access to medicine, access to generic drugs is not itself access to justice.

João Biehl, a medical anthropologist who works in Brazil, has pointed out that the "pharmaceuticalization of public health" in developing countries often involves state-led promotion of generic drugs—and even as this move becomes central to narratives of national self-determination, positing these drugs as the solution to dire health problems renders a very narrow concept of the scope of public health.[43] Impoverished people at the margins of social structures face exclusions much more systemic than the lack of treatment for their HIV status, and biological citizenship as access to antiretrovirals is not a fully inclusive form of citizenship.[44]

The elision of demands for social inclusion into demands for access to drugs is not limited to HIV. In Stefan Ecks's research on psychopharmaceutical marketing in India, what he calls "pharmaceutical citizenship" operates in a discourse in which being marginalized is framed as lacking pharmaceutical access, and thus provision of pharmaceuticals becomes the solution to marginalization—the biomedical promise becomes the promise of inclusion in middle-class consumer society.[45] Since, as Ecks and his coauthor Soumita Basu have pointed out, psychopharmaceuticals in India at the time were all generic, this promise that pharmaceuticals can solve marginalization cannot be sourced in any simple way to multinational corporations.[46] Similarly, part of thiazides' appeal for articulating pharmaceutical citizenship is that—even though multinational companies are among those that make them—enthusiasm for them as a site of intervening against disparities cannot necessarily be sourced to multinational corporations.

Indeed, "corporate interests" should be understood as heterogeneous. When efforts to promote generics are privately led, as Cori Hayden, an anthropologist who writes on Mexico, has pointed out, they make strong (albeit far from simple) claims to the public interest.[47] In the context she analyzes, private but Mexican-owned generic companies can articulate a compelling alternative to multinational companies, illustrating the slipperiness of private and public in generic drugs. Generics are an increasingly important segment of health care in the United States as well, and we should not assume that the only ones with a stake in their success are a pure public.

Even when the interests being served by the advocacy of generic drugs are not explicitly for profit, that does not mean that they are necessarily aligned with justice.[48] When inclusion in pharmaceutical consumption is fostered by global charities together with third-world states, it can bolster forms of medicalization that serve the interests of sectors of civil society that are broader than Big Pharma but hardly fully inclusive. Vinh-Kim Nguyen foregrounds the biopolitical stakes of what he calls "therapeutic citizenship" in the context of the "humanitarian/development complex that has emerged around HIV/AIDS."[49] There is a medical bureaucracy that has emerged around preventive health in the United States, not least in the NIH and Medicare (the federal governmental program that provides health coverage to Americans over age sixty-five), and pharmaceutical companies are not the only ones participating in the flows of resources around these drugs.

At the same time, there can be a volatile implicit analogizing between the first and third worlds when the generic drug is considered to be the best for blacks: in a context in which global licensing frameworks advocate the use of generics in "resource-limited countries" and free reign for Big Pharma elsewhere,[50] this can map troublingly onto disparities within the United States. Since participation in cardiovascular knowledge and pharmaceutical practice has become a mode of articulating citizenship demands, pharmaceutical distribution becomes a site for talking about aspirations of participation in American ways of life. Framings of hoped-for pharmaceutical practices might be either cutting-edge or accessible to all, differentiated or universal, near at hand or emerging at some future point once the science or the struggle for social justice has proceeded further. If the drug for blacks is the same kind of drug that is provided to "resource-limited countries," rather than the same kind of drug that is given to white Americans, that can both appeal and repel. Advocating thiazide diuretics for all Americans does not remove generic drugs' sanctimonious valence or their taint.

There is a tension here in advocating generic drugs as a solution to the needs of the masses, because it is never clear whether the elite of the Global North are part of those masses or distinct from them. If the former, this puts citizens of the Global South, African Americans, and white Americans all on equal footing. However, as the anthropologist and physician Paul Farmer has pointed out, demands for "cost-effectiveness" are often enrolled in ideologies of public health that favor efficiency over equity—which are "likely to be perverted unless social justice remains central to public health and medicine."[51] For Farmer, "the efficiency-equity trade-off" is antithetical to human rights: only if sickness and death among the poor are considered to be less important than among the rich can an "inegalitarian" system be "efficacious."[52] Farmer points out that the demand to be "cost-effective" is often applied to those who seek to help the poor, but for those who disregard the poor "the sky's the limit" on medical spending.[53] In this binary, where do African American patients stand? Given that "the masses" are often defined in contrast to global elites, these debates can spur anxiety about whether African Americans should be understood as part of the Global North participating in consumer capitalism, or the Global South deserving of public or philanthropic efforts priced at the whim of their financiers.

And yet, we cannot simply follow Farmer's implication that the gold standard of intensive medical response should be applied everywhere. Overtreatment and undertreatment have long coexisted in the United States, in ways that are racialized. As Nancy Tomes has pointed out, "the comparatively free-wheeling nature of American medical practice" "creates what economists quaintly term 'perverse incentives' for the overtreatment of affluent patients and the undertreatment of poor ones."[54] For Tomes, this is "the worst of both worlds," since it drives up costs while leaving out many people. If we take Farmer's critique seriously, the danger of increased costs is much less pressing than the harmful exclusions. Further incentives to treat black patients with the old, cheap drugs while giving the expensive new ones to white patients exacerbates a long-standing divide.

The coincidence of the cheap drug and the drug for blacks can be particularly irksome for those who support African Americans' integration into the science and art of cutting-edge medicine. Skepticism of the generic is continuous with that of earlier generations of African American physicians, who argued that blacks deserved scientific medicine in an era in which their needs were largely relegated to hygiene. At the same time, desire for the brand can be read as part of the history of African American consumption as a civil rights issue. The historian Lizabeth Cohen has persuasively argued that America should be understood as a "consumers' republic," and African Americans' struggle to participate fully in the allegedly "free" market has been part of claiming rights as citizens.[55] As the historian of advertising Jason Chambers argues, access to brand-name material goods has long been "a key means of communicating aspirations and showing that blacks were equal to whites in every possible way."[56]

And yet, the appeal of thiazide diuretics as a site of an inclusive public health has been a strong one. For example, the current director of the Framingham Study, Daniel Levy, together with his coauthor Susan Brink, wrote in their 2005 history of the Framingham Study of the potential value of thiazides for contributing to a broad social good:

> Despite the many new drugs available, and $15.5 billion spent annually on medications to lower high blood pressure, the ALLHAT study proved that diuretics, the drug class that was the cornerstone of Freis's clinical trial nearly four decades ago, were superior in blood pressure control and in preventing some of the most serious adverse consequences of cardiovascular disease than newer and much more costly medications. Using thiazide diuretics in the treatment of the 50 million people with hypertension in the United States would save billions of dollars each year. That money could be better spent on further research into the causes of heart disease and stroke,

or applied to additional clinical steps to prevent heart disease in those at greatest risk.[57]

A simultaneously zero-sum and remarkably social articulation of investment emerges here, in which it is imagined to be possible to shift money from consumer spending to basic research or public health. This kind of calculus imagines that money could be shifted from health care consumers (and their complex regime of payers, including insurance companies and Medicare) to investment in social good. The optimism here in the affordable quick fix that diuretics could provide is resonant with that described in previous chapters, in the mobilization around African American hypertension as a disease category since the 1960s and 1970s, as well as the twenty-first-century invocation of it by the economist Roland Fryer. Whether thiazides are a boon for affordable disease prevention for all Americans, or an available means to help African Americans catch up demographically, promoting them can be part of a democratic impulse.

This makes thiazide diuretics very different from the pharmacogenomic drugs that Anne Fausto-Sterling, among others, has criticized as being a diversion from focus on the possibilities of social progress against the effects of racism on disease states such as African American hypertension. Thiazides fit better into the model of "public health" that she champions rather than of pharmacogenomics that she criticizes when she writes:

> If . . . we already know how to solve a lot of the public health problems before us, including those that exact an excess toll from various minority communities, then why aren't we just doing it? And why are geneticists spending so much time on huge, multinational SNP and haplotype mapping projects, promising that their new definitions of race will help members of the newly defined racial groupings to improve their health? An analysis of our health care system's love of high-tech solutions for low-tech problems, of our national unwillingness to fund and carry out well designed public health measures, and of the force of the pharmaceutical industry as it drives for pill-based solutions to socially produced ills is much more than I can accomplish in this paper. Not here, not now, but . . .[58]

An old pill can play a different role in this kind of narrative than a new pill, and thiazides have been especially appealing for those interested in affordable health care for all and who believe that the state has a role in providing it. Promoting thiazides can be part of an egalitarian impulse. Thiazides' status as generic gives them a different valence than other drugs, and promoting them makes two moves. On the one hand, endorsing thiazides advocates an even more complete saturation of American publics with drugs. On the other, it frames participation in American pharmaceutical grammars in some ways rather than others. The future articulated through thiazides reflects a distinctive articulation of what American medical research and practice should be. As Sheila Jasanoff and Sang-Hyun Kim have argued, imagined possibilities matter; what they describe as "sociotechnical imaginaries" are vital sites for thinking through not just what technology should be, but also what the nation should be, because "technoscientific imaginaries are simultaneously also 'social imaginaries,' encoding collective visions of the good society."[59] A sociotechnical imaginary organized around diuretics articulates American medical research and practice in ways distinct from sociotechnical imaginaries of blockbuster drugs or pharmacogenomics.

The principal historian of thiazides, Jeremy Greene, has written the history of thiazide diuretics as tragedy, ending his 2005 narrative at a historical moment in which they were outshone by newer drugs even as ALLHAT "demonstrated" that they were superior. Greene's fascinating history describes how when the first thiazide, chlorothiazide, was launched as the brand-name revolutionary drug Diuril in 1958, it was a triumphant interplay of marketing and research, in fact the first blockbuster drug.[60] Its low toxicity profile made it possible to expand the definition of hypertension at a moment in which it was becoming an identifiable "prepathological" state of risk for future cardiovascular disease. After recounting a history that demonstrated the fluid boundaries between the knowledge of Diuril and of disease, Greene was suddenly declarative, as if the real value of diuretics can now be transparently ascertained: "Ironically, the recent publication of the National Institutes of Health's Antihypertensive and Lipid Lowering Therapy to Reduce Heart Attacks Trial (ALLHAT) places us at a moment when thiazide diuretics have recently been demonstrated to be the most efficacious and appropriate first-line antihypertensive therapy for most patients, though their actual prescription rates now lag far behind those of newer, more heavily advertised drugs."[61] Greene was more pessimistic about thiazides' future than many of the drugs' fans, including the economist Roland Fryer or the Framingham director Daniel Levy. Writing as if the story of thiazide diuretics was at its end, Greene lamented that the blockbuster drug model that Diuril ushered in became part of its class's ultimate decline, as ever newer blockbuster drugs have come to dominate the moment. Greene wrote:

Examination of Diuril's career, then, leaves us with some unsatisfying ambivalence toward the drug-promotion process: while we might applaud the fact that Diuril was launched into the world so effectively, it is clear that the same efficient machine of promotion was instrumental in the subsequent decline and neglect of the thiazide diuretics once they ceased to be a financial priority for the industry. Grasping this irony is essential to understanding the dual nature of pharmaceutical promotion as a process rooted in both education and salesmanship, a process that is now fundamental to the circulation of the knowledge and changing practice of American medicine.[62]

And yet by both opening the black box of ALLHAT and by attending to invocations of thiazide diuretics outside medicine, we can see that its story is not yet over.

Back when the thiazide was the brand-name cutting-edge Diuril, as Greene has described, it was enrolled in tropes of greatness and revolutionary medicine. Thiazide diuretics are now enrolled in tropes of mundane mediocrity and stalwartness, aspects I have suggested are inseparable from their familiarity and decreasing equivalent value. As the drug class lost its patent protection and its novelty, it lost its edge. But, as we will see in the next chapter, on BiDil, both novelty and stalwartness have their positive and negative valences. At stake is a tradeoff between risk and reliability, between being in on "the latest" and being at the mercy of fads. Drugs, like fashion, are amenable to retro-chic. When Roland Fryer and Henry Louis Gates Jr. styled diuretics' meaning in markedly different ways from those that its earliest marketers celebrated, or those that experts in ALLHAT emphasized, they were participating in meaning making of pharmaceuticals that exceeds that of marketers or medical experts. When medical experts advocate thiazides in a way that frames them as a site of resistance to high-cost medicine, thiazides operate as an interesting untrademarked brand of their own.

Indeed, other historians of thiazide diuretics have emphasized their resilience rather than their decline. Robert Kaiser concluded his 1997 account of the intersection of science and commerce in the creation of the first thiazide: "As an enduring staple of the therapeutic armamentarium, the thiazides today remain remarkable for their resilience. Once a symbol of corporate innovation and state-of-the-art science during a crucial decade in the history of therapeutics, they now represent reliable, sensible, inexpensive remedies for edema and hypertension. Far from anachronistic, they have retained a place in medical practice, even though their past symbolism has been forever altered in the present. They remain comfortable old warhorses in an age of cost-effective care."[63] Kaiser's account preceded but also presaged the reception of ALLHAT. The efficacy of thiazides as demonstrated in ALLHAT seemed to provide a refreshing counterpoint to pharmaceutical narratives focused on the private, new, and expensive.

If, as I have argued throughout this book, participation in cardiovascular disease knowledge and pharmaceutical practice has become part of articulating inclusion in American ways of life, we can read differing pharmaceutical grammars as differing articulations of that participation: placing hopes on new advances from Pharma, or on a democratic distribution of what is already at hand. Thiazides and generic drugs more broadly have been widely enrolled in narratives of inclusion at radically different scales: on the one hand, potentially providing a common ground of treatment for all people everywhere, and on the other, providing a way for those excluded from cutting-edge care to have access to medicines. In that tension between difference and inclusion in first-world medicine, African American health can be betwixt and between. Differences among U.S. populations also become sites of fraught debates about the meanings of racial prescriptions. Importantly, arguments situated around thiazides precede BiDil both conceptually and historically, revealing that articulations of racial difference in pharmaceuticals do not necessarily have marketing as their base.

The increasing prominence of pharmaceuticals has been part of a change in the center of gravity of medicine as a field. There has been a move away from the centrality of medical artistry, the unmasked human labor of the physician, toward a medical model centered on objects whose social relations are more hidden. It is into this terrain of medicine—a field of social relations that comes to be understood outside of social relations—that I see debates about thiazides both among medical experts and in broader public spheres. Interrogation of generics shows that our analysis of pharmaceuticals must attend not only to postwar innovations in marketing or their elaboration at the turn of the twenty-first century, but also to age-old commodity fetishisms.

No amount of clinical data has been able to settle thiazide diuretics—neither the drug class itself, nor its relationships with race. I argue, further, that data cannot do so. Meanings of both thiazides and race also draw from beyond the clinic as the drug class becomes a site of exchange among pharmaceutical-centered medicine, NIH politics, and emerging rearticulations of black identities. Social and economic conditions of differential access to pharmaceuticals are as much at stake as claims about differential biologies. The meanings of both this generic, old drug and of race are multiple and still in motion. Interrogating thiazides' intersections with race shows that to understand durable preoccupations with race and pharmaceuticals, attention to narrow economic interests of some players in the debate is not a full engagement with the generic drugs' broader appeal. This is an important foundation from which to go on to the next chapter, concerning the more blatantly racialized and controversially marketed drug BiDil.

CHAPTER 6

BiDil:
Medicating the Intersection
of Race and Heart Failure

The scene was a two-day conference in April 2006 that I had played a part in organizing with MIT's Center for the Study of Diversity in Science, Technology and Medicine. The conference, titled "Race, Pharmaceuticals, and Medical Technology,"[1] took place just months after the launch of BiDil, a new pill that combined two older drugs, hydralazine and isosorbide dinitrate. When it was approved by the U.S. Food and Drug Administration in 2005 for heart failure in "self-identified black patients," BiDil became the first drug ever to bear a racial indication. The explicitness of its racialization had attracted much critique from scholars, especially among the social scientists and historians of race and medicine who made up most of the conference attendees.

The critical race theorist and legal scholar Dorothy Roberts had just presented her paper on the diverse responses of African Americans to racial therapeutics such as BiDil, outlining frameworks that could foster or inhibit African American support for the drug.[2] After the talk, one questioner stood up. He identified himself as Juan Cofield, the president of the New England Area Conference of the National Association for the Advancement of Colored People, a major American civil rights organization. Cofield then declared: "There is consensus in the black community that this drug is good for black people." Roberts, after a beat, said: "There isn't consensus among the black people in *this room.*"

It was an exchange that would resonate through the rest of the conference.[3] It would seem in a formal logical sense that the disagreement among the African Americans who spoke at the conference would be enough to prove the lack of African American consensus generally. But, as the chair of the sessions, David Jones, would note in his closing remarks, it turned out to be more complicated than that.

Cofield's statement provides an opportunity to consider a few common rhetorical moves in the BiDil debates. First, he represented his moral stakes as exceeding those of himself as an individual conference participant. This rendered his intervention both more important and more explosive. In this move, he claimed an authority that both included (some of the) conference participants and exceeded them, opening questions of accountability both of himself and of us all. Second, his intervention denied the polyvalence of BiDil. Framing BiDil as pure salve, Cofield sought to dismiss many of the conference participants' concerns about the dangers of using racial categories in medicine. Third, he moved—unsuccessfully—to close the debate.

Claiming consensus in medicine—or anywhere—is never a practice of observation, but always a rhetorical strategy. If there had been consensus, this tense conference would have been a bland affair. As the theorist Chantal Mouffe highlights, in the politics of deconstruction it is precisely the impossibility of consensus that renders democratic debate lively.[4] Chaos underlies a provisional stabilization of consensus. This provides, in Derrida's terms, both a risk and a chance.[5] Many of the conference attendees spoke of the risk of racial reification, and Cofield was responding to another kind of risk: he was worried that any doubts about BiDil might hinder its distribution. But there was also a chance here in this debate, to make interlocutors' stakes in debates in race and medicine more explicit, and to mine BiDil as a new site for both academic analysis and political engagement.

There are inescapable ambivalences underlying both drugs and race, sets of what Derrida would characterize as undecidables, including whether this drug is fundamentally beneficent or maleficent. Cofield wanted to shove that undecidability to the side, render it secondary to the consensus about its clinical effectiveness. Of course there is not consensus, either in black communities or in medicine, about whether BiDil is a good thing. Yet the project for critical scholars is different: not to traverse or overcome undecidability, but to develop modes of engagement with unclosable undecidabilities. I argue that BiDil is irredeemably a *pharmakon*—a remedy and a poison. The pill is also irredeemably both material (stuff) and semiotic (meaning). Grappling with the polyvalence at this intersection of the material-semiotic categories of race and pharmaceuticals is key to understanding the simultaneous appeals and unpalatibilities of BiDil.

Situating BiDil: BiDil Is Not a Lifestyle Drug

BiDil has been remarkably unsuccessful in a commercial sense, estimated to have reached between 1 and 3 percent of its target market in the year after its release,[6] and it is no longer actively marketed.[7] And so my consideration of debates around BiDil is haunted by a curiosity about why this drug, which so many diverse groups found compelling and so many academic critics found threatening, has not been able to penetrate the pharmaceutical practices of African Americans with heart failure. The United States is a famously pharmaceutically saturated environment, and so there is something peculiar about BiDil's poor success in getting into bodies. BiDil initially seemed to many observers to be a good fit for consumerist market-driven medicine because of its high level of publicity and the fact that its patient population was defined around a specific market segment—even if they debated whether its market appeal was cause for celebration or alarm. I argue that its failure should be understood as inextricable from the story BiDil tells, both with regard to heart failure and niche drugs, and with regard to race.

Over the past decade, both science and technology studies work and popular debates about pharmaceuticals have been dominated by what have become called "lifestyle drugs," such as Viagra and Prozac, which are "life-enhancing" rather than "life-saving."[8] Drugs for the predisease categories of cardiovascular disease—such as hypertension and hypercholesterolemia—have also been prominently discussed, especially the way that they transform the focus of medicine from treating the sick to treating those at risk for becoming so, which is to say, most everyone,[9] through increased surveillance of the symptom-free body in processes of what Adele Clarke and her colleagues have termed "biomedicalization."[10] Yet precisely because BiDil is a drug that is actually effective for patients who are easily defined as needing it, it might be a poor fit for dominant contemporary pharmaceutical discourses, which have focused on the slipperiness of disease categories and potential risks. As a drug for a generally underserved population that is very sick, BiDil demands different analytical tools.

Considering Heart Failure as a Disease Category

BiDil's indication is for heart failure in "self-identified black patients," but discourse around it has been so overwhelmingly focused on the final words of that phrase that many observers inaccurately describe it as a drug for hypertension or vaguely define it as a drug for heart disease. On one level, this makes sense: although it is impossible to have an opinion about BiDil without having an opinion about race (even if that opinion is a disavowal), heart failure as a disease category does not operate that way. Just as it is possible to have an opinion about Vioxx without having an opinion about arthritis, it is possible to have an opinion about BiDil without having an opinion about heart failure. Critiques of BiDil have taken scant account of the particularities of heart failure. However, ignoring the specificities of heart failure is a missed opportunity to understand the drug's full context. What does it mean for hearts to fail?

The heart is emblematically responsive to load. It changes its rate and volume according to the demands of the body beyond it. It generally cannot grow new cells in order to repair itself—this is why heart cancer is so extraordinarily rare—and so its cells enlarge and "remodel" to accomplish more work.[11] For example, if blockages in the vessels or high peripheral pressure make it harder to circulate the blood, the heart's cells will increase in size—like any other muscle worked hard—and the capacity will also increase. But this is a temporary fix, called compensation. As soon as this cellular remodeling and hypertrophy starts, it's a sign of problems to come. Compensation is a symptom-free prelude to decompensation. Decompensation means that after the temporary respite offered by the heart's compensatory efforts, the success starts to break down. Either not enough blood can be accommodated by the chambers within the heart's now bulky muscle, or not enough can be expelled from the enlarged chambers, and insufficient oxygenization of the peripheral body leads to shortness of breath and fatigue, first with activity and then even at rest.

The diagnostic category "heart failure" has a contingent, technologically dependent history. That is, like myocardial infarction or hypertension, its clinical definition is confirmed on the basis of diagnostic tests and arbitrary dividing lines. For example, scans can show compensatory shape change in the left ventricle, and "ejection fraction."[12] Whereas normally a well-functioning heart relaxes to allow in fresh blood and has an ejection fraction of over 50 percent, a heart that either does not relax enough to fill or has an ejection fraction of less than 40 percent is considered failing.[13] These processes and fractions can only be determined through visualization technologies in a doctor's office.

Uncontrolled hypertension can cause heart failure, and so in some real sense heart failure can be considered to be the end of a line drawn from that starting point. Where hypertension is a way of understanding pre–heart disease, heart failure is a way of characterizing its conclusion. As the National Heart, Lung, and Blood Institute fact sheet on the topic puts it: heart failure "is often the end stage of cardiac disease."[14] However, unlike the stages of hypertension, the stages of heart failure are not determined numerically. Rather, symptoms define the stages: Classes I and II are defined by whether symptoms such as shortness of breath, palpitation, and fatigue cause no limitation on physical activity or slight limitation on physical activity, respectively. Classes III and IV are based on whether those symptoms occur only during normal physical activity or whether they are present even at rest.[15] Thus heart failure as a disease category is both a technical construct and a consciously embodied reality.

Consider how we might "make sense of" this illness in Robert Aronowitz's terms.[16] Aronowitz describes the tensions and interplay between ontological notions of disease rooted in doctors' expertise in identifying abstract disease categories, and holistic notions of disease rooted in the patient's idiosyncratic experience. Whereas hypertension is mainly ontological, heart failure is predominantly holistic. Heart failure is not (in Aronowitz's terms) as dominantly a "doctor's disease" as hypertension is; it is also a "patient's illness."

This difference in the holistic embodied reality of the conditions that they treat is one thing that makes BiDil very different from risk-averting drugs such as thiazide diuretics, which I described in the previous chapter. This matters for each drug's racialization: staking claims on abstract disease categories is different from doing so on experienced suffering. It also matters for each drug's role in contemporary pharmaceutical economies. Like thiazide diuretics, BiDil is imagined to be taken for the rest of a person's life, yet the prognosis for the length of that life is quite short. And unlike thiazides, lifestyle drugs, or potential future drugs for combinatorial categories of risk such as metabolic syndrome,[17] BiDil does not expand the category of the illness it seeks to treat. It is a drug for people who are sick, not for an infinitely expandable category of those at risk for becoming so.[18] It also often does make them feel better in the short term, and has impacts on prevention of hospitalization and death that can be on a scale that a patient can experience as a real improvement.

A drug for heart failure in blacks could never reach the scale of a blockbuster drug. Even if every single self-identified black patient with heart failure in the United States took the drug, the estimated 750,000 prescriptions would be a tenth of a percent of the 60 million annual prescriptions in this country for leading brand of statin at the time, Lipitor (or, for that matter, the tens of millions of prescriptions for thiazide diuretics).[19] Even if the racial indication were ignored, and every person with heart failure in the United States took BiDil, that would still be a relatively tiny market of 5.8 million.[20] Moreover, more than half of those diagnosed with heart failure will die within five years, and 80 percent will die within eight to twelve years.[21] Although the prevalence of heart failure as a diagnosis is growing, the potential for growth of the heart failure treatment market is hindered by the poor longevity of its sufferers (even with BiDil). The heart failure market is much more limited in terms of total patient-days of consumption than the market for "lifelong" drugs for young healthy people. Market expansion happens with antihypertensives and statins because more people become diagnosed with the risk factors than die with the diagnosis, but happens much more slowly with heart failure because time between diagnosis and death is limited. In order to increase the total number of patients living with the diagnosis, the increase in newly diagnosed patients would have to be of a greater scale than those who die of the diagnosis. As it is, heart failure remains far from the scale of pre–heart diseases such as hypertension and high cholesterol, which have become sites of blockbusters.

Of course, there is much money to be made in small markets and on what I have called elsewhere "drugs for short lives,"[22] but BiDil is also a poor fit for the niche model. It is not only easy to copy, it is a copy—a methods patent on combining two already existing generic drugs for a new indication. This is not to suggest that cheap ingredients should necessarily yield little revenue. Much is made of the high production cost of cancer biologics, but that is not actually the reason that they are so expensive. Prices are set not by production costs but by willingness to pay—and our willingness to pay has been extraordinarily high for remarkably ineffective end-stage cancer drugs. So why was it not for BiDil?

BiDil's Contingent History: V-HeFT to A-HeFT

BiDil's emergence did not follow a path typical for either blockbusters or niche drugs. It took the drug combination that would become BiDil a long time to get a trial that could show its success. Since the 1970s, the University of Minnesota cardiology professor Jay Cohn has believed for elegant physiological reasons that the combination of isosorbidedinitrate and hydralazine (I/H)—generic drugs already in wide use for other indications—would be highly beneficial for heart failure. He collaborated with Veterans Affairs, the U.S. government agency that provides health benefits to military veterans, to put his combination to the test in two cooperative studies between 1980 and 1991, called the Vasodilator in Heart Failure Trials (V-HeFT) I and II.[23] In the first trial, Cohn's combo did better than the placebo and the other agent, but not statistically significantly. In the second, the combo was not quite as effective as the ACE (angiotensin-converting enzyme) inhibitor with which it was put head to head.

Like many scientists confronted with evidence that fails to support their hypothesis, Cohn still believed that his idea worked.[24] He started to think that perhaps the combination of ACE inhibitors and his combo would provide the long-sought benefit, but could not find the commercial or governmental support to test his idea. A pharmaceutical benefit management company called Medco—a third-party administrator of prescription drug provision then owned by Merck, as it experimented with vertical integration[25]—secured property rights from Cohn and trademarked the drug combination as BiDil in 1995. Cohn went with Medco representatives to the FDA to seek a new drug application based on the data from the V-HeFT trials. But the FDA was not supportive of a new drug application based on the data amassed, especially since the components of the new drug were available generically, and it rejected the application.[26] Medco left the picture.[27]

But by the late 1990s, a time when focus on health disparities was growing at the FDA and beyond, two things had changed: ACE inhibitors were widely argued to be less effective in blacks, and Cohn and a colleague conducted a retrospective analysis of the few blacks in the V-HeFT trials. That analysis seemed to suggest that Cohn's combo showed a stronger benefit for them.[28] Cohn got a new methods patent for BiDil, this time for the race-specific benefit of the combination, and licensed it to a small biotech company called Nitro-Med. NitroMed had never developed or marketed drugs, but teamed up with Cohn's longtime colleagues at the Association of Black Cardiologists (ABC) to design a trial.[29] The FDA was supportive of the idea of a trial that would focus on this poorly served population. Thus emerged the trial that would lead to BiDil's approval: the African American Heart Failure Trial (A-HeFT).

A-HeFT began in 2001 with a cohort of 1,050 self-identified black patients with class III or IV heart failure.[30] It added BiDil or placebo to the current standard of care, which now included those ACE inhibitors that BiDil had gone head to head against in V-HeFT II. This combination proved to be very potent. By the time that the trial was ended two years later, in 2004 (early, because of the strength of the results), 43 percent fewer in the standard+BiDil group had died compared with the standard+placebo group, while 39 percent fewer had been hospitalized, and those in the treatment arm also reported better quality of life.[31]

The mechanism of BiDil is not completely understood. No one knows why BiDil was so much more effective in A-HeFT than it had been in the V-HeFT trials. Perhaps it was because of the synergistic effects of ACE inhibitors, with which it had not been previously combined.[32] Perhaps the synergy of drugs was even more comprehensive, by adding a fourth mechanism (nitrous oxide enhancement) to the mechanisms addressed by the standard of care, as several A-HeFT investigators have suggested.[33] Perhaps it had to do with other differences between the V-HeFT and A-HeFT populations: more hypertensive etiology, a younger cohort, the inclusion of women. But though there are questions, there seem to be few who contest the general efficacy of the drug combination.

In the A-HeFT trial, stakeholders who were not necessarily previously aligned came together around a practical project. The "pragmatism" here is like that which Joan Fujimura has theorized. To put this case in Fujimura's terms, heart failure in African Americans was a problem that was "ripe," or "both intellectually interesting and do-able."[34] As she points out, the doability does not rest only on the technical. Whether the A-HeFT trial was an optimal way to get at efficacy or not, it had been a way to make a "doable problem" out of a conundrum. Or perhaps three conundrums: a federal agency grappling with health disparities, a cardiologist and pharmaceutical company salvaging a drug, and a professional organization of African American cardiologists with particular professional needs and patient populations. A-HeFT is an "articulation," of both problems and potential solutions. What made African American heart failure "ripe" for the FDA, NitroMed, and ABC was rising interest in health disparities, the deluge of data around African American responses to ACE inhibitors, and the increasing capacity of African American cardiologists to do clinical trials.

The debate at the FDA hearing on BiDil's approval covered many questions about the study design and the role that the V-HeFT trials could play in approval based on the small A-HeFT trial, but discord focused not on whether BiDil should be approved, but squarely on whether it should receive the racially specific indication NitroMed desired.[35] That specification would allow a longer patent for the drug—since that indication was patented far later than the non-race-specific one.[36] Moreover, in the hearings, it became clear that the cardiologist Steven Nissen, the chair of the FDA committee, wanted to go on the record as doing something specifically for blacks to round out his tenure at the FDA.

In the lead-up to BiDil, there was alignment of interests by NitroMed and ABC, but they were not necessarily seeing BiDil as a solution to the same problem. For NitroMed, the principal problem was how to get approval for the drug combination in a way that would be profitable. They thought that the longer patent life of the race-specific indication would lead to that. For ABC, the problem was and is more diffuse: how to get the funding to run trials and thus participate in the production of evidence-based medicine, and how to find solutions for black morbidity and mortality from heart failure. In these senses, ABC is very much in the tradition of black practitioners in the early twentieth century who sought access to research hospitals. A-HeFT becomes a way for African American practitioners to participate in cutting-edge research and contribute to the communities that they serve at the same time. A-HeFT is not the only way that this tradition lives on; it is also present in the Jackson Heart Study, run by an ABC member under the auspices of the NHLBI. The association has always combined its interest in creating the social changes central to ameliorating health disparities with its efforts to participate in scientific medicine and distribute the best available medical treatment.

Many critics of BiDil highlighted—and as it turned out greatly exaggerated—the money that investigators stood to make, not quite claiming that it led to biased results per se, but suggesting that financial interests distorted the trajectory of the research.[37] This kind of implication is one that has fostered ill will in the debate, triggering doctors' defensiveness about whether the money they receive colors their expert judgment. Physicians often respond to critiques of their participation in gift exchange with pharmaceutical companies with righteous indignation, that *they* would never be swayed by such things. But what makes the gifts powerful is precisely this space: they might well believe, or they might not. Critics of BiDil often address ABC as if they are simply paid ventriloquists for NitroMed—in the account by the legal scholar and prominent BiDil critic Jonathan Kahn, ABC, the NAACP, the National Minority Health Month Foundation, and the Congressional Black Caucus are all evacuated of agency; they are portrayed simply as "able surrogates on hand to do the job for" NitroMed, who "put a 'black face' on BiDil as it went before the FDA" and, later, promoted off-label use.[38]

But gifts are more complicated than that. There should be room for some conceptual space here between being bought off and, in a limited way and with an independent voice, buying in. This is not to diminish the power of the gifts circulating here, but rather to capture the way that the gifts' power is actually more interesting than a simple purchase of support. Marcel Mauss taught us that there are no free gifts,[39] and funding for the physicians' organization that supports a drug trial comes at a cost for its recipient as well as for its giver. This critique applies not just to BiDil and ABC, but to the more general alliance of pharmaceutical funding (or government funding), clinician-scientists, and social justice organizations that campaign around health. For both physicians and their patients, the power of gifts is salient: the gift is something that should be received, yet is dangerous to take. When NitroMed and ABC align, the force of the objects of gift giving are both practical and mystical. More than mere utility circulates, and obligation and liberty intermingle.

Like the physicians engaged in contract research who are tracked by the sociologist Jill Fisher, ABC's role in A-HeFT straddles two distinct identities: "entrepreneurial agent" and "pharmaceutical emissary."[40] If we pay attention only to the latter element, we lose sight of the organization's agency. At the same time, because of the distinct role of African American cardiologists in advocating for African American patients, these ABC physicians also take on the role of what Alondra Nelson has called "bio-culture brokers," deploying "authentic expertise" "available to them as both minorities *and* community-minded professionals to forge consensus in and between biomedicine, scientific domains, policy circles, and the public."[41]

The FDA approved BiDil in June 2005. Its package insert describes its indications: "BiDil is indicated for the treatment of heart failure as an adjunct to standard therapy in self-identified black patients to improve survival, to prolong time to hospitalization for heart failure, and to improve patient-reported functional status. There is little experience in patients with NYHA class IV heart failure. Most patients in the clinical trial supporting effectiveness (A-HeFT) received a loop diuretic, an angiotensin converting enzyme inhibitor or an angiotensin II receptor blocker, and a beta blocker, and many also received a cardiac glycoside or an aldosterone antagonist."[42] This decision to target "self-identified black patients" rather than those with the presumably underlying markers for responsiveness to BiDil illustrates the broader applicability of the argument I made about African American hypertension as a disease category: physicians do not necessarily prefer to make decisions based on characteristics that they can *measure*, but rather on characteristics that they can *record*. It is easier to demonstrate and communicate a pragmatic application for "self-identified black patients" than it is to make complicated guidelines based either on test values or on alternative holistic characteristics such as long-standing poorly controlled hypertension.

Just because the population studied was "self-identified black patients," that did not necessarily mean that the indication had to be limited to that group. Consider a contrasting case of drugs believed to be more effective in whites: ACE inhibitors and angiotensin receptor blockers (ARBs) often include in their package inserts that their benefits have not been proven in black patients,[43] or are less effective in black patients.[44] This grammar is slightly but crucially different from that of BiDil. BiDil could have, like ACEs and ARBs, been approved for everyone while being accompanied by a package insert indicating that "this drug's benefit has not been proven in non-black patients." Instead, absence of evidence in nonblack patients was treated as tantamount to evidence of absence. The blackness of the subjects on whom the drug was tested could not be detached from the drug—neither for the FDA, nor for BiDil's critics.

Many have criticized the use of the unreliable category of race rather than sound medical indications in the design of the trial,[45] but Cohn has responded to criticisms that race is an arbitrary category by saying that age and presence/absence of ventricular abnormalities are arbitrary, too, but that does not mean that a study cannot be constructed around them.[46] But just because it is easier to target a drug this way does not mean that the enterprise is easy. The year after BiDil's release, a tiny percentage of eligible patients were taking the drug,[47] and NitroMed's stock had fallen by an order of magnitude from its high (from $27 per share to $2.50).[48] Critics of BiDil had not only reported its hype, but had also fueled it, using the highest possible estimates of projected revenue.[49] Real challenges confront a small pharma player in a Big Pharma field, and the polyvalence of the intersection of race and drugs exceeds Nitro-Med's control. The study around which the ABC, NitroMed, and the FDA intersected is not the complete articulation of BiDil, and BiDil's poor success may be connected to difficulties in articulating BiDil to broader publics.

Too High a Price?

If the power and meaning of gifts is not simple, neither is the power of price. Many critics took for granted that NitroMed could receive any price it demanded, even long after it became clear that BiDil was a commercial failure.[50] Critics used asking price as a straightforward stand-in for patient cost. For example, the anthropologist and historian of science Duana Fullwiley has put BiDil into a framework of pharmacogenomics: "In its first instance (the African American heart medication called BiDil), race-tailored therapy has dramatically increased cost for the racial group it claims to benefit."[51] But although the FDA hailed BiDil as a step toward "personalized medicine,"[52] and many analysts have situated their critique in terms of pharmacogenomics,[53] BiDil is not a pharmacogenomic drug,[54] and the members of the "racial group it claims to benefit" are overwhelmingly not receiving the drug at all, at any price.

The conventional wisdom on the commercial failure of BiDil is that it was priced too aggressively, especially since its components are available as generics.[55] But why was BiDil not able to command ten dollars per day? That is a bargain compared to hospitalization,[56] and orders of magnitude below the price point of the niche biotech drugs that are a primary source of profit for the pharmaceutical industry today. High price might have even added to the allure of the drug, since, as we saw in the previous chapter, commodity fetishism often results in more value being imputed to that which is more expensive. The market's willingness to pay is up for debate, and could change in response to political pressure. But the pharmaceutical company's sponsorship of physicians and civil rights organizations turned out not to be able to buy sufficient political pressure to force insurers and the government to pay.

NitroMed did try to prop up BiDil's high price by using a common technique: having a drug donation program for patients who could not afford the drug, called "NitroMed Cares."[57] As Stefan Ecks has shown in his analysis of Glivec in India, drug donation programs should be understood as part of "a global pricing strategy" that "should not be disguised through a rhetoric of good citizenship."[58] Yet this drug donation strategy has been ineffective in BiDil's case, either in propping up price or in widely distributing the drug. A key element that NitroMed's drug donation program ignored is something that anthropologists of pharmaceuticals in the Global South have pointed out: even when the drug is free, the place of labor in the distribution of drug donations is complex.[59] Since BiDil's patient population is already often underserved by overstretched doctors, it is unrealistic to expect those doctors to take the uncompensated time to do the paperwork necessary to get patients the free drugs.

Even if the brand's value-added over the generic is not deemed to be worth it, BiDil's failure does not even end there. As of 2006, not only was just a small percentage of the African American heart failure population receiving BiDil, only 6 percent of patients were receiving the combination of isosorbide dinitrate and hydralazine at all, including generic equivalents.[60] If physicians' reluctance to prescribe BiDil had been due only to its price, they would have been adopting generics in droves. That they have not done so suggests that there are resistances unaccounted for by price.

Resistances to BiDil certainly do come from willingness to pay—by the complicated regimes of payers we have in the United States, and by consumers themselves. But one of the lessons of BiDil is that catering to a well-defined market of first-world consumers is not always enough to secure a high price.

The assumption made by both BiDil's makers and its critics, that patients would hear the publicity about BiDil and successfully demand it from their physicians, suggests that they underestimated how structurally underserved the population treated with BiDil is. Reports in the *Wall Street Journal* did better at capturing this than ones in more traditionally liberal venues, such as National Public Radio. Whereas NPR's report noted that the low prescription rate for BiDil "hasn't sat well with the NAACP," their report effectively dismissed this dissatisfaction by following that claim with the observation that the NAACP received a grant from NitroMed.[61] In contrast, the *Wall Street Journal* wrote: "The drug's unavailability, say some medical experts, may also be symptomatic of a deeper problem in the health-care system, where issues affecting minorities and the poor sometimes fall through the cracks."[62]

The *Wall Street Journal* quotes Gary Puckrein, who is noted as a NitroMed shareholder as well as a health activist: "If that were white patients, nobody in America would tell them, 'Excuse me, I want you to go buy a drug for angina and another for hypertension, and I want you to go home and cut them, and I want you to take multiple pills a day on top of all the [other drugs] you got.'"[63] For Puckrein, claiming value for convenience for black patients becomes a consumerist citizenship demand. This differentiates Puckrein from more publicly oriented leaders in race and medicine such as Charles Curry, the recently retired head of cardiology at Howard University (and founding member of the Association of Black Cardiologists), who described BiDil as one of the "most valuable" drugs to come along but criticized NitroMed's pricing and spoke of "practical" doctors using generics instead.[64]

And yet the kinds of consumerist demands that Puckrein wants to make are not easy to make for BiDil's target population, which is both sick and generally underserved. The implicitly white, middle class may be well positioned to make these kinds of demands, but in the context of what Clarke and her colleagues have termed "stratified biomedicalization,"[65] not everyone in the United States is so well positioned. Drugs do not simply naturally reach their markets, but do so in a complex and stratified terrain.

Neither BiDil's proponents nor its opponents seemed to grasp that a drug "for heart failure in self-identified black patients" is a poor fit for consumerist logics developed for iconic lifestyle drugs. Given the wide range of physicians who deal with heart failure with already intensive drug regimens, it has not been easy for BiDil to find its way in this terrain. Most general practice physicians keep their patients on whichever drugs they were prescribed in the hospital where their heart failure diagnosis was most likely received, meaning that advertising to hospitals is particularly important. But for a tiny company like NitroMed, getting hospitals and insurance formularies to change their practices was a huge challenge.

It's worth reflecting upon the poor resemblance between BiDil and a brand name that has been rhetorically attached to it from disparate quarters: Viagra. Jonathan Kahn has invoked it this way in describing NitroMed's success in raising money: "Where drugs such as Viagra may target one sex or another, BiDil promises to lead the way in ethnic niche marketing of pharmaceuticals."[66] Viagra was also invoked by Juan Cofield to situate BiDil at the New England Conference of the NAACP, where he introduced the presentation by a NitroMed spokesperson with a half-joke that induced some giggles: "I would like to see the name BiDil as common in our community as Viagra is in the general public."[67] The NitroMed speaker, Gerald Bruce, came back around to Viagra after a speech in which he emphasized the importance of grassroots education because insurers' refusal to cover BiDil would change in the face of demand. "What you can do to help is just building awareness in the community," Bruce said. "Talk to your family members, your constituents, your friends, your neighbors. Tell them you heard about a lifesaving medication that makes patients feel better and be able to function better. Let's, as Juan said, make BiDil as commonly known in the African American community as Viagra is in the broader community."[68]

There is a slippage here between whether BiDil should be "as common" or "as commonly known" as Viagra. In drugs' mobilization in cultural debate, these can become something of the same thing. The audience is described as laughing. In a sense, Cofield seems to be making fun of their knowledge of erectile dysfunction drugs. Taunting them a little: why do you know more about restoring sexual function than about heart function? BiDil and erectile dysfunction drugs are actually contraindicated—the combination of them can cause dangerous hypotension. The heart failure population is made up of more women than men, yet recurring references to Viagra evoke a sense that patients have to choose whether to salvage their erection or their heart. Preoccupation with that lifestyle drug makes it difficult to grapple with BiDil's own stakes.

And as it happened, although BiDil generated a good deal of publicity, it generated very little advertising that could have provided patients with scripts for making demands on doctors.[69] Its patient and provider education website mobilized some of the typical grammars of pharmaceutical websites, with the evocative URL—www.hearthealthheritage.com—but NitroMed was slow to focus on "elite" cardiovascular experts, health plans, and medical centers.[70] These experts are normally the first line of marketing for any drug, since sales generated by direct-to-consumer advertising are small as a percentage of investment (even if still profitable for blockbusters). This traditional approach might be more in tune with who actually has more determining power in the prescribing patterns of African Americans. A limitation of relying on this website, direct-to-consumer ads in black newspapers, and community education in black churches is that they rest on the assumption that doctors listen to their black patients in the same way that they do to their white patients, that "patient empowerment" to demand drugs works whether the patient in question is imagined to be a "compliant" one or a "drug-seeking" one. The challenge of configuring a "typical black patient" within grammars of an unmarked "typical patient" applies as much here as it did in treating coronary disease or hypertension.

Willingness to pay and price both become sites of narratives of pharmaceuticals, which can resonate or repel. Heart failure may be a ripe category for pharmaceutical research, but it is a challenging site for integration into contemporary pharmaceutical narratives of either blockbusters on the one hand—risk reduction or capacities for limitless health—or high-margin niche biotech drugs on the other. And articulation of a drug for African American heart failure may be compelling to actors as diverse as the FDA, the Congressional Black Caucus, the Association of Black Cardiologists, and a small pharmaceutical company, but unpalatable to public and private payers and to black publics long skeptical of medicine's beneficence.

Pharmakon

The meaning of any drug exceeds that given by its marketers or medical experts.[71] In the case of BiDil, the meanings that have circulated around the drug have been polarized and volatile. This situation is not, of course, unique to BiDil. As Asha Persson has pointed out, "For all their innocuous appearance, every pill is a potent fusion of ingredients, including scientific practices, political agendas and commercial interests, along with social activism and media spin."[72] She turns to the concept of *pharmakon* to understand not "misuse" of drugs—in her case antiretrovirals—but precisely how "correctly" used drugs "have the capacity to be beneficial and detrimental *to the same person at the same time*."[73] The pharmakon is also a useful theoretical tool for considering BiDil.

Derrida, writing about the polyvalent meanings of the Greek term *phar-*

makon, criticizes the translation of it as "remedy," with its sense of inherent beneficence.[74] He argues, rather, that the pharmakon cannot be so constrained. The word "remedy" excludes what he characterizes as "the magic virtues of a force whose effects are hard to master, a dynamics that constantly surprises the one who tries to manipulate it."[75] But hard-to-master forces and surprising dynamics are key to understanding BiDil.

BiDil has promised remedy on (at least) three registers: survival and quality-of-life benefit of the pill for individual patients, a potential mechanism in progress toward the alleviation of health disparities, and as a path toward pharmacogenomics. Similarly, the danger associated with BiDil has been on (at least) three registers: that of potential literal toxicity of the pill, that of harm to the cause of antiracism in medicine and society, and that of profits for amoral drug companies at the expense of suffering patients. A good deal of discursive boundary work has gone into trying to address BiDil's remedy and harm separately. For example, commentators such as Jonathan Kahn want to accept the physical benefit of the pill for individual patients while arguing that its racial indication leads away from progress in race relations and medicine. Perhaps part of the reason that Kahn so often gets criticized for wanting to deny the pill to patients in need is that these registers cannot quite be separated.

The potential unpalatability of a black drug was not predicted by many critics or proponents of BiDil, even though warnings about the risk of unpredictable market acceptance and the potential difficulty of convincing third-party payers to accept BiDil was already present in NitroMed's 2004 financial disclosures.[76] Right from the early stages of the A-HeFT trial, the prominent sociologist of race and medicine Troy Duster lamented in the popular press that although "it is difficult to bring anti-discrimination to the market," BiDil showed that the future of drug development was about "population aggregates that become the target market."[77] In 2005, the sociologist George Ellison characterized the drug's racial specification as "highly palatable" in that political and market context:

> There is a political demand for treatments for African Americans in America that makes the production of an ethnic drug for African Americans a highly palatable political event. At the same time, as we're well aware within our racialised societies, African Americans have a social and political identity that makes them a powerful lobbying group and a powerful market in their own right. So it's possible to develop a drug for African Americans because we can identify them, we can market to them, we can sell it to them,

we can justify it to them, and that makes it a commercially sensitive, commercially successful enterprise.[78]

Yet, as its poor market performance should alert us, BiDil's "palatability" is not so clear. Indeed, I argue, some unpalatability of a "black drug" is overdetermined, as a cartoon in the weekly syndicated comic strip *The K Chronicles* begins to illustrate (figure 5).

Associations between blackness and drugs are overwhelmingly illicit. Black drugs connote black markets. In the context of Tuskegee and rumors that crack was a government invention to suppress Black Power, there is a sinister connotation to "a drug for black people." All of this inhibits palatability. Moreover, black patients are stigmatized in medical literature for their distrust, and as noncompliant and refractory,[79] and so drugs for black people bear a taint. We even have the peculiar situation in which a drug that combines two banal old generics to treat a disease with high morbidity and mortality generates references, especially in black media, to doubts about whether BiDil is "safe."[80] All of this suggests that there may actually be, in Nathan Greenslit's terms, a "symbolic mistake"[81] in targeting drugs at African Americans.

Approval by the FDA does not by itself determine drug palatability in a differentiated society. We might read FDA approval as certification of edibility, albeit one not always trusted. Yet edibility alone does not determine what is "good to eat," which as we learn from Claude Lévi-Strauss is inextricable from what is "good to think."[82] It is not altogether clear, a priori, whether evidence of discrimination is to be found in greater access to drugs—as it is in the distribution of crack sales, or in excessive prescriptions for the antipsychotic drug Haldol[83]—or in less access to drugs, as it is generally understood in medical disparities literature. Indeed, both kinds of access can operate together: less access to antihypertensives and statins leads to more heart failure—and hence, potentially a role for BiDil. Although BiDil was "good to think" from the perspective of turn-of-the-millennium biotech investors and the FDA, not many rushed to swallow the black pill.

This is not to suggest that these dangerous connotations themselves explain BiDil's failure. The inability of a pharmakon to shed its toxic aspects does not always impede its spread. Sense of toxicity can add to the appeal of a pharmakon. The dangers pointed to in raising the specter of race and drugs together are not necessarily understood as a contraindication for a racial drug. When Kahn describes the ABC and Congressional Black Caucus support for the "purportedly benign" use of race as biology in BiDil, he operates on the

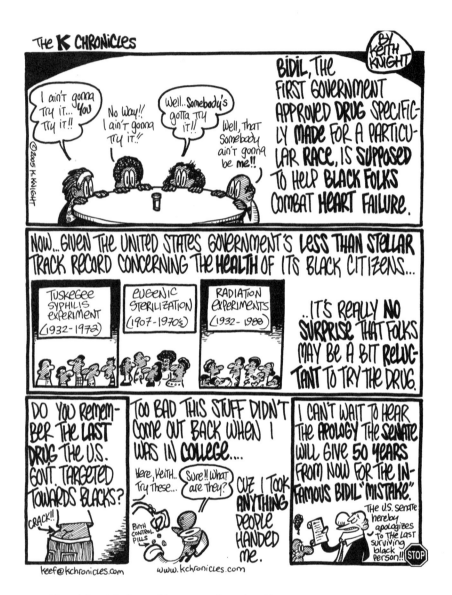

5. Keith Knight, "BiDil Me This, Man," *The K Chronicles*.

At http://www.buzzle.com/. Reprinted with permission from the author.

assumption that if its malignance were known it would be rejected.[84] But many leaders of the ABC were concerned from the outset about dangers of racial profiling in medicine, and participated anyway because of their commitment to serving the immediate needs of their very sick patients.[85]

Moreover, the poison that is part of the pharmakon is not separate from its efficacy, but immanent with it. This helps to understand why a low side-effect profile does not guarantee that a drug will be taken. Indeed, as we saw with thiazides, a low side-effect profile for a drug for an asymptomatic condition can inhibit compliance. If a drug causes no harm, it may not have any effect at all. Side effects, then, can either inhibit or inspire compliance. We can see a lateral but evocative parallel with antiretrovirals, as described by Persson:[86] for some people the evidence of the drug's toxicity on their bodies is evidence of its effectiveness against an otherwise invisible virus.

The relationship between a drug and its side effects is analogous to the relationship between BiDil as a pill and its location in debates about race. Sense of toxicity can add to the appeal of a pharmakon. The toxicity of the connection between drugs and blackness suggests, for some, that the unease must be worth it. Some of the calls to tackle fear and pursue racial medicine come across like disingenuous right-wing arguments,[87] but others do seem genuinely interested in keeping the focus on black well-being.[88] The problem of black disease is widely recognized as serious, and yet hard to get a handle on. If the problem is considered intractable, a risky discursive intervention can hold a powerful appeal.

Even though the poles of the pharmakon are inseparable, many of BiDil's supporters shared the desire of Juan Cofield in the vignette at the start of this chapter, to ignore or deny dissent. Many supporters expressed anxiety that social science and other critiques of the drug would make people afraid of it, and thus prevent access to the remedy it offers. They wanted to suppress expression of the poison aspects of this pharmakon. This rhetorical strategy suggests that the danger comes not from the drug itself, but from the lack of consensus about its unqualified beneficence.

The Material-Semiotic

There is a second, interrelated undecidable in addition to the pharmakon: the material-semiotic. Drugs are a clear case for Haraway's "material-semiotic": they are generally accepted as having both physical and social aspects. They are a ready example of the capacity of objects to carry both matter and meaning.

Moreover, their ability to move between the material and the semiotic renders drugs appealing objects for boundary work with regard to other categories on that divide. Just as arguments over the "reality" of mental illness are sometimes staked out in terms of antidepressants, the "reality" of race has been staked out in terms of BiDil. Yet the attempt to use BiDil to put race onto one side or the other of a material-semiotic divide ultimately fails because both BiDil and race keep their dual aspect. Critique of BiDil's role in the "biological basis" of race is insufficient; we should attend to the productive work it is doing at the social-biological boundary.

As we have seen throughout this book, pharmaceutical-centered medicine is an excellent site for critique of race because it intervenes on the boundaries between the social and the biological, the material and the semiotic. Race operates on precisely these boundaries. Racial difference in heart disease is material: early mortality of African Americans relative to whites takes place in actual bodies in the world and, despite caveats about the trickiness of data and etiology, death is a material event and the terrain is necessarily in part about biology. Yet racial difference in heart disease is also semiotic: the data cannot be extricated from lenses of difference-oriented preoccupations, and arguments about race and disease become ways to articulate difference in other aspects of society and individual identity.

It is helpful to consider the relationship between BiDil and race-as-biology by thinking through what it means for race to be fixed, as I did when thinking about the intersection of thiazide diuretics and the slavery hypothesis. If black heart failure is to be "fixed" through this pharmacological intervention, it is in at least three ways: by rendering race identifiably stable, by focusing attention upon it, and by promising easy repair. Pharmaceuticals are mobilized not only on the basis of existing biological categories, but also on their capacity for changing biology. One aspect of this process is that race is a difference that is imagined to be fixed enough for action, but that is at the same time potentially able to be medically mitigated. This is key to understanding the support for BiDil from such antiracist actors as the Association of Black Cardiologists. Pharmaceuticals can provide a basis for argument not only for essential racial difference, but also for mutability. As the anthropologist Jonathan Xavier Inda has argued, part of BiDil's potent appeal was its ability to "materialize hope."[89]

Genes cannot change in the medical encounter, but biologies can and do. Troy Duster has characterized the FDA approval of BiDil as marking the "reversal" of the idea that black hypertension is a biological problem with social causes, and its replacement with a model that locates both the origin and the solution in the biological.[90] However, the FDA is notably agnostic about the causes of differences in heart failure rates and drug response.[91]

Several critics have responded to BiDil by advocating regulatory efforts to separate material from semiotic categories in race research, for example through guidelines that would require distinguishing between "race as a sociopolitical category" and "race as a biological and/or explicitly genetic category."[92] But as Latour teaches us, modern science is not capable of creating pure categories without creating hybrids, and analysts are in error if we take modernism at its reductionist word.[93] When BiDil's critics want to make a choice for social justice against biology, they are solidifying the validity of that boundary in the sense that, as Nancy Krieger points out, "the notion that scientific thinking and work must somehow 'choose' between social justice and biology is itself an ideological stance."[94] Trying to separate out that nexus of race as social/biological and material/semiotic will not lead to a better account of race in medicine or the world, and the undecidabilities will remain. Scientific medicine is not even capable of fully purifying and rationalizing its objects of study into piles of genes—the human organisms that are the necessary intersection between genes and society continually get in the way.

It is BiDil's critics, not NitroMed or ABC, who reduce race-as-biological to race-as-genetic.[95] Although much criticism has debunked BiDil on the lack of a genetic basis of disparity, this is not actually a direct engagement with Nitro-Med or ABC. Paul Underwood, former president of ABC, responded to Kahn categorically: "I think there's no implication at all that genetics has anything to do with BiDil's mechanism of action. In fact, there's no claim that there's genetics at all. I believe that race in the United States is a social construct, not really a genetic construct."[96] This disconnect over the stakes of the debate should alert us that we have more work to do than simply, repeatedly and in each case reiterating that "race is not genetic." Only a few scholars have taken seriously why the drug was supported by many antiracist actors who explicitly reject race as a genetically deterministic category.[97] Many in the ABC have a deeper engagement with the complexly material-semiotic character of race than do their critics. To grapple with the alliance of ABC and NitroMed, we should not assume that "value" and "values" are necessarily in opposition, and should instead seize the opportunity for "transcending dichotomies between the economic and the moral."[98]

Rather than operating on the assumption that participating in a commercial trial is at odds with a social vision of caring for African American patients, we should pay attention to how these two impetuses can operate together. Notwithstanding the individualistic context of the United States more broadly, ABC is strikingly social in its vision. During the time period being described here, ABC's slogan was "Children Should Know Their Grandparents"; it is now "Saving the Hearts of Diverse America."[99] The organization has always used varied means toward its mission of the "elimination of cardiovascular disparities through education, research and advocacy."[100] The work of Keith Ferdinand, one of the principal investigators in A-HeFT, exemplifies this. Ferdinand is now the chief science officer for ABC, engaged in both scientific research and advocacy. Until his HeartBeats Life Center in the Ninth Ward of New Orleans was destroyed in Hurricane Katrina, it was the organizational center of diverse programs ranging from high-tech scans and clinical trials to the training of church cooks in making tasty food according to the NHLBI's blood-pressure-lowering "DASH diet."[101] The mission of Ferdinand's center was grounded as much in community engagement as it was in medical innovation. It may well be that participating in clinical trials added resources to his practice's holistic engagement with African American health and community. That is, it is more plausible that A-HeFT redirected resources to HeartBeats that would have otherwise gone to less socially committed practices, than that A-HeFT siphoned resources away from HeartBeats's social mission. In this way, clinical trial funding might have diverted resources to a more holistic practice, not from it.

It is academic critics of BiDil, not the NAACP or ABC, who are preoccupied with genetics above all other arguments about race. Historians and social scientists of race and science have made this preoccupation with the relationship between race and genetics a principal part of our occupation, such that insofar as science and technology studies as a field has focused on race it has focused overwhelmingly on genetics and critique thereof.

For ABC, participating in clinical research on BiDil was precisely a way to renegotiate the social imbalance of biologies, and in this sense they were not at odds with NitroMed. NitroMed's CEO Michael Sablonski was quick to say, "We know that skin pigmentation is at best a poor surrogate marker for looking at responses to medication."[102] This poor correlative potential was simply not threatening to BiDil as a solution, because even a poor proxy could be used "in the meantime."[103] Kahn thinks that the "caveats" about race being a rough proxy were somehow buried and insufficient, and characterized BiDil researchers' caution about using race as a surrogate marker for genetics as "ironic,"[104] but it is actually part of a racial narrative that exceeds any narrow reliance on genetics as determinative.

Just after the drug's release, BiDil's patient education website answered the question: "Why are African Americans at greater risk?" by agnostically pointing toward plural nongenetic possibilities: high blood pressure, diabetes, nitric oxide, and "other possible causes" that include less access to health care, more exposure to environmental risks such as pollution, and a greater tendency toward being overweight and sedentary.[105] On one level, this explanation is "performative and generative," exhibiting a "value and usefulness to uncertainty" that is a common feature in pharmaceutical debates as described by Linsey McGoey: uncertainty cannot be disproved, and it implies a call for further research.[106] On another level, it points toward the inherent ambiguity of bodily experience. The eclecticism in this etiology confounds easy divisions between the genetic material of the lived body and the history of the lived body.[107] As Judith Butler reminds us, nature itself is not a given: matter has a history.[108] The stuff of our bodies does not exist before or separate from the layers of meaning in which they emerge—and the regulatory norms that are sometimes contested, sometimes reached, sometimes resisted in the performance of identity. The racialized medical history is both discursive and lived, and when it is mobilized as a treatment indication it is a site of both labeling and negotiating race. For physicians in the field, there is no necessary conflict between social causes and medical solutions, and drugs can be a way to renegotiate the social imbalance of biologies. Arguing against BiDil on the basis that racial differences are "not biological" sets up the debate in an unuseful way, because it reinforces an artificial binary between originary states and living bodies.

Pharmaceutical research is a central project of American medicine, and pharmaceutical consumption an important site of American biological citizenship. This renders problematic critics' complaints that BiDil "not only . . . biologizes race but also . . . create[s] the impression that the best way to address health disparities is through drug development."[109] Kahn, for example, makes drug development sound preposterously easy, suggesting that "the appeal of taking a predominantly biomedical approach to addressing health disparities is undeniable—instead of fixing social inequality you simply fix molecules."[110] The FDA is a better target for this line of criticism than ABC is—and it is to the FDA that Kirsten Bibbins-Domingo and Alicia Fernandez, for example, direct their critique that focusing on drugs "reframes" the discussion of disparities away from social inequalities.[111] But given the explicit drug focus of the FDA, it's hard to see how that agency could do otherwise. Similarly, as Robert Sade has pointed out in the *Journal of the National Medical Associa-*

tion, government policy has been structured to incentivize research that brings drugs to market for profit, and criticizing the behavior of an individual company for following those incentives rather than pure science or abstract public good mischaracterizes the role that private companies play in this system.[112] Analytically collapsing the FDA, NitroMed, and ABC shirks the opportunity to take ABC's much more comprehensive mission seriously.

There should be conceptual space between drug development as "a way" to address disparities and drug development as "the best way" to do so—though ABC and NAACP were prominent in promoting BiDil, the drug certainly never come to dominate their work as a whole. Further, to participate in medical responses to injustice is not necessarily to abdicate commitment to social change. As Alondra Nelson has tracked, social movements can recontextualize medical ideas in diverse ways, and can be tactical rather than necessarily consistent.[113] Moreover, drug development is a node of progress and power in America, and suggestions that the NAACP and ABC have no business being there is to suggest a less democratic debate. If we assume that conducting clinical trials is generally an endeavor in which diverse researchers should be involved, A-HeFT was not in vain: it did build capacity among members of the Association of Black Cardiologists to conduct clinical trials, a capacity that continues even after the drug's promise of profit recedes.

Conclusion

Efforts to close down the heterogeneous meanings of BiDil opened this chapter, and BiDil's critics' efforts to segregate BiDil's acceptable molecules from its unacceptable meanings bring it to an end if not a close. Both are attempts to pin down the slipperiness of BiDil and race in order to make a clear embrace or denunciation on one register. If the NAACP's Juan Cofield wanted the only thing at stake to be African American access to drugs as remedies, many of BiDil's critics wanted the only thing at stake to be the purging of race from drug development and marketing. But BiDil retains what we can characterize in Derrida's terms as undecidability. The goal of critical scholars should not be to claim the decision, but to engage with the tenacity of undecidabilities.

The poor economic performance of BiDil has been explained away too quickly with reference to structural and market aspects (availability of generic versions, resistance from formularies, too small a marketing force), as well as tactical errors (price, too little marketing to hospitals). If we let these explanations rest, we miss an opportunity to use BiDil to extend not only critical scholarship of race but also of pharmaceuticals. Exploring the case of BiDil, then, is an opportunity to open up the contingency of pharmaceuticals more generally. Drugs do not always reach their markets, and we can use analysis of BiDil to destabilize notions of the inevitability of drugs' capacity for infinite expansion. Where much scholarship has attended to the expansive potential of drugs, this chapter seeks to understand what sites of resistance might impede complete saturation of American publics with drugs.[114]

BiDil's racialization has attracted considerable scholarly critique, but this has almost all been reluctant to grapple with why prominent civil rights and black health actors have backed the drug, typically resorting to implicit suggestions that they have been bought off. Yet the involvement of organizations long critical of the genetic reification of race should spur further analysis. Engaging those who invoke racialized pharmaceuticals to indict injustices and articulate aspirations can disrupt assumptions of the superiority of "natural" bodies over pharmaceutically enrolled ones, and the privileging of the sameness of "natural" bodies over lived inequalities. The NAACP and ABC articulate a sense of the racialized diseased body as the site not only of genetics, but also of history—and of both hope and hype.[115]

Considering race to be fixed enough for action is one part of the process we could call "medicating race." Yet since pharmaceuticals are mobilized not only on the basis of existing biological categories, but also on their capacity for changing biology, we can see their appeal for those with a stake in the very malleability of race. At the same time, the commercial failure of BiDil can allow us to reflect upon how both BiDil's proponents and its opponents overestimated the ease of drugs reaching their markets and underestimated the unpalatability of a "black drug" in the current historical moment.

CONCLUSION

On one level, this book tells a very specific story: the durable preoccupations with difference at intersections of race, heart disease, and pharmaceuticals in the United States over the course of a century. That itself is a broad and vital account, and the argument and approach of the book are also relevant well beyond those spheres. Here, I will underscore the value of this mode of attention to medicating race, for both race and medicine and for medical ethics.

Too often, engagement with topics of race and medicine uses a grammar of lamentation, adopting an aggrieved subject position and mourning the racialization perpetuated by pharmaceuticalized medicine. Paradoxically, part of the problem with this approach is that it is too comfortable. Medicine appears far more stable than it is, and the analyst far less implicated. I argue that accounts of race and medicine, and of ethics in medicine, should endeavor to leave the terrain more unsettled than it was when we found it. This requires deep engagement with the world as it is, resisting quandary ethics and engaging in ethical noninnocence.

Consider one final vignette. It was the end of March 2007, almost two years after the FDA approval of BiDil for heart failure in "self-identified black patients." The scene was the second annual conference of the MIT Center for the Study of Diversity in Science Technology and Medicine, which I had helped to organize. This conference followed up on the previous year's theme of "Race, Pharmaceuticals, and Medical Technology," and marked something of a shift, now focusing on "The Business of Race and Science."[1] After a morning dedicated to such topics as population genetics and genetic ancestry testing, and a break for lunch, it was my turn to moderate the panel "Debating Race in Biomedicine."

The three papers were rather disparate—one on the scope of genetic correlations by race, another on physicians' responses to race-based therapeutics, and a third on race in Alzheimer's genetics research. After the panel's presentations, I called on questions from the audience. The first several questions came from academics I knew and could call on by name, and were the regular order of the day for an academic conference—standard questions about methodology and clarification. But then I called on someone standing in the back of the room by the door, a middle-aged African American man in a brown suit whom I did not know by sight. Familiar with his voice and his take from radio appearances and newspaper articles, I was able recognize him as soon as he started to speak: Gary Puckrein, a disparities activist who was a strong public voice in support of BiDil. His comments were unrelated to the specifics discussed in the panel, and slipped as he spoke from an individual panelist to the general audience.

Puckrein's tone was belligerent from the outset, and he performed a crescendo with both his words and body language directed against a "you" that seemed to include everyone in the room. He said that coming from his position "down with the people," he was having a hard time containing his outrage that we were "up here" at MIT debating these issues. He said that we should be ashamed of indulging in academic conversation when people are dying. Insurance companies were refusing to cover BiDil, and they cited our academic debate as a justification. Thus, he declared, we were responsible for killing people. Pointing out that his mother had died of heart failure, and that of the 750,000 African Americans with heart failure only a few percent were getting the potentially life-saving drug, he said it was unethical to deny access to this drug, and demanded to know: "Do you want people to live or die?"

Puckrein went on for minutes, and it was only with great difficulty that I cut him off to attend to other comments and questions. Even as other audience members and panelists joined in on the debate, Puckrein maintained a good share of the floor with an expertly performative denunciation.

I closed the session with a plea for common ground. I said that everyone in the room was concerned about health disparities and dedicated to ameliorating them, and that it was important to realize that BiDil is not the only drug to which African Americans are being denied access. In fact, lack of access to antihypertensives is part of what leads to heart failure, and thus a need for BiDil. So I suggested that we could best proceed from that starting point: our shared commitment to reducing health disparities.

On reflection, this was just part of Puckrein's common ground with us "up at MIT." In addition to sharing concern about health disparities, Puckrein shared other things with the majority of those in the room, including indirect engagement with medical practice, noninnocence, and a desire to separate arguments about the approval of BiDil from arguments about its distribution.

First, Puckrein's engagement in medical practice and advocacy, like ours, was primarily indirect. Contrary to the impression he gave of being a medical practitioner, his title "doctor" was not that of a doctor of medicine; he has a Ph.D. in history from Brown University,[2] and has published a book about Barbados under British rule.[3] That training could well have led him on a path to a career in the academic study of the history of race, and so the kind of conference we were having "up at MIT" was not nearly as alien to his experience as he would have us think. At the same time, since he had left academia and shifted his life work to activism, he did forge a distinct position. His engagement with medical advocacy and practice was not quite the same as academic engagement, but neither was it the same as that of a doctor or a patient. It, too, was indirect.

Second, Puckrein's position, like ours, was not disinterested. It was noninnocent. His alliance was not only "down with the people," but also "up" with the pharmaceutical company behind BiDil: according to the *Wall Street Journal*, he was a shareholder in NitroMed and his nonprofit organization also received grants from it.[4] This makes his "interest" in the market for BiDil far more literal than that of the academic analysts. But conventional academic frameworks provide their own kind of "interest." The disinterestedness of academic analysis in any narrow economic sense can mask the incentives to reproduce conventional disciplinary frameworks in the building of academic careers. For neither Puckrein nor academics is an alliance with "the people" simple or complete.

Third, like BiDil's critics, Puckrein wanted to separate arguments about BiDil's approval from those about its distribution. Although he claimed that academics opposed the provision of BiDil to patients in need, to a person everyone had supported the distribution of the chemical compound to blacks with heart failure (among others), even if there was some disagreement about peripheral questions such as the appropriateness of prescribing generic equivalents.

Puckrein's framing of the antagonism between those "down with the people" and those "up in the academy" was one that would resonate throughout the rest of the conference. Attending to Puckrein's own plural interests behind his stance does not discredit his intervention. Innocent engagement with race is not possible, and race is a topic about which neither academics nor activists should ever feel comfortable. Puckrein's intervention was an important reminder to consider not only the residue of a horrific history and the specter of an unacceptable future, but also the unbearable present. The kernel of truth in what he said was that social justice as such was not on the table in the academic discussion, and it should be.

Moreover, Puckrein was by no means alone in refusing to acknowledge all of his own stakes or to engage with what is at stake for his interlocutors, or in his preference for denunciation over engagement. Most of BiDil's advocates, including Puckrein, were quick to disavow race as a genetic category. Yet academic critique of BiDil has focused heavily on genetic reification of race. That fits BiDil into the main framework of scholarship about race and medicine in the humanities and social sciences, but is not quite engagement.

One way to frame what was at stake in this impasse over race and biomedicine is in terms of *medicating race*: what aspect of medicating race is the most important subject of discussion. Medicine can best be understood as a heterogeneous field that is both a science and a practice—one that does not merely reify difference but also seeks to act on it in plural ways. Medicine *both* represents *and* intervenes on racialized bodies. A central theme of this book involves tracking the ways that diverse medicating processes are implicated in two aspects of mediating race: mediating in the sense of arbitrating, and mediating in the sense of intervening. Whether the arbitration or the intervention is primary is one source of the disconnect between Puckrein and many of BiDil's critics. Whereas the preponderance of academic interest has been in how BiDil mediates race in the sense of arbitrating, Puckrein's call was for attention to the role BiDil could have in mediating race in the sense of intervening.

At the same time, this particular argument points to something else that exceeds BiDil's role in supporting pernicious racial profiling in medicine or in extending the lives of people with heart failure. For everyone in this tense conversation, BiDil provided opportunities to *meditate upon* race. When we argued about how to medicate race, one thing that we were doing was meditating upon race, articulating emergent theories of a differentiated world through languages of medical terminology and data.

Putting the meditations about BiDil's implications for race in medicine into the context of the intersection of race, heart disease, and pharmaceuticals over the past century allows us to see the ways that it is neither a mere repetition of older racial discourses nor a brand new one. This contextualization illuminates both BiDil's appeal to many parties as a site in which to express diverging articulations of race, as well as its unpalatabilities in the continuing volatility of debates about the drug.

Connecting This Impasse with Those of the Past Century

In this vignette, we can see connections with and reverberations of the debates about race and medicine of the past century. At the time of the conference, the name of Puckrein's organization was the National Minority Health Month Foundation.[5] This is an evocative name, which explicitly invokes the lineage of Booker T. Washington's "National Negro Health Week," and thus provides an opportunity to return to questions raised in the era of early cardiology. The National Negro Health Week was founded by Booker T. Washington in 1915, remained important as the Public Health Service took it on in the 1930s, and continued until 1951. It was with Washington's movement's historical precedent in mind that Puckrein's organization framed its goals and means. Like the earlier movement, the National Minority Health Month Foundation sought uplift through black mass mobilization supported by black health professionals and business leaders, as well as the federal government and the philanthropy of major corporations. Thus a minority health month is not quite new, it is also renewed.

Puckrein's approach is also vulnerable to critiques like those leveled at the National Negro Health Week. For example, we should remember that the NAACP physician Louis T. Wright admonished in the 1930s that black health is not a separate problem needing separate solutions but an American problem that should be solved through integration. Whether attention to African American health as a segregated enterprise is inevitably flawed remains an open question. At the same time, then, as now, absolutism in holding out for integration garnered justifiable critique as elitist, because it disregarded the immediate needs of suffering black patients. It also undercut work done by black physicians striving to bring their practices and patient populations into modern medicine on their own terms.

This exchange also reopens questions about representation and extrapolation in the Framingham and Jackson heart studies. Debates about whether research conducted in one racial group are applicable "beyond" them are not new. Tensions between representation and extrapolation remain open problems in the application of medical science. Though the earliest reports of the Framingham Study suggested that its results could be extrapolated only as far as "the white race," over time the Framingham findings have been used to account for both white stories and universal ones. It is still not clear whether research conducted on black patients can, as the Jackson Heart Study investigators hope, tell both black stories and universal ones. At stake in BiDil, as in this book as a whole, is both whether studies by black doctors in black patients can provide knowledge that has the capacity to be as mobile and extrapolatable as studies done by white doctors in white patients, and whether the work of black doctors and the health of black patients matter for their own reasons independent of that extrapolation process. One audience member who objected to Puckrein's insinuation that idle academic fretting had prevented BiDil from being available to patients in need said that, on the contrary, one harm of BiDil's race-specific approval was that it was not indicated widely enough: since it was indicated only for "self-identified black patients," it would not be made available to as many people as it should be. This line of argument is troubling because preoccupation with what BiDil means for white people turns again away from the needs of suffering black patients.

Like the black health advocates mobilized around African American hypertension as a disease category, Puckrein both supports scientific medicine's continuing investigation into racialized difference, and argues to close the debate so that treatment known to work can be given. He wants black heart failure to be durable enough to command intervention. He blames etiological ambiguity for its failure to do so. Yet we can tell from the etiological ambiguity that underlies African American hypertension that debate over the nature of race does not preclude but rather bolsters the durability of that disease category. Diverse actors accommodate considerable epistemological eclecticism underlying what is recorded as status as African American. That recorded status is then employed to tell stories about difference and make demands for medical intervention and social change. Thus, explanations for BiDil's commercial failure cannot rest on the ambiguity provoked by our academic debates.

Puckrein's intervention at the conference was an example of performative identity practices and citizenship claims around a drug, practices and claims that exceed the literal in ways that resonate with the discussion of thiazide diuretics. As illustrated in the performative intervention by Henry Louis Gates Jr. with regard to the generic drug hydrochlorothiazide, drugs' relationships to preoccupations with difference both include and exceed their role in narrow economic interests or medical data, and we should preserve some conceptual space between being *bought off* by pharmaceutical companies and *buying in* to pharmaceutical grammars. Looking at debates over BiDil in light of those over thiazide diuretics shows that there is not just one way that pharmaceuticals can articulate participation in racialized American ways of life, but rather plural ways. When Puckrein objected to the prescription of generic equivalents, he was quibbling not only about bioequivalence but also about the scope of African American participation in consumer capitalism.

This exchange also opens up an opportunity to return to larger ideas around BiDil, especially the ineffectiveness of attempts to separate BiDil's beneficence from its dangers. Puckrein was as unsuccessful as BiDil's critics were in closing down the irredeemable polyvalence of a "black drug," but he was wrong that academic meddling alone sowed doubt about this drug or impeded its rush to its markets. Using BiDil to track plural noninnocent discourses about race and medicine is an endeavor that is more productive than attempts to decry racist villains. Discourses of BiDil are racial discourses not because they support particular political or commercial interests, but rather because it is impossible to talk about BiDil without talking about race. We should not try to use this drug to put the material-semiotic category of race to one side (material) or the other (semiotic), but rather to engage with race as material-semiotic in both academic and social justice spheres.

Resisting Quandary Ethics

Puckrein's rhetorical intervention centered on the question "Do you want people to live or to die?" This framework can be read as an attempt to force the question of BiDil into a mode of ethical inquiry that the philosopher Kwame Anthony Appiah has pointed out has become extremely popular in moral philosophy: "quandary ethics."[6] Appiah's critique of quandary ethics is very useful for opening up questions of ethics and technology. Sherry Turkle has invoked Appiah's interrogation of this topic in order to reframe questions about contemporary information technology beyond yes-or-no questions.[7] As she points out, the conversation should not be about whether or not to live with technology, but *how* to live in our technology-infused world. This is also an urgent question for medical technology.

Quandary ethics has become the dominant way of asking ethical questions about medicine, especially in the field of bioethics. Why is it so appealing to put BiDil into a binary question of whether to accept or reject the technology, and why is this ultimately unsatisfying? I will explore this issue in order to highlight in relief the value of this book's mode of inquiry. A wide-ranging historically and socially engaged account has much to offer to both scholars and publics who want to engage with ethical questions in medicine more broadly conceived.

Appiah draws on Edmund Pincoffs to define quandary ethics: "Quandary ethics, as the name suggests, took the central problem of moral life to be the resolution of quandaries about what to do. One of its favorite methods was to examine stylized scenarios, like the trolley problem, and figure out what we should do and why."[8] Questions such as: if a train is speeding along a path where it will hit and kill five people, and you are positioned by a switch that allows you to divert the train and hit only one person, wouldn't you do it?[9] If a train is rushing along a path where it will hit five people, and you are standing on a bridge next to a fat man, would you push him in front of the train to prevent the train from killing five people? These kinds of questions posit ethical decision making as a moral emergency.

According to Appiah, moral emergencies operate on a few key assumptions: limited time, clear choices, high stakes, and optimum placement.[10] The train is moving quickly, the choices will definitely lead to the survival of some and death of other(s), and the ethical thinker is the one making the decision. Like many academics in this area, I want to have a less binary conversation than whether or not to push the fat man on the train tracks to save the five people, a less constrained case where more is up for grabs. Yet Puckrein's intervention is an opportunity to consider: is BiDil a good fit for this kind of moral emergency?

"Limited time" is an aspect of moral emergencies that is relevant for the problem of African American heart failure. "Clear choices" are not quite: the choices are less clear than Puckrein would have them—the pills delay death, they don't prevent it, and by the time someone is taking BiDil they are taking an extensive drug regimen and are quite sick. BiDil decisions do qualify as "high stakes"—life or death—but not in a simple way: BiDil's benefit is statistical and probabilistic rather than binary and sure (BiDil is not penicillin). "Optimum placement" is perhaps the component of moral emergencies that applies the least. Academic analysts are not the ones standing by the trolley tracks deciding whether race-based therapy is a moral good. Although it is true that those who seek to deny insurance coverage might cite us, we are really not making the decision.

One element in Puckrein's intervention that is distinct from traditional quandary ethics is that the decontextualization was not quite complete. We were told about the death of a specific African American from heart failure—Puckrein's own mother—before we were told about 750,000 people, who were in turn racially marked rather than completely abstract. But then Puckrein's frame retreats from context. There was a striking decontextualization involved in Puckrein's climactic question "Do you want people to live or to die?" We were not talking about pure abstractions here. The patients being denied BiDil —the people that Puckrein wanted to put onto quandary ethics' trolley track, whose fate would be decided by whether we intervened—were incompletely decontextualized.

However, the other key decontextualizing aspect of quandary ethics—the decontextualization of the decision maker—remained in full force. Puckrein's intervention sought to force us to have the ethical argument over BiDil not as ourselves in our ongoing disciplinary conversations with our conventional and individual preoccupations and commitments, but as abstract agents with the power to decide whether BiDil should be prescribed. Collapsing the distance between our public conversation and that within insurance companies' interior spaces, Puckrein wanted to argue against us as if we were the ones making the insurance companies' decisions. Like the person to whom a trolley problem is posed, this puts us in the role of umpire. Appiah argues that quandary ethics often starts with the mistaken picture that he calls the "umpire fantasy," that denies that we are involved in making rules as well as following rules, and imagines that we are outside of the game.[11] Puckrein was frustrated that no one wanted the role of umpire in those terms.

Puckrein framed his quandary—"Do you want people to live or to die?"—in a very loaded way, invoking his dead mother and hundreds of thousands of inadequately treated African Americans with heart failure before boiling it down to a yes-or-no question. This exemplifies what Appiah calls the "package problem": "In the real world, situations are not bundled together with options. In the real world, the act of framing—the act of describing a situation, and thus determining that there's a decision to be made—is itself a moral task. It's often *the* moral task."[12] If Puckrein's packaging is not optimal, how *should* we package BiDil? Abstractions about the dangers of genetic reification and lamentations about the preference for medical treatment over social justice in a neoliberal era cannot compete with the large-scale embodied suffering that Puckrein's packaging evokes. Any alternative packaging of BiDil should be at least as concrete as his packaging, and so it must provide a fuller account of the terrain of medical treatment and embodied suffering. The historical and contemporary context of injustice and political struggle need to be not just invoked, but fleshed out.

Calling attention to the baseline situation that we take for granted is a key element of quandary ethics that Puckrein's intervention helps us to pay attention to. One thing that quandary ethics can highlight is the fraught nature of the principle of dual effect. While this principle holds that allowing someone to die and killing someone are morally distinct, Puckrein tries to blur that in his effort to make the only BiDil question on the table one of how to provide it as widely as possible. Puckrein wants us to accept those with heart failure who are not receiving BiDil as our moral responsibility.

As Appiah points out, moral intuition tends to be risk-averse, and so taking action to prevent the loss of a present situation seems less significant than taking action to take a risk for a gain.[13] When presented the baseline of five people on the track, most people respond with willingness to take switch-flipping action to prevent their loss (even though another will die in the process). When the baseline is expanded to include the fat man on the bridge, most people are not willing to kill him (even though it might result in a net gain). Puckrein wants to shift us from seeing BiDil as a risk for a gain, to a loss-of-life prevention measure. He wants us to see that losing nothing is not one of the options available here: people are dying every day, and that has moral import, too.

As Paul Farmer has pointed out, posing ethical questions as quandaries dominates discussions of medical ethics, especially the decision whether to pull the plug on life support. In contrast, the everyday passively caused deaths of masses of poor people through denial of care are considered almost beyond the scope of medical ethics. Farmer writes:

> In the face of unprecedented bounty and untold penury, where are the prophetic voices in medicine? Instead of forthright demands for access to care, we have foggy-minded critiques of technology. Take a look at "medical ethics," a staple of medical school curricula. What is defined, these days, as an ethical issue? End-of-life decisions, medicolegal questions of brain death and organ transplantation, and medical disclosure issues dominate the published literature. In the hospital, the quandary ethics of the individual constitute most of the discussion of medical ethics. The question "When is a life worth preserving?" is asked largely of lives one click of the switch away from extinction, lives wholly at the mercy of the technology that works to preserve some. The countless people whose life course is shortened by unequal access to health care are not topics of discussion.[14]

It is hard for questions of broad-based access to medicine to gain traction in this framework, but Puckrein makes a provocative gesture in that direction. Puckrein's maneuver tries to move the question of BiDil into a quandary-type, bioethics-type model. As compelling as this move is, it also points toward a fallacy at the center: heart failure remains an end-of-life issue, and BiDil is not a cure. The package is compelling, but almost completely empty. By staking so much on access to one pill rather than social justice or access to care more broadly, it does not broaden the frame enough.

But vague reference to social justice will not solve the problem here. Of course, simply answering Puckrein's question in narrow terms is not sufficient: as we saw, that was ineffective in this instance. That is, insistence by academic critics of BiDil that the drug should be widely available did nothing to quell the accusation that dwelling on epistemological shortcomings was a diversion from addressing the needs of "the people." The way forward is to take much more seriously what it would look like to put the ethics at stake here into a broader frame. That would require taking heart failure seriously, bringing it in to the frame of analysis of BiDil, so that we do not cede the high-stakes life-or-death questions to simplistic ethical puzzles.

But I think that we have gotten stuck in this model because of the way that we have engaged with BiDil, jumping onto it like a hot-button issue rather than putting it into its concrete contexts. It becomes logical to address our conversation in terms of traditional bioethics when we are acting like the ethicists who sweep in and tell the world what to do about an ethical problem, rather than engage with broader questions of what it is to live a good life or construct a just society. As Appiah argues, "In the quandary paradigm that has come to shape 'applied ethics,' moral discourse has effectively been relegated to instances of conflict, to 'problems.' A problem arises (what shall we do with the frozen embryos? shall euthanasia be authorized?) and ethicists spring into action. Here, morality has been reduced to something like a clinical intervention: a moral dispensary for the afflicted."[15] This approach may be appropriate terrain for traditional bioethicists, but it is not sufficient for those of us who strive to be engaged in broader questions of the social and cultural context of medicine and inequality. The historical context of sensational abuses, such as the diagnosis of "drapetomania" or the Tuskegee Syphilis Study, is not enough. We need to put BiDil into the context of normal medicine, past and present. If critics of race in medicine let decrying the alarming racial reification of the day sets our agenda—whether debunking BiDil, or the slavery hypothesis for hypertension, or whatever else might be on the pages of the New York Times Magazine or abuzz in the blogosphere at that moment—we should not be surprised to be drawn into a trap of quandary ethics, called upon to answer questions in these narrow terms.

Toward Ethical Noninnocence

In this book, my goal has been not to settle race and heart disease generally or BiDil in particular, but rather to open up these emergent processes for analysis. A consequence of this process of opening and unsettling, I hope, is that the productivity of race in medicine emerges as more difficult to come to terms with after reading the book than before doing so. Attempts to settle both drugs and disease categories and their intersections with race are productive of new ambiguities.

My mode of critique is not to render a verdict, but to engage in a process that could be characterized as one of ethical noninnocence, that acknowledges the impossibility of innocent engagement without abdicating the imperative to strive to work toward justice. In embracing noninnocence, I am inspired by Donna Haraway, who points out that it was because the United States decided that teaching American girls science would bolster its militaristic interests that she was able to receive the training that would foster her radical critique.[16] In her own biographical case, the military industrial complex did not get what it sought. Similarly, as Cathy Griggers points out, the same reproductive technologies that generally serve to reinforce the repressive maternal economy of straight reproduction also allow a lesbian to bear her partner's genetic child.[17] Although the goals of racialized biocapitalism do infuse processes of medicating race, that biocapitalism does not always get what it wants.

Articulating the noninnocence of the plural discourses of race and pharmaceuticals is not the end of the inquiry, but a condition of continuing engagement. Haraway's argument to move beyond deconstructing oppressive knowledge claims to participate in creating more faithful accounts of the world is relevant not only to questions of epistemology in science, but also to medicating race: "So, I think my problem, and 'our' problem, is how to have *simultaneously* an account of radical historical contingency for all knowledge claims and knowing subjects . . . *and* a no-nonsense commitment to faithful accounts of a 'real' world, one that can be partially shared and that is friendly to earthwide projects of finite freedom, adequate material abundance, modest meaning in suffering, and limited happiness."[18] Pointing out that any given present or future injustice in medicine emerges from a historical context of racial oppression or serves the interests of those in power is only one component of critique. Paying attention to the partial and contingent, noninnocent sites of resistance is also vital to avoiding the error of decontextualization. So is leaving space open for surprise.

With Haraway, my goal has been not to reject one side of the boundary between the technical and the political, between the social and the biological, but to put those boundaries into permanent question.[19] Attending to this with regard to race opens up a possibility that is analogous to Sandra Harding's call to get "beyond spontaneous feminist empiricism" (which simply takes the standards of scientific rigor for granted and then measures a claim against those).[20] Harding urges feminist science studies to move toward a successor science that considers perspectives from those with diverse interested stakes, not only to criticize the science but also to make it better—more answerable to both truth and justice. In this book, I hope to have situated my argument in a place "beyond antiracist empiricism," even if making science better is less central to my stakes. As Evelynn Hammonds and Rebecca Herzig have argued, moving beyond sorting good racial science from bad is part of "resisting visions of salvation as well as damnation."[21]

Interventionist medicine, too, must be held answerable to questions of truth and justice, both for its practitioners and for its publics. Yet we need to remember that answerability is not the same as an answer. This is the most insidious problem of puzzle-oriented philosophizing like quandary ethics: that a definitive answer is the goal. If an analysis of race and medicine ever leaves a settled feeling, in which it is possible to feel comfortable that an unjust racial discourse has been taken down and a just racial discourse characterized, that is a symptom that the critique has strayed from engagement. Any particular racial discourse that seems to crumble in the hands of a sharp critique could not possibly be fundamental to racial discourse itself, because as we have seen, racial discourse is extraordinarily resilient. Contents shift, but durable preoccupation endures, and engagement with that preoccupation should remain uncomfortable for as long as injustice remains.

This project of ethical noninnocence might be allied with that of the prophetic pragmatism theorized by Cornel West, that "promotes the possibility of human progress" even as it acknowledges the "impossibility of human paradise."[22] Analysis of race and medicine is not a project that can perfect the world. There is no place of engagement that is above the fray, but abstention is not the solution. If there is hope for progress in both the social justice and academic debates about race and medicine, it comes from the recognition of the inevitability of injustice combined with the commitment to engage in the pursuit of justice.

Race in Medicine as Hydra

Invoking the hydra is a common way of describing the tenacity of race in science. If we take the cliché seriously, we have an opportunity to rethink strategy. For example, one conventional invocation of the hydra appears in a 2006 issue of the magazine of the nonprofit GeneWatch, a critique of genetic determinism with the title "The Hydra and Its Many Heads."[23] After noting that genetic arguments keep reappearing after being vanquished, the counter-argument provided merely recites the history of the dangers of genetic determinism. BiDil has garnered many responses along these lines as well. The alarm around BiDil has often configured the drug as a specter of genetic re-ification of race, and the response has been to slash at it as if with a sword.

I want to suggest that we should take the myth of the hydra more seriously. We might imagine race in medicine as a multiheaded hydra. Several of the heads might be specters of the etiology of racial disparities—genetics, socio-economic status, stress, culture. Other heads might be manifestations of racial profiling in medical research, racialized pharmaceuticals among them. These are each resilient components that are both hard to impede individually and independent enough to take over if another component is temporarily weakened. In Greek mythology, the hydra was a many-headed creature that was difficult to kill because the heads had the capacity to regrow if severed. Heracles and his nephew were able to kill the hydra only after they went beyond merely cutting off individual heads and used fire to cauterize each of the wounds to prevent regeneration. (The last head of the hydra was immortal, but, after a bludgeoning, Heracles buried it under a rock where it was no longer a threat.)

There is no technology for cauterizing the hydra heads of race in medicine. Without that capacity, when arguments are leveled at any individual head, that head can be battered or removed momentarily but not destroyed, and the others remain unfettered. When critics keep antiracist focus so resolutely on genetics, they refuse both to grapple with the constant regeneration of race and genetics and to acknowledge the larger beast behind that particular head. Continually holding up the severed head of race and genetics, they seem uncomprehending when others are not convinced that the monster of race and medicine is dead. Relatedly, there is no satisfaction in the commercial failure of BiDil. Holding up that severed head is uncommon precisely because it is even less convincing as a victory for the fight against racism in medicine.

The assault on any hydra is a difficult venture, and in the case of race and medicine it is not necessarily the right fight. Attempts to kill race in medicine have left it with undead uncanny power. As the sociologist Troy Duster has compellingly argued, attempting to implement a "radical surgical removal" of race from science is not the best alternative to uncritically accepting old taxonomies—excision ignores the "reciprocal interplay of biological outcomes that makes it impossible to disentangle the biological from the social."[24] Critique of race in medicine can better proceed by engaging with the hydra for as long as it remains vital. If it dies, it will die not from the force of argument against its individual heads, but from a shift in the preoccupations of race in society.

Weakening of the generativity of race in medicine can only follow its irrelevance to our preoccupations. We saw in the case of intra-white difference in Framingham that the concept did not die because of data or logical argument but because it became a less salient way for Americans to talk about racial difference. Interest in such distinctions as Italian versus non-Italian withered away rather than dying in an assault. Vestiges of such distinctions (perhaps an analogue to the hydra's immortal head buried under a rock) remain in old books and old data but have lost their power to inspire or terrorize. As long as black-white difference remains a preoccupation in America, there will not be a fire or ice capable of cauterizing discourses of race and medicine, to once and for all stop the productivity of connections between race and culture, race and genetics, and the others. Even if there were, cauterizing is a technology with plural implications: cauterizing might prevent regeneration of the monster's head, but it would also deaden feeling in the discourse of race and medicine. Cauterizing an open wound is not an appropriate tool for those who want to remain morally engaged.

Consideration of the hydra can be an opportunity to consider an ethical praxis. I want to suggest that the affective experience of debunking biological race is precisely as seductive as it is diverting. Forever severing the head of race and genetics gives critical scholars of race and medicine something to hold up as a mantle of the battle being waged, but it is not plausibly a victory in that battle. I argue that if we ever leave an argument about race and medicine with a feeling of satisfaction, that is a symptom of error. I hope that the reader of this book is uncomfortable, both with the story told and about the stakes going forward.

Generative Dissonance

One resource for a better alternative approach to analysis of BiDil—or any other problem in race and medicine that emerges down the line—is to pay attention to generative dissonance. It is striking that so many academic critics of BiDil have focused their critique so heavily on the writings of the right-wing blowhard Sally Satel, who writes egregious things about a wide range of topics in medicine, rather than on those who were more centrally involved in BiDil's creation and promotion. I suspect that part of the appeal of focusing on Satel is that there is no need to grapple with generative dissonance. Leaving aside any question of whether Puckrein himself has reflected deeply on the competing priorities of scientific truth and service to patients, certainly many of those he allied himself with in the Association of Black Cardiologists were well aware of the competition among goals. Whereas many of my fellow academics talked about medical researchers in the area of race and medicine as if they were unreflective about the tensions within medical work on health disparities, I found many of the researchers to be well aware of the dissonance produced by a recognition that disparities are principally caused by structural inequalities but that medical practice strives to modify individual bodies.

Indeed, as the economic sociologist David Stark has found with regard to those working in diverse entrepreneurial fields, for physicians committed to social justice having "multiple evaluative processes in play" can "foster a generative friction."[25] As in Stark's case, for medical practitioners working in the area of disparities research, "dissonance" among regimes of valuation can be uncomfortable, but this is not seen as something to be avoided at all costs. In the case of medicating race, conflicts among career goals, clinical goals, and social goals can be resources for reflective engagement rather than causes of paralysis. Far from needing an outsider like me to point out what is obscured by the clinical gaze, many of the leading researchers are epistemologically sophisticated and deeply politically engaged. For many, medical research is a component of rather than a substitute for commitment to much broader social change.

At the same time, we should heed generative dissonance in our own work as well. We should feel uncomfortable when we as academics involved in questions of race and justice find ourselves on a different side of an issue from major civil rights organizations. We should not assume that they are right, or innocent, but we should take their points of view seriously.

Foregrounding heart disease as a specific site of racialized medicine led me to take a different starting point from those that have become conventional in the field of science and technology studies of race and biomedicine. Rather than starting from the UNESCO Statement on Race or the Human Genome Project, I started from the professionalization of cardiology as a field. Indeed, I think that the routine rehearsing of the Human Genome Project before analysis of any specific topic in race and medicine leads us astray. This is especially true for analysis of pharmaceuticals, since vanishingly few drugs have emerged from the Human Genome Project. The historical and material origins of BiDil are not in genetic research, but in clinical trial research, and that distinction matters. Starting from the field of heart disease rather than genetics, I found myself particularly intrigued by the ways that African American physicians' arguments for their own inclusion at the table of modern scientific medicine—whether in research hospitals in the early twentieth century, in risk factor research after the Second World War, or in clinical trial design and participation in the early twenty-first century—often enroll arguments for the need to include black patients. I do not presume that this is a cynical move. On the contrary, attending to the competing and complementary professional and social justice goals of physicians dedicated to the treatment of African American patients provides a rich window into the field for anyone who wants to take both scientific claims and social justice arguments seriously. The productivity of medicating race, then, has a reach that exceeds the medical practitioners. Attending to their meditations, mediations, and diverse medication practices is a rich site for race and medicine critique.

If a new claim about race and medicine emerges, we should be suspicious if it falls too easily into a framework of critique that we already have at hand. The disease category "heart failure in self-identified black patients" is not the same as that of African American hypertension or of syphilitic heart disease, and even as my account has highlighted continuities, it has been necessary to draw on distinctive analytical frameworks to account for each in turn. Reading an account of medicating race and heart disease across time and category hopefully provides insight that is not only discretely applicable to its particular category, but speaks to larger processes of medicating race. Thus, even though none of these disease categories can be mapped neatly onto other racialized disease categories such as sickle cell anemia, schizophrenia, or drapetomania, attention to heart disease hopefully provides a richer reading of other diseases that become enrolled in preoccupations with racial difference, past or future. Each time that we grapple with race and a disease category or pharmaceutical we should seek to explore the generative dissonance provoked by seeing ways in which race is simultaneously new and renewed, a site of medical intervention and political contestation that is fascinating to track.

NOTES

Introduction

1 Berg and Mol, *Differences in Medicine*, 3; see also Löwy, *Between Bench and Bedside*.

2 Hacking, *Representing and Intervening*.

3 Nathan Greenslit has rendered the immanence of *medication for* and *mediation of* mental illness as "medi(c)ating illness." Greenslit and Dumit, *Medi(c)ating Illness*.

4 Callon, "Some Elements of a Sociology of Translation."

5 Jasanoff, *States of Knowledge*, 18.

6 Most archetypally, Illich, *Medical Nemesis*; see also Zola, "Medicine as an Institution of Social Control"; Conrad, "Medicalization and Social Control."

7 See, for example, Kleinman, *What Really Matters*, 9–10.

8 Clarke et al., "Biomedicalization," 172.

9 Skinner, "Groundhog Day?," 939.

10 Williams, *Eliminating Healthcare Disparities in America*, 46.

11 Nelson, *Body and Soul*, 44.

12 Omi and Winant, *Racial Formation in the United States*, 56 (emphasis in original).

13 Stoler, "Racial Histories and Their Regimes of Truth"; see also Stoler, *Race and the Education of Desire*.

14 Petryna, *Life Exposed*, 6.

15 Rose and Novas, "Biological Citizenship"; Rose, *The Politics of Life Itself*, 178.

16 Roberts, "Race and the New Biocitizen."

17 Stefan Timmermans, "Suffering and Hope: A Warrant for STS," paper presented at the Presidential Plenary, Society for the Social Studies of Science, Vancouver, B.C., November 4, 2006.

18 Archives that I visited included the National Library of Medicine, the Framingham Heart Study, the Jackson Heart Study, and the National Heart, Lung and Blood Institute.

19 I attended the ISHIB meetings in Detroit (2004), San Juan, Puerto Rico (2005), Atlanta (2006), New Orleans (2008), and Chicago (2009). I also attended related conferences with overlapping characters: an Association of Black Cardiologists symposium in New York (2005); the annual meeting of the American Society for Hypertension in San Francisco (2005), which hosted a special full-day symposium cosponsored by the ISHIB on African American hypertension; the Amer-

ican Heart Association Scientific Sessions in Dallas (2005); and a National Medical Association meeting in Atlanta (2008).

20 Anderson, "Teaching 'Race' in Medical School," 788.

21 Jasanoff, *States of Knowledge*, 276.

22 The 2006 conference "Race, Pharmaceuticals and Medical Technology" and the 2007 conference "Business of Race and Science." I also attended the final conference in the series, the 2008 "What's the Use of Race?"

23 Stoler, "Racial Histories and Their Regimes of Truth," 187.

24 Ernst and Harris, *Race, Science and Medicine*, 7.

25 Fields, "Ideology and Race in American History," 150 (first quotation) and 144 (second quotation).

26 Hammonds and Herzig, *The Nature of Difference*, xiii.

27 Metzl, *The Protest Psychosis*, xxi.

28 Wailoo, *How Cancer Crossed the Color Line*, 181.

29 Roberts, *Fatal Invention*; see especially 81–82. See also Kahn, for example, "From Disparity to Difference," 125.

30 Hacking, "The Self-Vindication of the Laboratory Sciences," 42–43; Latour and Callon, "Unscrewing the Big Leviathan"; Latour, *Science in Action*

31 Latour, "Opening Pandora's Black Box," 1–17. See especially 14.

32 Michael Hardt, "What Affects Are Good For," in Clough and Halley, *The Affective Turn*, ix.

33 Patricia Ticineto Clough, "Introduction," in Clough and Halley, *The Affective Turn*, 2; See also Massumi, *Parables for the Virtual*.

34 Pollock, "Reading Friedan."

35 Lerner, *The Breast Cancer Wars*; Hartman, "Reading the Scar in Breast Cancer Poetry."

36 Lorde, *The Cancer Journals*.

37 Klawiter, *The Biopolitics of Breast Cancer*.

38 Weiner, "Exploring Genetic Responsibility."

39 Epstein, *Inclusion*.

40 Jones, *Rationalizing Epidemics*, 3.

41 MacKinnon, "Difference and Dominance."

42 Aronowitz, *Making Sense of Illness*; Jones, "Visions of a Cure"; Mol, *The Body Multiple*; Timmermans, "Making the Case for Heart Disease"; Weiner and Martin, "A Genetic Future for Coronary Heart Disease?"

43 Bridges, *Reproducing Race*; Roberts, *Killing the Black Body*; Williams, "Spare Parts."

44 On genetics, see Rapp, "Cell Life and Death"; Wailoo and Pemberton, *The Troubled Dream of Genetic Medicine*; Parthasarathy, *Building Genetic Medicine*. On neuroscience, see Dumit, *Picturing Personhood*; Littlefield, "Constructing the Organ of Deceit"; Vrecko, "Birth of a Brain Disease"; Wilson, *Psychosomatic*.

45 On gender, see Birke "The Heart"; Emslie, Hunt, and Watt, "Invisible Women?";

Riska, "The Rise and Fall of Type A Man"; Riska, "From Type A Man to the Hardy Man." On race and class, see Aronowitz, *Making Sense of Illness*; Shim, "Constructing 'Race' across the Science-Lay Divide."

46 Kawachi and Conrad, "Medicalization and the Pharmacological Treatment of Blood Pressure."

47 Aronowitz, *Making Sense of Illness*, 84.

48 Ibid.

49 On atherosclerosis in Egyptian mummies, see Bing, *Cardiology*, 118. On the ancient history of heart disease, see also Acierno, *A History of Cardiology*; see especially "Earliest Concepts: Theories and Myths," 3–16; Leibowitz, *The History of Coronary Heart Disease*.

50 Michaels, *The Eighteenth-Century Origins of Angina Pectoris*.

51 Bynum, Lawrence, and Nutton, *The Emergence of Modern Cardiology*, ix.

52 Some other categories of heart disease beyond those that I consider are congenital and valvular, but these are less prominent in medical research and are outside the scope of this book.

53 Howell, "The Changing Face of Twentieth-Century American Cardiology," 780.

54 On blockbuster drugs, see Greene, *Prescribing by Numbers*. On making normality drug-dependent, see Dumit, "Drugs for Life."

55 Williams, Martin, and Gabe, "The Pharmaceuticalisation of Society?"; Conrad, "The Shifting Engines of Medicalization."

56 Weiner, "Exploring Genetic Responsibility."

57 On postgenomic biology and science and technology studies, see Fujimura, "Postgenomic Futures," and Rajan, *Biocapital*.

58 Keller, *The Century of the Gene*, 147.

59 Wailoo, *Dying in the City of the Blues*; see also Tapper, *In the Blood*.

60 Lock, "Eclipse of the Gene."

61 Reardon, *The Postgenomic Condition*.

62 Fausto-Sterling, "Refashioning Race."

63 Blackman, "Psychiatric Culture and Bodies of Resistance"; Dumit, "Is It Me or My Brain?"; Greenslit, *Pharmaceutical Relationships*; Healy, "Shaping the Intimate"; Martin, *Bipolar Expeditions*; Martin, "The Pharmaceutical Person"; Metzl, *Prozac on the Couch*; Wilson, "The Work of Antidepressants."

64 On the Pill, see Hester, "Bricolage and Bodies of Knowledge"; May, *America and the Pill*; Tone, *Devices and Desires*, especially part 3, "The Medicalization of Contraceptives," 203–92. On gendered diseases, see Fishman, "Manufacturing Desire"; Greenslit, "Dep®ession and Consum♀tion"; Taylor, *Rock-a-By Baby*; Mamo and Fishman, "Potency in All the Right Places." On HIV/AIDS, see Epstein, *Impure Science*; Race, *Pleasure Consuming Medicine*; Rosengarten, *HIV Interventions*.

65 Greene, *Prescribing by Numbers*; Rasmussen, "The Moral Economy of the Drug Company."

66 Dumit, "Drugs for Life"; Dumit, "Pharmaceutical Witnessing"; Dumit, *A Pharmaceutical Grammar*.

67 Race, *Pleasure Consuming Medicine*, 9.

68 Nelson, "Bio Science."

69 Reardon, *Race to the Finish*; Hamilton, "The Case of the Genetic Ancestor"; Tallbear, "Narratives of Race and Indigeneity."

70 On the role of forensic DNA in incarceration, see Aronson, *Genetic Witness*; Lynch, Cole, and McNally, *The Truth Machine*; on human rights, see Smith, *Subversive Genes*; Wagner, *To Know Where He Lies*.

71 Geest et al., "The Anthropology of Pharmaceuticals," 154.

72 Roberts, "Nervous and Mental Influences in Angina Pectoris."

73 For insightful attention to the ways that American healthy citizenship has been articulated in a contrast with Asian disease, see Shah, *Contagious Divides*.

74 See, for example, the NHLBI's initiative "Salud para su Corazon," described on "Latino Cardiovascular Health Resources," http://www.nhlbi.nih.gov/. Montoya, *Making the Mexican Diabetic*.

75 Brown et al., *Whitewashing Race*, xi.

76 Ibid., x.

77 Anderson, *The Cultivation of Whiteness*.

78 Lauretis, *Technologies of Gender*.

79 Foucault, *Archeology of Knowledge*.

80 Eagan, "The Invention of the White Race[s]."

81 Trask, "Guide to Punctuation."

82 Žižek, "Dialectical Clarity versus the Misty Conceit of Paradox," 297.

83 Derrida, *The Gift of Death*.

84 Haraway, *Modest_Witness*.

Chapter 1: Racial Preoccupations

1 American Society for Hypertension Annual Meeting, Scientific Sessions, "Special Symposium: Hypertension in the African American Population," San Francisco, Calif., May 14, 2005.

2 Thompson, "Population"; for discussion, see Kirk, "Demographic Transition Theory."

3 Omran, "The Epidemiologic Transition," 510.

4 Weisse, *Heart to Heart*, xxxi.

5 White, *My Life and Medicine*, 14.

6 Ibid., 20.

7 Ibid., 19.

8 Howell, "The Changing Face of Twentieth-Century American Cardiology," 773.

9 These events appear on the AHA's version of its own history, at http://www.heart

.org/HEARTORG/General/History-of-the-American-Heart-Association_UCM_ 308120_Article.jsp#.TxMJe4FWJS8. For reflections by early AHA leaders on rheumatic heart disease, see Moore, *Fighting for Life*, 5. Contemporary press coverage included attention to infectious causes as well: "Move to Combat Heart Disease," *New York Times*, November 18, 1916. The first campaign of the American Heart Association, in 1946, was against rheumatic fever.

10 Munly, "Problems in the Prevention and Relief of Heart Disease."

11 Ibid., 1101.

12 Roberts, "The Larger View of Heart Disease," 392.

13 Ibid., 394.

14 "Says Heart Disease Can Be Headed Off: Has Taken Place of Tuberculosis in Mortality: Dr. Emerson Lectures before Massachusetts Medical Society," *Boston Globe*, June 1, 1921, 6.

15 "Uses New Method in Heart Research: U. of P. Foundation Photographs Pulse Waves and Records Cardiac Disturbances: 150 Executives Studied: Many, Apparently Sound, Are Found to Have Ailments in Early Stages," *New York Times*, September 29, 1930, 17.

16 Wald, "Imagined Immunities: The Epidemiology of Belonging," in *Contagious*, 28–67; Anderson, *Imagined Communities*.

17 Gieryn, "Boundary-Work and the Demarcation of Science from Non-science."

18 Haraway, *Modest_Witness*, 222.

19 Aronowitz, "From the Patient's Angina Pectoris to the Cardiologist's Coronary Heart Disease," in *Making Sense of Illness*, 84–110.

20 Fye, *American Cardiology*, 34.

21 White, *Heart Disease*, 99.

22 Roberts, *Life and Writings of Stewart R. Roberts*.

23 Ibid.

24 "Dr. Stewart R. Roberts," *New York Times*, April 15, 1941, 23.

25 Weatherford, *Negro Life in the South*.

26 Roberts, "The Larger View of Heart Disease," 395.

27 Roberts, "Nervous and Mental Influences in Angina Pectoris," 23.

28 Ibid.

29 Ibid., 32.

30 Ibid., 30.

31 Ibid., 33.

32 Aronowitz, *Making Sense of Illness*, 100.

33 Herzberg, *Happy Pills in America*, 49–51.

34 Wailoo, *How Cancer Crossed the Color Line*.

35 Roberts, "Nervous and Mental Influences in Angina Pectoris," 34.

36 Agamben, *Homo Sacer*.

37 West, "On Prophetic Pragmatism," 165.

38 Schwab and Schulze,"Heart Disease in the American Negro of the South," 717.

39 Jones, *Rationalizing Epidemics*.

40 Aronowitz, *Making Sense of Illness*, 99.

41 McBride, From *TB* to *AIDS*.

42 See Baker, *From Savage to Negro*, especially "Progressive Era Reform: Holding On to Hierarchy," 81–98, and "Rethinking Race at the Turn of the 20th Century: W. E. B. Du Bois and Franz Boas," 99–126. On Hoffman's theory, see Roman, "Vitality of the Negroes."

43 Jones, *Rationalizing Epidemics*, 4.

44 Du Bois, *The Philadelphia Negro*, 106.

45 Birnie, "The Influence of Environment and Race on Diseases."

46 Du Bois, *The Health and Physique of the Negro American*.

47 On these three proposals, see respectively: Taylor, "Remarks on the Health of the Colored People"; *JNMA*, "On Dr. Taylor of Philadelphia," 208; and Allen, "The Negro Health Problem."

48 Woodward, "Racial Health," 177.

49 See Stocking, "The Turn-of-the-Century Concept of Race," 4–16; Holmes, "The Principal Causes of Death among Negroes."

50 Bousfield, "Reaching the Negro Community."

51 On AIDs, see Patton, "Migratory Vices"; on public health efforts, see Briggs and Mantini-Briggs, *Stories in the Time of Cholera*, 10.

52 Haraway, *Modest_Witness*, 233.

53 Terry, "The Negro."

54 For an excellent overview of this topic, with a comprehensive introduction and primary sources, see Gamble, *Germs Have No Color Line*. See also Smith, *Sick and Tired of Being Sick and Tired*.

55 Brunner, "The Negro Health Problem in Southern Cities."

56 Wailoo, "Stigma, Race, and Disease in 20th Century America."

57 Hammonds and Herzig, *The Nature of Difference*, xii.

58 Allen, "The Negro Health Problem," 194.

59 Embree, "Negro Illness and Its Effect upon the Nation's Health," 50.

60 See Brown, "The National Negro Health Week Movement."

61 Petryna, *Life Exposed*, 5.

62 Gager, "Changing Conditions in Medical Practice," 76.

63 This advertisement appeared in USA Today on January 18, 2007, and was airing in Edwards Cinemas at the same time. It also was shown during the Super Bowl, February 4, 2007.

64 Smith, *Health Care Divided*, 44–46.

65 Lawrence, "'Definite and Material'"; see also Fye, "A History of the Origin, Evolution, and Impact of Electrocardiography."

66 Fleming, *A Short History of Cardiology*, 156.

67 On the ascendency of the rational, see Acierno, *The History of Cardiology*. On change in medical practice, see Reiser, *Medicine and the Reign of Technology*.

68 Foucault, *Birth of the Clinic*.

69 Stevens, *In Sickness and in Wealth*, 12.

70 Flexner, "The Medical Education of the Negro." A point-by-point critique of Flexner's chapter can be found in Hunt, "The Flexner Report and Black Academic Medicine"; see also Savitt, "Abraham Flexner and the Black Medical Schools."

71 Smith, *Health Care Divided*, 16.

72 Gamble, *Making a Place for Ourselves*.

73 Bethea, "Some Significant Negro Movements to Lower Their Mortality," 87.

74 Wright, "Health Problems of the Negro," 6–8. See also Gamble, *Germs Have No Color Line*, and Smith, *Sick and Tired of Being Sick and Tired*.

75 Gamble, *Germs Have No Color Line*, ix.

76 "Report of the Committee on Medical Education in Colored Hospitals," 283.

77 Jackson, "Public Health and the Negro," 258.

78 Kenney, "The Negro Hospital Renaissance," 112.

79 Gamble, *Germs Have No Color Line*, ix.

80 Crenshaw, "Race, Reform, and Retrenchment."

81 Woodward, "Racial Health," 178.

82 Rothstein, *Public Health and the Risk Factor*; Postel-Vinay, *A Century of Arterial Hypertension*.

83 Jones, *Rationalizing Epidemics*.

84 Ibid., 5.

85 Lilienfeld, "Louis I. Dublin and the Development of the Observational Study."

86 Dublin, "The Health of the Negro," 79.

87 Dublin, "The Problem of Negro Health as Revealed by Vital Statistics," 271.

88 Ibid., 273.

89 Ibid., 274.

90 Ibid., 274, 270.

91 Holmes, "The Principal Causes of Death among Negroes," 295.

92 On rates of syphilis among blacks, see Hazen, *Syphilis*, 22–24; Hazen, "A Leading Cause of Death among the Negroes"; and Hindman, "Syphilis among Insane Negroes." On rates of syphilitic heart disease, see France, "Cardio-Vascular Syphilis," and Baker, "Certain Aspects of Syphilitic Cardiac Disease," 471.

93 Vonderlehr, "Untreated Syphilis in the Male Negro."

94 Stoler, *Along the Archival Grain*, 248.

95 "Dr. B. T. Washington, Negro Leader, Dead: Founder of the Tuskegee Institute Expires of Hardening of Arteries after Brief Illness: Taken to His Home to Die," *New York Times*, November 15, 1915, 1.

96 Harlan, *Booker T. Washington*, 451–53.

97 Harlan and Smock, "Introduction," xxv.

98 Wright, Brundage, and Mackowiak, "A 59-Year-Old Man with 'Racial Charac-teristics.'" The original case discussion took place at a conference sponsored by the Department of Veterans Affairs Maryland Health Care System and the Uni-versity of Maryland School of Medicine in Baltimore, Md., on May 5, 2006, and further discussion of the investigation appeared in a collection of examinations of mysterious deaths of a dozen prominent historical figures ranging from Alex-ander the Great to Edgar Allan Poe: Mackowiak, "Racial Characteristics."

99 Landecker, "Immortality, in Vitro."

100 Wright, Brundage, and Mackowiak, "A 59-Year-Old Man with 'Racial Charac-teristics,'" 128–29. Other details given in the account included the limited knowledge of his family history; lack of oedema; and lack of abnormalities of external genitalia.

101 Ibid., 132.

102 Ibid.

103 Ibid., 130.

104 Ibid.

105 Ibid., 131.

106 Ibid., 132.

107 Fields, "Ideology and Race in American History," 146.

108 Smith, "Coronary Atherosclerosis in the Negro"; Mihaly and Whiteman, "Myo-cardial Infarction in the Negro"; Peniston and Randall, "Coronary Artery Dis-ease in Black Americans."

109 Williams, *Textbook of Black-Related Diseases*, 377.

110 Byrd and Clayton, *An American Health Dilemma*, vol. 2, 537.

111 Susser, "Epidemiology in the United States after World War II," 158.

Chapter 2: Making Normal Populations

1 Herman Taylor, "The Jackson Heart Study," paper presented at the session "The Evolution of Hypertension and Cardiovascular Risk: A 20-Year Perspective," In-ternational Society for Hypertension in Blacks Annual Conference, Atlanta, Ga., June 23, 2006.

2 Ibid.

3 Ibid.

4 NHLBI, "Framingham Heart Study."

5 Marks, "You Gotta Have Heart," in *The Progress of Experiment*, 164–96.

6 Gilcin Meadors, letter to Surgeon General Bert R. Boone, July 19, 1947, Papers of the NHLBI, Bethesda, Md., Epidemiology Correspondence Folder, 1947.

7 Oppenheimer, "Profiling Risk"; Aronowitz, "The Social Construction of Coro-nary Heart Disease Risk Factors," in *Making Sense of Illness*, 111–43.

8 Canguilhem, *The Normal and the Pathological*.

9 Dumit, "Drugs for Life."

10 Moore, "Committee on Design and Analysis of Studies," S10.

11 Dawber, Moore, and Mann, "Coronary Heart Disease in the Framingham Study," 4.

12 Gilcin Meadors, "Descriptions of the H.D.E.S. 1947–1949," n.d. (undated draft), Folder, Papers of the NHLBI.

13 Dawber and Moore, "Longitudinal Study of Heart Disease in Framingham, Massachusetts"; for more on the selection of Framingham as the study site, see Gilcin Meadors to Bert Boone, letter, September 8, 1947, Epidemiology Correspondence Folder, 1947, Papers of the NHLBI.

14 Epstein, "Bodily Differences and Collective Identities."

15 Dawber, The Framingham Study, 59–60; Rothstein, Public Health and the Risk Factor, 281; Blackburn, "Oral History."

16 C. P. Gillmore, "The Real Villain in Heart Disease," New York Times Magazine, March 25, 1973, 72.

17 Levy and Brink, A Change of Heart, see especially chapter 2, "The Dawn of Peace and Prosperity—and a Deadly Lifestyle," 22–34, and chapter 4, "A Struggle for Identity," 50–66.

18 Ibid., 24.

19 Lynch, The Broken Heart, 19.

20 Ibid., 19 and 21.

21 Ibid., 50.

22 Ibid., 53.

23 Jacobson, Whiteness of a Different Color; McDermott and Samson, "White Racial and Ethnic Identity in the United States."

24 See, for example, Castelli, quoted in Levy and Brink, A Change of Heart, 210.

25 "General Statement of Plans," November 11, 1949, in the Heart Disease Epidemiology: Manuals of Operation Folder, Papers of the NHLBI.

26 Dawber, Meadors, and Moore, "Epidemiological Approaches to the Heart Disease," 282.

27 Ibid., 281.

28 Ibid.

29 Ibid. (emphasis added).

30 Dawber, The Framingham Study, 21–22.

31 Ibid., 59–60.

32 For more on the homogenizing processes that comprise whiteness out of heterogeneous bits, see Hartigan, "Establishing the Fact of Whiteness."

33 Oppenheimer, "Profiling Risk," 722.

34 Scott, Seeing Like a State.

35 "Brief Cardiovascular History for Survey Screening," PHS-1030(SR) 9–48, from the file "Coding—First Examination," at the Framingham Heart Study, Framingham, Massachusetts.

36 "Proposed detail coding of Exam I, not used. Only Card 9 (the Summary card) of this series was actually punched," from the file "Coding—First Examination," at the Framingham Heart Study.

37 On mechanical means, see Blackburn, "Oral History"; on computational means, see Dawber, Kannel, and Friedman, "The Use of Computers in Cardiovascular Epidemiology"; Kahn, "Use of Computers in Analyzing Framingham Data."

38 Agar, "What Difference Did Computers Make?," 878.

39 Oppenheimer, "Becoming the Framingham Study," 607.

40 "Code Sheet Framingham Heart Study Abstract," PHS-1583, National Heart Institute Biometrics 1-15-51. From the file "Cohort Code Sheets 1–12," Papers of the NHLBI.

41 The 1950 Census, for example, had ninety-eight categories of "Foreign Country or Outlying Area" that could be listed as place of birth, including such specifics as Ireland separate from northern Ireland, as well as (this categorization is mine) each European, Latin American, and Middle Eastern, Pacific country separately, though the whole continent of Africa was in one category. U.S. Department of Commerce Bureau of the Census, *Census of the Population, 1950 [United States]: Public Use Data Microsample,* "Appendix A3: Foreign Country and Outlying Area Codes," accessed through the Inter-University Consortium for Political and Social Research.

42 The absence of a line for race would be a source of consternation later, when the researchers were asked about the racial makeup of their samples. In 1954, Philip Person wrote to McElholm: "After talking with various members of the staff I have compiled the list of case numbers shown below which are remembered to be negroes. It is unlikely that there are more than two or three others. However we will be glad to search the full list of case numbers if it is considered necessary." He goes on to list "case numbers of known negroes," and there are handwritten notes on the paper that say "another noted 9/02/57," "another noted 3/16/60," "another noted 6/29/60 (Portuguese + Negro)." Letter from Philip Person to D. M. McElholm, August 26, 1954, from the file "Coding—First Examination" at the Framingham Heart Study.

43 "National Heart Institute Office of Biometric Research Framingham Epidemiological Study," from the file "Coding Manuals," Papers of the NHLBI.

44 According to a 1958 letter from the director of the Biometrics Research Branch of the NHLBI, 7.8 percent of the Framingham cohort was born in Italy and 20.2 percent had at least one grandparent born in Italy, compared to the white population of the whole United States, of which only 1.4 percent was born in Italy and 4.5 percent had at least one parent born in Italy. Letter from Tavia Gordon to Dr. Kagan, June 4, 1958, in "General Correspondence File: Jan 1, 1958—June 3, 1958," Papers of the NHLBI.

45 Mann et al., "Diet and Cardiovascular Disease in the Framingham Study," 224.

46 Dawber et al., "Environmental Factors in Hypertension."

47 Oppenheimer, "Becoming the Framingham Study," 605.

48 Porter, *Trust in Numbers*, 42.

49 Dawber et al., "Some Factors Associated with the Development of Coronary Heart Disease."

50 Kannel et al., "Factors of Risk in the Development of Coronary Heart Disease."

51 Paul Sorlie, personal communication, October 19, 2006.

52 "Deck 06 Coding Manual," from the *Tape Coding Manual Book 2 (of 3)*, from the Papers of the NHLBI.

53 Bowker and Star, *Sorting Things Out*.

54 Chun, *Control and Freedom*, 18.

55 Conroy, "From Epidemiological Risk to Clinical Practice by Way of Statistics," 19–20.

56 Bowker and Star, *Sorting Things Out*, 7.

57 Epstein, "Bodily Differences and Collective Identities."

58 NHLBI and Boston University, *You Changed America's Heart*, 14–15.

59 Hadden, "Holidays in Framingham?," 544.

60 Epstein, *Inclusion*.

61 NHLBI and Boston University, *You Changed America's Heart*, 14–15.

62 Allen and Turner, "Boston's Emerging Ethnic Quilt."

63 Memo from George O'Connor and Daniel Levy to All FHS Staff, June 14, 1994, from the Omni Overview Binder, Framingham, Massachusetts.

64 Email from Emelia Benjamin to Phil Wold and Raph (?), April 25, 1996. From the Omni Overview Binder.

65 Williams, "Cardiology," 381–82.

66 Ibid.

67 Daniel Levy, personal communication, October 30, 2006.

68 Francis Henderson, personal communication, November 13, 2006.

69 Taylor, "The Jackson Heart Study."

70 NHLBI, "Jackson Heart Study."

71 ARIC Investigators, "The Atherosclerosis Risk in Communities (ARIC) Study."

72 Wyatt et al., *Community-Driven Model of Recruitment*. A shorter report from this material was published as "A Community-Driven Model of Research Participation."

73 Form A-113, "Fasting/Tracking Form Instructions," from the "Cohort Component Procedures," Manual 2, Appendix 9, p. 4, at http://www.cscc.unc.edu/aric/pubuse/form/cohort/exam1/FTRA.pdf.

74 Oppenheimer, "Becoming the Framingham Study"; Levy and Brink, *Change of Heart*.

75 Paul Sorlie, personal communication, October 19, 2006.

76 Sempos, Bild, and Manolio, "Overview of the Jackson Heart Study."

77 Bill Kannel, personal communication, September 29, 2006.

78 NHLBI, "Jackson Heart Study."

79 Taylor, "Toward Resolution of Cardiovascular Health Disparities in African Americans," S6 8–9.

80 "Cardiovascular Examination Code Sheet," Federal Security Agency Public Health Service, PHS-1446-4 (NIH) 8–50. From the file "Cohort Code Sheets 1–12," with handwritten note at top stating "used for Exam I; beginning case #3375." Papers of the NHLBI.

81 Payne et al., "Sociocultural Methods in the Jackson Heart Study," S6-42.

82 Ibid., S6-44.

83 On participants' access to medical care, see William B. Kannel, letter to *British Medical Journal* 2, no. 6046 (November 20, 1976): 1255; on participants' access to their personal physicians, see Dawber, *The Framingham Study*, 86–87.

84 For an overview of the study and its implications, see Brandt, "Racism in Research"; for comprehensive analysis, see Reverby, ed., *Tuskegee's Truths*.

85 Carole Cannon, "The Un-Tuskegee Experiment," *Jackson Free Press*, March 24, 2004, at http://www.jacksonfreepress.com/.

86 Epstein, "The Rise of 'Recruitmentology' "; Wyatt et al., *Community-Driven Model of Recruitment*.

87 Taylor et al., "Toward Resolution of Cardiovascular Health Disparities in African Americans," S6-5.

88 See http://www.jacksonmedicalmall.org/.

89 See Brandt and Sloane, "Of Beds and Benches"; Sloane and Sloane, *Medicine Moves to the Mall*.

90 Millman, "Going Nativist."

91 Taylor, "The Jackson Heart Study: An Overview."

92 Paulina Drummond, "Omni Cohort of the Framingham Heart Study," from the Omni Overview Binder.

93 Wyatt et al., *Community-Driven Model of Recruitment*, 26.

94 Ibid.

95 Ibid., 26–27.

96 Ibid., 49.

97 Bhabha, *The Location of Culture*, 128.

98 Mitchell and Waldby, "National Biobanks," 337.

99 Levy and Brink, *A Change of Heart*.

100 For more on scientists of color in the United States, see Fullwiley, "The Biologistical Construction of Race"; for postcolonial scientists, see Benjamin, "A Lab of Their Own."

101 Dawber, *The Framingham Study*, 11.

102 Thomas, "In the Trenches of Framingham," 69–70.

103 Dawber, *The Framingham Study*, 16.

104 Nelkin and Tancredi, *Dangerous Diagnostics*, 9.

105 Postel-Vinay and Corvol, *Le retour du Dr Knock*.

Chapter 3: A Durable Disease Category

1 American Society for Hypertension Annual Meeting, Scientific Sessions, "Special Symposium: Hypertension in the African American Population," San Francisco, Calif., May 14, 2005.

2 Interview with Elijah Saunders, San Juan, Puerto Rico, July 18, 2005.

3 Greene, *Prescribing by Numbers*; Greenlee, *Biomedicine and Ideology*; Kawachi and Conrad, "Medicalization and the Pharmacological Treatment of Blood Pressure."

4 Byrd and Clayton, *An American Health Dilemma*, vol. 1, 329.

5 Kaufman and Hall, "The Slavery Hypertension Hypothesis," 111; quotation from Adams, "Some Racial Differences in Blood Pressure and Morbidity in Groups of White and Colored Workmen."

6 Bays and Scrimshaw, "Facts and Fallacies Regarding the Blood Pressure of Different Regional and Racial Groups"; Moser, "Epidemiology of Hypertension with Particular Reference to Racial Susceptibility."

7 Cited in Farmer, "The Incidence of Heart Disease among Negroes," 202.

8 Holloway, "Approach to Cardiac Diagnosis," 59.

9 Postel-Vinay, *A Century of Arterial Hypertension*, 31; Rothstein, *Public Health and the Risk Factor*.

10 Page, *Hypertension Research*.

11 Cited in ibid., 126.

12 Postel-Vinay, *A Century of Arterial Hypertension*, 6–7.

13 Greene, "Releasing the Flood Waters."

14 Dawber et al., "Environmental Factors in Hypertension," 256.

15 Stoler, "Racial Histories and Their Regimes of Truth," 191.

16 Abu-Jamal, *We Want Freedom*, 185; Zane and Jeffries, "A Panther Sighting in the Pacific Northwest," 84.

17 Welsing, "Blacks, Hypertension, and the Active Skin Melanocyte"; Welsing, *The Isis Papers*.

18 Harry Aubin, "Victims of High Blood Pressure in Inner City Sought by Doctor," *Washington Post*, July 19, 1971, C1.

19 Metzl, *Protest Psychosis*.

20 Wailoo, *Dying in the City of the Blues*.

21 Rosenberg, "What Is Disease?," 503.

22 "Report of the Joint National Committee on Detection, Evaluation, and Treatment of High Blood Pressure," 257.

23 Greenlee, "Discourse, Foucault, and Critical Medical Anthropology"; see also Greenlee, *Biomedicine and Ideology.*

24 Braithwaite, Taylor, and Austin, *Building Health Coalitions in the Black Community,* 69; West, "Honoring the Body."

25 Williams, *Textbook of Black Related Diseases,* 363.

26 Helen Hammer, Richard Allen Williams, and Deborah Gould, and Kaiser Audio Visual Center (Calif.), and Permanente Medical Group (Oakland, Calif.), Staff Education, *African American Health Issues,* videorecording, a coproduction of the Regional Audio Visual Center and Physician Education and Development (Oakland, Calif.: Kaiser Foundation Health Plan, ca. 1995).

27 Association of Black Cardiologists, "About Us: Our History." At http://www.ab cardio.org/history.htm.

28 DHEW, *National High Blood Pressure Education Program,* 22.

29 Ibid.

30 Ibid., 24.

31 DHEW, *Diagnosis and Management of Hypertension.* For all physicians, the full statistics are as follows: family history: 69 percent; being black: 61 percent; obesity: 54 percent; high-salt diet: 50 percent; diabetes: 39 percent; increasing age: 33 percent; environmental stress: 32 percent; nervous personality: 25 percent; high-cholesterol diet: 15 percent; lack of exercise: 9 percent; low income: 6 percent.

32 DHEW, *Diagnosis and Management of Hypertension,* 10–11. For physicians under thirty-five, the full statistics are as follows: family history: 74 percent; being black: 73 percent; obesity: 58 percent; high-salt diet: 46 percent; diabetes: 44 percent; increasing age: 51 percent; environmental stress: 25 percent; nervous personality: 15 percent; high-cholesterol diet: 10 percent; lack of exercise: 6 percent; low income: 5 percent.

33 Interview with Elijah Saunders, July 18, 2005; "A 20 Year ISHIB Perspective," part of the session "The Evolution of Hypertension and Cardiovascular Risk: A 20-Year Perspective," International Society for Hypertension in Blacks Annual Conference, Atlanta, Ga., June 23, 2006.

34 Hall, Saunders, and Shulman, *Hypertension in Blacks.*

35 Epstein, "Bodily Differences and Collective Identities."

36 See Greene, *Prescribing by Numbers.*

37 Shim, "Constructing 'Race' across the Science-Lay Divide."

38 Benjamin, "Organized Ambivalence," 447.

39 Braun, "Race, Ethnicity, and Health," 170.

40 See, for example, Rankins, Wortham, and Brown, "Modifying Soul Food for the Dietary Approaches to Stop Hypertension Diet (DASH) plan." Also see, for example, Jackson T. Wright quoted in Walter Brooks, "Hypertension Expert on Research, Recruitment, and Soul Food," February 10, 2004, at http://app1.unmc .edu/.

41 Shim, "Constructing 'Race' across the Science-Lay Divide," 411–12.

42 Osborne and Feit, "The Use of Race in Medical Research."

43 Klag et al., "The Association of Skin Color with Blood Pressure in US Blacks with Low Socioeconomic Status."

44 Aronowitz, *Making Sense of Illness*.

45 Din-Dzietham et al., "Perceived Stress Following Race-Based Discrimination at Work."

46 One provocative example of this that explicitly engaged many of the health professionals and academics who have critiqued race as genetic was the documentary film *The Angry Heart: The Impact of Racism on Heart Disease among African Americans* (dir. Jay Fedigan, Boston: Jay Fedigan Video, 2001). I saw it at the Boston Social Forum, University of Massachusetts, Boston, July 25, 2004. Nancy Krieger, Cornel West, and Camara Jones all participate as commentators on the compelling documentary of a particular Roxbury man's struggle with heart disease and its interventions.

47 See Aronowitz, *Making Sense of Illness*.

48 Jones, "Levels of Racism." See also Wyatt et al., "Racism and Cardiovascular Diseases in African Americans."

49 Krieger, "Does Racism Harm Health?," 195. See also Peters, "Racism and Hypertension among African Americans."

50 Krieger, quoted in Amersbach, "Through the Lens of Race."

51 Gravlee, "How Race Becomes Biology"; see especially Gravlee, Non, and Mulligan, "Genetic Ancestry, Social Classification, and Racial Inequalities."

52 Fausto-Sterling, "Refashioning Race," 26.

53 Ibid., 27–28.

54 Watson and Fonarow, "Adherence to Best Practices"; Smedley, Stith, and Nelson, *Unequal Treatment*.

55 Flack et al., "Management of High Blood Pressure in Blacks."

56 AHA (American Heart Association), "Am I at Risk?," April 1, 2009. Formerly at http://www.americanheart.org/ (accessed August 11, 2009). Also available at http://www.idph.state.il.us/public/hb/hbhype.htm.

57 Krieger, "Embodying Inequality," 296.

58 Althusser, *For Marx*. See also Rajan, *Biocapital*, 6.

59 Shim, "Understanding the Routinised Inclusion of Race, Socioeconomic Status and Sex in Epidemiology," 138.

60 Elijah Saunders, International Society for Hypertension in Blacks Conference, Detroit, Mich., June 2004.

61 Hertz et al., "Racial Disparities in Hypertension Prevalence, Awareness, and Management."

62 Hoberman, "Medical Racism and the Rhetoric of Exculpation."

63 Douglas et al., "Management of High Blood Pressure in African Americans."

64 Hoberman, "Medical Racism and the Rhetoric of Exculpation," 514.

65 Paul Rabinow has described this shift under the heading "From Stigma to Risk: Normal Handicaps" in his "Artificiality and Enlightenment," 98.

66 Aronowitz, *Making Sense of Illness*, 144.

67 Ibid.

68 Hammonds, "New Technologies of Race," 306.

69 Timmermans and Berg, *The Gold Standard*.

70 Berg, "Practices of Reading and Writing," 501.

71 Garrety, "Social Worlds, Actor-Networks and Controversy," 754.

72 Whitmarsh, "Biomedical Ambivalence," 52.

73 Dumit, "Drugs for Life."

74 Omi and Winant, *Racial Formation in the United States*, 56.

75 Stoler, "Racial Histories and Their Regimes of Truth," 199.

76 Ibid.

Chapter 4: Beyond Genetic Determinism

1 Fryer later became more widely known because of a front-page profile of him in the *New York Times Magazine*: Stephen J. Dubner, "Toward a Unified Theory of Black America," *New York Times Magazine*, March 20, 2005, 54.

2 Roland G. Fryer, "Understanding the Racial Difference in Life Expectancy," paper presented at the W. E. B. Du Bois Institute for African American Research Colloquium, October 20, 2004.

3 Wilson and Grim, "Biohistory of Slavery and Blood Pressure Differences in Blacks Today."

4 Work Fryer did with his advisor, Steven Levitt, on *Freakonomics*—which also involves economists reaching well out of bounds of their own discipline to find surprising answers to social problems from other fields—has also found broad appeal.

5 This refutation was published in 1992: Philip D. Curtin, "The Slavery Hypothesis for Hypertension among African Americans."

6 A concise representation of the larger field of discourse on this theory in relationship to psychosocial theories can be found in Postel-Vinay's elegant history of hypertension: "Black Hypertension: A Questionable Entity," in *A Century of Arterial Hypertension*, 148–49.

7 There have also been debates on the theory in other venues. For example, in *Transforming Anthropology: Journal of the Association of Black Anthropologists*, there was an exchange between Fatimah Jackson and George J. Armelagos in which Jackson argues that the problem with the theory is dilution: see Jackson, "Anthropological Science and the Salt-Hypertension Hypothesis," and "A Response to

George Armelagos' Commentary." Armelagos argues that the genetic bottleneck never existed to be diluted: Armelagos, "The Slavery Hypertension Hypothesis."

8 Kaufman and Hall, "The Slavery Hypertension Hypothesis," 112.

9 Interview with Clarence Grim, July 15, 2005.

10 McDonough et al., "Cardiovascular Disease Study in Evans County, Georgia." This study is a touchstone for race and cardiovascular disease, and purported to provide evidence for the widely held clinical impression that after controlling for such factors as education, income, and smoking, whites have more coronary disease than blacks and explored possible reasons for that incidence. Grim's work investigating dietary sodium and racial differences—which suggested that sodium intake was similar in blacks and whites and thus not an explanation for the differences in hypertension—became part of the large literature that emerged out of that biracial longitudinal study; see, for example, Grim et al., "Racial Differences in Blood Pressure in Evans Co., Georgia."

11 See Kempner, "Treatment of Heart and Kidney Disease and of Hypertensive and Arteriosclerotic Vascular Disease with the Rice Diet."

12 For simplicity, this chronology skips a few steps. Grim was also inspired by the work of Dr. Oscar Helmer in Indiana, who found that blacks were more salt-sensitive than whites, and he spent time with physiologist Arthur Guyton in Mississippi, who emphasized the role of salt in kidney function and hypertension.

13 Michener, Hawaii.

14 See Grim et al., "Blood Pressure in Blacks."

15 Interview with Clarence Grim, July 15, 2005.

16 Ibid.

17 Stoler, "Racial Histories and Their Regimes of Truth," 192.

18 Kaufman and Hall, "The Slavery Hypertension Hypothesis," 116.

19 Grim and Robinson, "Salt, Slavery and Survival," 120–22.

20 Stoler "Racial Histories and Their Regimes of Truth," 196.

21 Kaufman and Hall, "The Slavery Hypertension Hypothesis," 116.

22 Ibid.

23 Cooper et al., "The Prevalence of Hypertension in Seven Populations of West African Origin"; Cooper and Rotimi, "Hypertension in Populations of West African Origin"; Cooper and David, "The Biological Concept of Race."

24 Cooper and David, "The Biological Concept of Race," 113.

25 Cooper and Rotimi, "Hypertension in Blacks," 804.

26 Wade, Race, Nature and Culture, 37.

27 Skinner, "Racialised Futures," 474.

28 Dimsdale, "Stalked by the Past."

29 Ibid., 162.

30 Ibid., 162–63.

31 Ibid., 169.

32 Kaufman, "No More 'Slavery Hypothesis' Yarns," 324.

33 This claim of a righteous position of truth against naiveté on the part of opponents in a debate over the relationships between biology is of course also often made by those supporting race-as-biological, as noted by Hammonds, "Straw Men and Their Followers."

34 Kaufman, "No More 'Slavery Hypothesis' Yarns," 324.

35 Dimsdale, "Stalked by the Past," 166.

36 Dunklee, Reardon, and Wentworth, "Race and Crisis."

37 Jenks, "What's the Use of Culture?"

38 For more discussion of how both social and genetic explanations for racial difference effectively root difference in individual bodies, see Shim, "Bio-power and Racial, Class, and Gender Formation in Biomedical Knowledge Production."

39 Stoler, "Racial Histories and Their Regimes of Truth," 187.

40 "Ask Doctor Oz II," *Oprah Winfrey Show*, April 26, 2007: http://www.oprah.com/.

41 Ibid.

42 Obasogie, published under two titles: "Hypertension: What Oprah Doesn't Know: Blacks' Higher Average Blood Pressure May Have an Obvious Cause That Doesn't Involve Genetics or Slavery," and "Oprah's Unhealthy Mistake." *Los Angeles Times*, May 17, 2007. Available at the website of Obasogie's organization, the Center for Genetics and Society: http://www.geneticsandsociety.org/downloads/Obasogie_LATimes_0507_F2.pdf.

43 Ibid.

44 Ibid.

45 For a womanist invocation, see Townes, *Breaking the Fine Rain of Death*, 63; for a self-help invocation, see Duhart, "Killing Us Softly," 6.

46 Reardon, "The Democratic, Anti-racist Genome?"

47 Obasogie, "Hypertension."

48 Dumit, "Drugs for Life"; Greenslit, "Dep®ession and Consum♀tion"; Lakoff, "The Anxieties of Globalization"; Mamo and Fishman, "Potency in All the Right Places"; Martin, "The Pharmaceutical Person"; Metzl, *Prozac on the Couch*, especially "Prozac and the Pharmacokinetics of Narrative Form," 165–94.

49 Marx, *Capital*, vol. 1, 125–77.

50 Ibid., 165.

51 Turkle, "Whither Psychoanalysis in Computer Culture?," 18. See also "Introduction," in Turkle, *Evocative Objects*, 1–7.

52 See Clarke et al., "Biomedicalization."

53 Dumit, "Pharmaceutical Witnessing."

54 Althusser, "Ideology and Ideological State Aparatuses," 171.

55 Haraway, *Modest_Witness*, 50.

56 Dumit, "Pharmaceutical Witnessing," 40.

57 See, for example, Gates, *Figures in Black*; Gates, "*Race*," *Writing, and Difference*.

58 Gates, *The Signifying Monkey*.

59 Dumit, *Drugs for Life*.

60 Žižek, *The Puppet and the Dwarf*, 7.

61 Ibid., 7–8.

62 Žižek, *The Sublime Object of Ideology*, 28–30.

63 Haraway, *Modest_Witness*, 144.

64 Barthes, *Mythologies*.

65 Nelson, "Bio Science."

66 Ibid., 763.

67 Rose, "Race, Risk and Medicine in the Age of 'Your Own Personal Genome,'" 430.

68 Ibid.

69 Patricia Williams, "Salt in the Wound," *The Nation*, June 6, 2005.

70 Barthes, *Mythologies*, 116–31.

71 Ibid., 128.

72 Petryna, *Life Exposed*, 5.

73 Rose, *Politics of Life Itself*, 110.

74 Of course, as Jenny Reardon persuasively argues, the work of racial projects in genomics and their contestation is also much more complicated than simply propping up as opposed to exposing racism in natural science: Reardon, "Race and Biology."

Chapter 5: Thiazide Diuretics

1 The reduction of fluid was itself the original aim of the drug class, hence its moniker "diuretic," and it continues to be used for this indication. For the history of thiazides in this trajectory, see Maren, "Diuretics and Renal Drug Development."

2 For an overview of this literature, see Glieberman, "Sodium, Blood Pressure, and Ethnicity."

3 Diamond and Rotter, "Evolution of Human Genetic Diseases," 59.

4 Jones, "Virgin Soils Revisited."

5 Lewontin, "The Apportionment of Human Diversity."

6 Kahn, "Misreading Race and Genomics after BiDil."

7 Mokwe et al., "Determinants of Blood Pressure Response to Quinapril in Black and White Hypertensive Patients."

8 For the Joint National Committee guidelines, see National High Blood Pressure Education Program, *The Seventh Report of the Joint National Committee*; for ISHIB'S, see Douglas et al., "Management of High Blood Pressure in African Americans."

9 Materson, "Variability in Response to Anti-hypertensive Drug Treatment."

10 Davis et al., "Rationale and Design for the Antihypertensive and Lipid Lowering Treatment to Prevent Heart Attack Trial."

11 Grimm et al., "Baseline Characteristics of the 42,448 High Risk Hypertensives Enrolled in the Antihypertensive and Lipid Lowering Treatment to Prevent Heart Attack Trial."

12 Wright et al., "Outcomes in Hypertensive Black and Nonblack Patients Treated with Chlorthalidone, Amlodipine, and Lisinopril."

13 National Institutes of Health, "ALLHAT Study Findings for Racial Groups Show Diuretics Work Better Than Newer Medicines for High Blood Pressure," press release, April 5, 2005, at http://www.nhlbi.nih.gov/.

14 Wright et al., "Outcomes in Hypertensive Black and Nonblack Patients."

15 Epstein, Inclusion.

16 Steenburgh, "Diuretics for Hypertension Get a Big Boost."

17 Ibid.

18 The piece references prices at www.drugstore.com: "At drugstore.com, diuretics cost $22 to $36 per year, ACE inhibitors range from $282 to $532, and calcium channel blockers cost between $584 and $679 per year." Ibid.

19 Ibid.

20 Annual meeting of International Society for Hypertension in Blacks, Atlanta, Ga., June 23, 2006.

21 The risk of new-onset diabetes on diuretics has been the subject of much literature that seeks to redeem the new expensive drugs in the wake of ALLHAT. See, for example, Ando and Fujita, "Anti-diabetic Effect of Blockade of the Renin-Angiotensin System."

22 Fleck, "Some Specific Features of the Medical Way of Thinking."

23 Angell, The Truth about the Drug Companies; Rodwin, "Drug Advertising."

24 Greene and Podolsky, "Keeping Modern in Medicine," 331.

25 Postel-Vinay, A Century of Arterial Hypertension, 164–65.

26 Bud, Penicillin, 2.

27 Carruthers and Babb, Economy/Society, 26.

28 Marx, Capital, 125–77.

29 Ibid.

30 Mamo and Fishman, "Potency in All the Right Places," 27.

31 Davis, Quarells, and Gibbons, "Hypertension in African American Communities," 246–47.

32 For discussion of the earlier debates, see Tobbell, "Allied against Reform"; Greene, "What's in a Name?"

33 Meltzer, "A Specialist in Clinical Hypertension Critiques ALLHAT."

34 Moloney, Rethinking Public Relations.

35 Postel-Vinay, *A Century of Arterial Hypertension*, 164. The citation they provide is J. Menard, "Oil and Water?"

36 Benjamin, "The Work of Art in the Age of Mechanical Reproduction," 233.

37 Petryna, *Life Exposed*, 5.

38 Ibid., 6.

39 Rose and Novas, "Biological Citizenship," 440.

40 Ibid., 458.

41 Ibid., 451.

42 Roberts, "Race and the New Biocitizen."

43 Biehl, "Pharmaceuticalization." See also Das and Das, "Pharmaceuticals in Urban Ecologies."

44 Biehl develops this further in his book *The Will to Live*.

45 Ecks, "Pharmaceutical Citizenship."

46 Ecks and Basu, "The Unlicensed Lives of Antidepressants in India."

47 Hayden, "A Generic Solution?"

48 Pollock, "Transforming the Critique of Big Pharma."

49 Nguyen, "Anti-retroviral Globalism, Biopolitics, and Therapeutic Citizenship," 126.

50 Universities Allied for Essential Medicines, *Global Access Licensing Framework*, February 2009, updates at http://essentialmedicine.org/.

51 Farmer, *Pathologies of Power*, 18–19.

52 Ibid., 19.

53 Ibid., 177.

54 Tomes, "The Great American Medicine Show Revisited," 661.

55 Cohen, *A Consumers' Republic*; see especially 83–109.

56 Chambers, "Equal in Every Way."

57 Levy and Brink, *A Change of Heart*, 148.

58 Fausto-Sterling, "Refashioning Race," 30.

59 Jasanoff and Kim, "Containing the Atom," 123.

60 Greene, "Releasing the Flood Waters."

61 Ibid., 791–92.

62 Ibid., 792–93.

63 Kaiser, "Introduction of Thiazides," 133.

Chapter 6: BiDil

1 The conference "Race, Pharmaceuticals, and Medical Technology," at Massachusetts Institute of Technology Center for the Study of Diversity in Science, Technology and Medicine, Cambridge, Mass., April 7–8, 2006.

2 Roberts's paper "Is Race-Based Medicine Good for Us?" was among several of

those from the conference published in a special issue of the *Journal of Law, Medicine and Ethics*.

3 Roberts has written about the exchange in her article "Race and the New Bio-citizen," 269.

4 Mouffe, "Deconstruction, Pragmatism, and the Politics of Democracy," 9.

5 Derrida, "Remarks on Deconstruction and Pragmatism," 77–88.

6 See Sylvia Pagan Westphal, "Tough Prescription: Heart Medication Approved for Blacks Faces Uphill Battle; As Insurers Debate Costs and Generics Loom, BiDil Fails to Reach Needy; The Role of Medicare Part D," *Wall Street Journal*, October 16, 2006, A1; Dan Devine, "Cost Prevents Heart Patients from Receiving Adequate Care," *Bay State Banner*, August 3, 2006; and Steven Syre, "NitroMed's Challenge," Knight Ridder Tribune Business News, *Boston Globe*, August 10, 2006, 1. Westphal gives the figure 1 percent; Devine, "less than two percent"; Syre, 3 percent. I have not seen any estimates higher than 3 percent.

7 David Armstrong, "NitroMed Halts Marketing of Drug," *Wall Street Journal*, January 16, 2008.

8 Mamo and Fishman, "Potency in All the Right Places." See also Fox and Ward, "Pharma in the Bedroom."

9 Greene, *Prescribing by Numbers*; Dumit, "Drugs for Life."

10 Clarke et al., "Biomedicalization."

11 Dyer and Lilly, "Heart Failure."

12 Shamsham and Mitchell, "Essentials of the Diagnosis of Heart Failure."

13 Cleveland Clinic, "What Is Heart Failure?," http://my.clevelandclinic.org/heart/disorders/heartfailure/hfwhatis.aspx.

14 National Heart, Lung, and Blood Institute [NHLBI], "Data Fact Sheet."

15 Dyer and Lilly, "Heart Failure."

16 Aronowitz, *Making Sense of Illness*.

17 See Hatch, "The Politics of Metabolism."

18 This is not to say that BiDil did not have the potential to transform into a larger preventive drug: the compensation stage may be that eventually we will all be defined as suffering from "pre–heart failure," which is in any case analogous to (and could even be synonymous with) our status as people with "high" cholesterol and hypertension as well as "abnormalities" that appear on visual diagnostic technologies. We might be imagined to be all "compensating" for the pathologies unknown to us, ready to decompensate unless we are protected by pharmaceuticals. If this had happened, BiDil would have fallen into the "dependent normality" along the lines described by Dumit, "Drugs for Life."

19 An estimated 63,219,000 Lipitor prescriptions were dispensed in the United States in 2005, and 42,757,000 for the top thiazide (hydrochlorothiazide) as well as many more for other thiazides. See http://www.rxlist.com/top200.htm.

20 American Heart Association, *American Heart Disease and Stroke Statistics*.

21 NHLBI, "Data Fact Sheet."

22 Pollock, "Transforming the Critique of Big Pharma."

23 Cohn et al., "Effect of Vasodilator Therapy on Mortality in Chronic Congestive Heart Failure"; Cohn et al., "A Comparison of Enalapril with Hydralazine-Isosorbidedinitrate in the Treatment of Chronic Congestive Heart Failure."

24 After BiDil's approval, Cohn said: "This has been 30 years. I have to feel that I am finally vindicated" (quoted in Andrew Pollack, "Drug Approved for Heart Failure in Black Patients," *New York Times*, July 20, 2004). Cohn's belief remains that the combination works as he always predicted, rather than just for a smaller group: "Dr. Cohn said that despite any flaws in the first studies, the similar findings in the new trial suggest the original data was accurate. 'The replication gives me confidence that this combination is more likely to be effective in people who call themselves black than in people who call themselves white,' he said. 'Do I believe this drug should work in whites? Biology would tell me it should'" (Stephanie Saul, "US to Review Drug Intended for One Race," *New York Times*, June 13, 2005).

25 Bloomberg Business News, "Merck Profits Were Higher in Second Quarter," *New York Times*, July 19, 1996; Harvard Business School, "Merck-Medco."

26 "Panel Recommends FDA Reject BiDil Application," *Wall Street Journal*, February 28, 1997, 3.

27 Pollack, "Drug Approved for Heart Failure in Black Patients."

28 Carson et al., "Racial Differences in Response to Therapy for Heart Failure."

29 Cohn is among the couple of white physicians whose hand-painted portraits are included in the portrait gallery of dozens of notable cardiologists at the Association of Black Cardiologists headquarters in suburban Atlanta.

30 Taylor et al., "Combination of Isosorbide Dinitrate and Hydralazine in Blacks with Heart Failure."

31 Ibid.

32 Bloche, "Race-Based Therapeutics."

33 Ghali et al., "Exploring the Potential Synergistic Action of Spironolactone on Nitric Oxide-Enhancing Therapy," 257.

34 Fujimura, "Constructing 'Do-Able' Problems in Cancer Research."

35 Department of Health and Human Services, Food and Drug Administration Center for Drug Evaluation and Research, "Cardiovascular and Renal Drugs Advisory Committee, Volume II," Gaithersburg, Md., June 16, 2005. Transcript available at http://www.fda.gov/ohrms/dockets/ac/05/transcripts/2005-4145T2.pdf. See also Nissen, "Report from the Cardiovascular and Renal Drugs Advisory Committee."

36 Kahn, "How a Drug Becomes 'Ethnic.'"

37 Sankar and Kahn, "BiDil."

38 Kahn, "Exploiting Race in Drug Development," 750–51.

39 Mauss, *The Gift*.

40 Fisher, *Medical Research for Hire*, 40–65.

41 Nelson, "Inclusion-and-Difference Paradox," 742–43. See also Nelson, "The Factness of Diaspora."

42 BiDil package insert, http://www.bidil.com/PI.pdf.

43 For example, the patient product information for the ARB COZAAR suggests that one reason to prescribe it may not apply to blacks: "to lower the chance of stroke in patients with high blood pressure and a heart problem called left ventricular hypertrophy. COZAAR may not help Black patients with this problem." See http://www.merck.com/product/usa/pi_circulars/c/cozaar/cozaar_ppi.pdf.

44 For example, the package insert for the ACE inhibitor ALTACE notes that "although ALTACE was antihypertensive in all races studied, Black hypertensive patients (usually a low-renin hypertensive population) had a blood pressure lowering response to monotherapy, albeit a smaller average response, than non-Black patients" and that "in considering the use of ALTACE, note that in controlled clinical trials ACE inhibitors cause a higher rate of angioedema in Black patients than in non-Black patients." See http://www.altace.com.

45 Hoffman, " 'Racially-Tailored' Medicine Unravelled."

46 Cohn, "The Use of Race and Ethnicity in Medicine."

47 Westphal, "Tough Prescription."

48 Syre, "NitroMed's Challenge."

49 The most glaring example of this is Sankar and Kahn, "BiDil," 458. Sankar and Kahn not only uncritically quote the sales projections of $1 billion from Nitro-Med's CEO, but use the price once released to ratchet up the projection to $3 billion.

50 Kahn has continued to use the highest possible projections of revenue—in order to decry their egregiousness—long after it was clear that BiDil was a commercial failure. Kahn, "Exploiting Race in Drug Development," 754.

51 Fullwiley, "The Molecularization of Race," 2–3.

52 FDA, "FDA Approves BiDil Heart Failure Drug for Black Patients," http://www.fda.gov/NewsEvents/Newsroom/PressAnnouncements/2005/ucm108445.htm.

53 See, for example, Kahn, "Exploiting Race in Drug Development," and Lee, "Racializing Drug Design."

54 That is, unlike drugs such as Herceptin and Gleevec, it is not targeted according to protein or biogenetic markers. See Haga and Ginsburg, "Prescribing BiDil," 12–13.

55 Huggett, "BiDil Flops," 252.

56 See Angus, et al., "Cost Effectiveness of Fixed-Dose Combination Therapy for Blacks with Heart Failure."

57 "BiDil: Patient: Coverage and Assistance: Programs," http://www.nitromed.com/pnt/programs.php.

58 Ecks, "Global Pharmaceutical Markets and Corporate Citizenship," 178.

59 For a particularly rich account, see Samsky, "Since We Are Taking the Drugs."

60 Devine, "NAACP Goes to the Grassroots for BiDil," *Bay State Banner*, October 5, 2006, 7.

61 Sarah Varney, "A Drug Just for Blacks?," *National Public Radio: News and Notes*, December 13, 2006. At http://www.npr.org/.

62 Westphal, "Tough Prescription."

63 Ibid.

64 Silberner, "Race-Specific Drug Comes In at High Cost," *All Things Considered*, July 12, 2005, National Public Radio.

65 Clarke et al., "Biomedicalization."

66 Kahn "How a Drug Becomes 'Ethnic,'" 24.

67 Devine, "NAACP goes to the grassroots for BiDil."

68 Ibid.

69 Even within the category of "patient education" marketing by NitroMed, most of the resources have targeted black churches and communities on a low-budget grassroots level. There was a print advertisement that appeared in black newspapers in Houston, Detroit, and the District of Columbia in October and November 2006, that looked like a copy-cat of major pharmaceutical campaigns, made on the cheap. The half-page advertisement is dominated by a photograph of an old man and a young girl, smiling together. They appear to be grandfather and granddaughter, which resonates with the campaign by the Association of Black Cardiologists, framing the importance of heart health around "Children Should Know Their Grandparents." The large print ad copy under the picture reads "Live Longer . . . Live Better." Also in prominent typeface is "BiDil®" and underneath is its chemical name "isosorbidedinitrate/hydralazine HCI" and the slogan "More Life to Live." The basic promise of the ad is indistinguishable from one for arthritis or some other condition—"Life is made for living. And you deserve to enjoy every moment of it"—before discussing specifics. There was also a radio ad that played in black stations in Houston, Washington, and Detroit, that dramatized the potential need for BiDil in a conversation in which a grandfather was too tired to play. See Mark Jewell, "Ad Campaign for Blacks-Only Heart Drug Touches Lightly on Race," *Associated Press*, September 1, 2006.

70 Devine, "Heart Pill Maker Slashes Sales Staff," *Bay State Banner*, October 19, 2006.

71 Pollock, "Pharmaceutical Meaning Making."

72 Persson, "Incorporating *Pharmakon*," 46.

73 Ibid., 49.

74 Derrida, "Plato's Pharmacy." There are even more definitions than Derrida fully explores. The pharmakon is also, according to the Tufts *Greek-English Lexicon*: (1) drug, whether healing or noxious; (2) healing remedy, medicine; (3) enchanted potion, philter, hence charm, spell; (4) poison; (5) lye for laundering; II generally remedy, cure; (2) means of producing something; (3) remedy or consolation in; III Dye, paint, color; IV chemical reagent used by tanners.

75 Derrida, "Plato's Pharmacy," 99.

76 See Tutton, "Promising Pessimism."

77 Duster, "Medicine and People of Color: Unlikely Mix—Race, Biology, and Drugs," *San Francisco Chronicle*, March 17, 2003, B7.

78 George Ellison on Kenan Malik, "A Colour Coded Prescription."

79 On alleged distrust, see Byrd and Linda, *An American Health Dilemma*; on noncompliance, see Smith, *Health Care Divided*.

80 Chepesiuk and Jones, "Are Race-Specific Drugs Unethical?," 37; Kimberley, "Rx for Black Hearts."

81 Greenslit, "Dep®ession and Consum♀tion," 478.

82 Lévi-Strauss, *Totemism*.

83 For a compelling account of racism in antipsychotic prescribing practices, see Metzl, *The Protest Psychosis*.

84 Kahn, "How a Drug Becomes 'Ethnic.'"

85 Charles Curry, quoted in Wheelwright, "Human, Study Thyself."

86 Persson, "Incorporating *Pharmakon*."

87 Sailer, "Race Flat-Earthers Dangerous to Everyone's Health." See also Carlson, "The Case of BiDil." These are among the many of the race-embracers that narrate what Dunklee, Reardon, and Wentworth, in "Race and Crisis," describe as "Galilean victimization narrative in which a small vanguard group or individual is cast as being persecuted by the powerful Orthodox forces for their/his allegiance to the Truth."

88 Leah Sammons, "Racial Profiling: Not Always a Bad Thing," *Jacksonville Free Press*, February 16–23, 2006, 4.

89 Inda, "Materializing Hope."

90 Duster, "Comparative Perspectives and Competing Explanations."

91 Food and Drug Administration, "FDA Label for BiDil Approved on 6/23/05," http://www.accessdata.fda.gov/drugsatfda_docs/appletter/2005/020727ltr.pdf; Temple and Stockbridge, "BiDil for Heart Failure in Black Patients."

92 Kahn, "How a Drug Becomes 'Ethnic,' 44.

93 Latour, *We Have Never Been Modern*.

94 Krieger, "Stormy Weather," 2155.

95 The most categorical equations of biology with genetics go so far as to say that any race-based medical claim fails unless "each individually-defined or self-declared race would have to have a 100% pure and homogenous gene pool" (Hoover, "There Is No Scientific Rationale for Race-Based Research"). Harriet Washington discusses BiDil in a chapter titled "Genetic Perdition: The Rise of Molecular Bias" in her book *Medical Apartheid*). In equating race-as-biological with race-as-genetic, BiDil's critics are like BiDil's right-wing fans rather than like the ABC.

96 Amy Goodman, "The FDA Approves a Race-Specific Drug for the First Time in History," *Democracy Now!*, August 1, 2005.

97 Yu, Goering, and Fullerton, "Race-Based Medicine and Justice as Recognition"; Inda, "Materializing Hope."

98 Kelly and Geissler, "The Value of Transnational Medical Research," 7.

99 At the home page of ABC, http://www.abcardio.org/.

100 "Our Mission," at http://www.abcardio.org/about.htm.

101 Ferdinand's center's mission is founded as much in community engagement as in medical innovation: see, for example, Ferdinand, "Lessons Learned from the Healthy Heart Community Prevention Project in Reaching the African American Population." Since Katrina, Ferdinand has led efforts by the Association of Black Cardiologists to assist New Orleans. Ferdinand's compelling life story, including building the HeartBeats Life Center and its loss, are told in the volume he coedited: Penner and Ferdinand, *Overcoming Katrina*.

102 Fard Johnmar, "Conversations about Race-Based Medicine: NitroMed's Michael L. Sabolinksi," July 27, 2006, at http://fardj.prblogs.org/2006/06/27/conversations-about-race-based-medicine-nitromeds-michael-l-sabolinski-md/.

103 Fortun, "Race in the Meantime."

104 Kahn, "How a Drug Becomes 'Ethnic,'" 25.

105 The website has since altered the wording somewhat, so that as of 2012 it gave the reasons for African American risk as: "Two well-known contributors to the increased risk are much higher rates of high blood pressure and diabetes in the African American community. Other potential risk factors being explored are African Americans' lower access to and use of health care services, greater exposure to environmental pollutants, and greater tendencies to be overweight and to get less exercise" (http://www.hearthealthheritage.com/pnt/questions.php #18).

106 McGoey, "Pharmaceutical Controversies and the Performative Value of Uncertainty," 155.

107 In the case of BiDil, the history of the lived body is framed as both individual and ancestral. That black history is both social and biological has been important to some commentators sympathetic to BiDil (especially Crawley, "The Paradox of Race in the BiDil® Debate," who argues against waiting until these questions are all sorted out before using BiDil).

108 Butler, *Bodies That Matter*.

109 Sankar and Kahn, "BiDil," 462.

110 Kahn, "How a Drug Becomes 'Ethnic,'" 7.

111 Bibbins-Domingo and Fernandez, "BiDil for Heart Failure in Black Patients," 55.

112 Sade, "What's Right (and Wrong) with Racially Stratified Research and Therapies."

113 Nelson, *Body and Soul*, 48.

114 See also Pollock, "Transforming the Critique of Big Pharma."

115 This alliterative framing was used by Tavis Smiley, "Dr. Ian Smith: Race-Specific Drugs," *Tavis Smiley Show*, November 17, 2004, National Public Radio.

Conclusion

1   MIT Center for the Study of Diversity in Science, Technology and Medicine, Second Annual Conference, "The Business of Race and Science," Cambridge, Mass., March 30–31, 2007.

2   Puckrein, *The Acquisitive Impulse.*

3   Puckrein, *Little England.*

4   Westphal, "Tough Prescription."

5   The name has since changed, to the National Minority Quality Forum, http://www.nmqf.org/.

6   Appiah, *Experiments in Ethics,* 193.

7   Turkle, *Alone Together,* 291.

8   Appiah, *Experiments in Ethics,* 193.

9   Appiah discusses these at length in *Experiments in Ethics,* especially chap. 3, "The Case against Intuition," 73–120.

10   Ibid., 96–97.

11   Ibid., 195–96.

12   Ibid., 196.

13   Ibid., 90–92.

14   Farmer, *Pathologies of Power,* 174.

15   Appiah, *Experiments in Ethics,* 197–98.

16   Haraway, "Manifesto for Cyborgs."

17   Griggers, "Lesbian Bodies in the Age of (Post)Mechanical Reproduction."

18   Haraway, "Situated Knowledges," 579.

19   Haraway, *Modest_Witness.*

20   Harding, *The Feminist Standpoint Theory Reader.*

21   Hammonds and Herzig, *The Nature of Difference,* xi–xii.

22   West, "Prophetic Pragmatism," 167.

23   Allen, "The Hydra and Its Many Heads."

24   Duster, "Buried Alive," 259, 262.

25   Stark, *The Sense of Dissonance,* 16.

WORKS CITED

Abu-Jamal, Mumia. *We Want Freedom: A Life in the Black Panther Party*. Boston: South End Press, 2004.

Acierno, L. J. *The History of Cardiology*. Pearl River, N.Y.: Parthenon Publishing Group, 1994.

Adams, J. M. "Some Racial Differences in Blood Pressure and Morbidity in Groups of White and Colored Workmen." *American Journal of the Medical Sciences* 184 (1932): 342–50.

Agamben, Georgio. *Homo Sacer: Sovereign Power and Bare Life*. Palo Alto, Calif.: Stanford University Press, 1998.

Agar, Jon. "What Difference Did Computers Make?" *Social Studies of Science* 36 (2006): 869–907.

Allen, Gerald E. "The Hydra and Its Many Heads." *GeneWatch* 19, no. 5 (September–October 2006): 3–8.

Allen, James P., and Eugene Turner. "Boston's Emerging Ethnic Quilt: A Geographic Perspective." Paper presented at the annual meeting of the Population Association of America, Boston, April 1, 2004. At http://paa2004.princeton.edu.

Allen, L. C. "The Negro Health Problem." *American Journal of Public Health* 5 (1915): 194–203.

Althusser, Louis. *For Marx*. Translated by Ben Brewster. New York: Pantheon Books, 1965.

——. "Ideology and Ideological State Apparatuses." In *Lenin and Philosophy and Other Essays*, translated by Ben Brewster, 127–86. New York: Monthly Review Press, 1971.

American Heart Association. *Heart Disease and Stroke Statistics: 2010 Update At-a-Glance*. December 2009. At http://circ.ahajournals.org/.

Amersbach, Gabriele. "Through the Lens of Race: Unequal Health Care in America." *Harvard Public Health Review*, Winter 2002. At http://www.hsph.harvard.edu/review/.

Anderson, Benedict. *Imagined Communities: Reflections on the Origin and Spread of Nationalism*. London: Verso, 1983.

Anderson, Warwick. *The Cultivation of Whiteness: Science, Health, and Racial Destiny in Australia*. New York: Basic Books, 2003.

——. "Teaching 'Race' in Medical School." *Social Studies of Science* 38 (2008): 785–800.

Ando, Katsuyuki, and Toshiro Fujita. "Anti-diabetic Effect of Blockade of the Renin-Angiotensin System." *Diabetes, Obesity and Metabolism* 8 (July 2006): 396–403.

Angell, Marcia. *The Truth about the Drug Companies: How They Deceive Us and What to Do about It.* New York: Random House, 2004.

Angus, Derek, et al. "Cost Effectiveness of Fixed-Dose Combination of Isosorbide Dinitrate and Hydralazine Therapy for Blacks with Heart Failure," *Circulation* 112 (2005): 3745–53.

——. "Heart Failure; Study Finds That African-American Heart Failure Drug Is Cost Effective." *Heart Disease Weekly*, January 8, 2006, 84.

Appiah, Kwame Anthony. *Experiments in Ethics.* Cambridge: Harvard University Press, 2008.

ARIC Investigators. "The Atherosclerosis Risk in Communities (ARIC) Study: Design and Objectives." *American Journal of Epidemiology* 129 (1989): 687–702.

Armelagos, George J. "The Slavery Hypertension Hypothesis—Natural Selection and Scientific Investigation: A Commentary." *Transforming Anthropology* 13 (2005): 119–24.

Aronowitz, Robert A. *Making Sense of Illness: Science, Society and Disease.* Cambridge: Cambridge University Press, 1998.

Aronson, Jay. *Genetic Witness: Science, Law, and Controversy in the Making of DNA Profiling.* Piscataway, N.J.: Rutgers University Press, 2007.

Baker, Benjamin M. "Certain Aspects of Syphilitic Cardiac Disease." *Venereal Disease Information* 12 (September 20, 1931): 471.

Baker, Lee. *From Savage to Negro: Anthropology and the Construction of Race, 1896–1954.* Berkeley: University of California Press, 1998.

Barthes, Roland. *Mythologies.* Translated by Annette Levers. New York: Hill and Wang, 1972.

Bays, Robert P., and Nevin S. Scrimshaw. "Facts and Fallacies Regarding the Blood Pressure of Different Regional and Racial Groups." *Circulation* 8 (1953): 655–63.

Benjamin, Ruha. "A Lab of Their Own: Genomic Sovereignty as Postcolonial Science Policy." *Policy and Society* 28, no. 4 (2009): 341–55.

——. "Organized Ambivalence: When Sickle Cell Disease and Stem Cell Research Converge." *Ethnicity and Health* 16, no. 4–5 (August–October 2011): 447–63.

Benjamin, Walter. "The Work of Art in the Age of Mechanical Reproduction." In *Illuminations: Essays and Reflections*, translated by H. Zohn, 217–52. New York: Schocken, 1968.

Berg, Marc. "Practices of Reading and Writing: The Constitutive Role of the Patient Record in Medical Work." *Sociology of Health and Illness* 18, no. 4 (1996): 499–524.

Berg, Marc, and Annemarie Mol. *Differences in Medicine: Unraveling Practices, Techniques, and Bodies.* Durham: Duke University Press, 1998.

Bethea, Dennis A. "Some Significant Negro Movements to Lower Their Mortality." *Journal of the National Medical Association* 22, no. 2 (1930): 85–88.

Bhabha, Homi. *The Location of Culture.* New York: Routledge, 1994.

Bibbins-Domingo, Kirsten, and Alicia Fernandez. "BiDil for Heart Failure in Black Patients: Implications of the U.S. Food and Drug Administration Approval." *Annals of Internal Medicine* 146 (January 2007): 52–56.

Biehl, João. "Pharmaceuticalization: AIDS Treatment and Global Health Politics." *Anthropological Quarterly* 80, no. 4 (Fall 2007): 1083–126.

———. *The Will to Live: AIDS Therapies and the Politics of Survival.* Princeton: Princeton University Press, 2008.

Bing, Richard J. *Cardiology: The Evolution of the Science and the Art.* 2nd ed. New Brunswick: Rutgers University Press, 1999.

Birke, Lynda. "The Heart: A Broken Metaphor?" In *Feminism and the Biological Body,* 112–34. Edinburgh: Edinburgh University Press, 1999.

Birnie, C. W. "The Influence of Environment and Race on Diseases." *Journal of the National Medical Association* 2, no. 4 (1910): 243–51.

Blackburn, Henry. "Oral History: Interview with Felix Moore." August 8, 1989, Granlibakken, California. At http://www.epi.umn.edu/.

———. "Oral History: Interview with Dr. William Kannel." February 23, 2002, Palm Beach Florida. Excerpts at http://www.epi.umn.edu/.

Blackman, Lisa. "Psychiatric Culture and Bodies of Resistance." *Body and Society* 13, no. 2 (June 2007): 1–23.

Bloche, M. Gregg. "Race-Based Therapeutics." *New England Journal of Medicine* 351 (November 11, 2004): 2035–37.

Bousfield, M. O. "Reaching the Negro Community." *American Journal of Public Health* 24 (1934): 209–15.

Bowker, Geoffrey C., and Susan Leigh Star. *Sorting Things Out: Classification and Its Consequences.* Cambridge: MIT Press, 1999.

Braithwaite, Ronald L., Sandra E. Taylor, and John N. Austin. *Building Health Coalitions in the Black Community.* Thousand Oaks, Calif.: Sage, 2000.

Brandt, Allan M. "Racism and Research: The Case of the Tuskegee Syphilis Study." *Hastings Center Report* 8 (December 1978): 21–29.

Brandt, Allan M., and David C. Sloane. "Of Beds and Benches: Building the Modern American Hospital." In *The Architecture of Science,* edited by Peter Galison and Emily Thompson, 281–308. Cambridge: MIT Press, 1999.

Braun, Lundy. "Race, Ethnicity, and Health: Can Genetics Explain Disparities?" *Perspectives in Biology and Medicine* 45 (Spring 2002): 159–74.

Bridges, Khiara. *Reproducing Race: An Ethnography of Pregnancy as a Site of Racialization.* Berkeley: University of California Press, 2011.

Briggs, Charles, and Clara Mantini-Briggs. *Stories in the Time of Cholera: Racial Profiling during a Medical Nightmare.* Berkeley: University of California Press, 2003.

Brooks, Walter. "Hypertension Expert on Research, Recruitment, and Soul Food." February 10, 2004. At http://app1.unmc.edu/publicaffairs/.

Brown, Michael K., Martin Carnoy, Elliott Currie, Troy Duster, David B. Oppenheimer, Marjorie M. Shultz, and David Wellman. *Whitewashing Race: The Myth of a Color-Blind Society*. Berkeley: University of California Press, 2003.

Brown, Roscoe C. "The National Negro Health Week Movement." *Journal of Negro Education* 6 (July 1937): 553–64.

Brunner, William F. "The Negro Health Problem in Southern Cities." *American Journal of Public Health* 5 (1915): 183–90.

Bud, Robert. *Penicillin: Triumph and Tragedy*. Oxford: Oxford University Press, 2007.

Butler, Judith. *Bodies That Matter: On the Discursive Limits of "Sex."* New York: Routledge, 1993.

Bynum, William F., Christopher Lawrence, and Vivian Nutton, eds. *The Emergence of Modern Cardiology*. London: Wellcome, 1985.

Byrd, W. Michael, and Linda A. Clayton. *An American Health Dilemma: A Medical History of African Americans and the Problem of Race, Beginnings to 1900*. New York: Routledge, 2000.

——. *An American Health Dilemma*, vol. 2, *Race, Medicine, and Health Care in the United States, 1900–2000*. New York: Routledge, 2002.

Callon, Michel. "Some Elements of a Sociology of Translation: Domestication of the Scallops and the Fishermen of St Brieuc Bay." In *Power, Action and Belief: A New Sociology of Knowledge?*, edited by John Law, 196–223. London: Routledge, 1986.

Canguilhem, Georges. *The Normal and the Pathological*. New York: Zone Books, 1991.

Carlson, Rick J. "The Case of BiDil: A Policy Commentary on Race and Genetics: The Debate between Sociologists and Biologists Is Just the Beginning, When It Comes to Genomics and Race." *Health Affairs* 24 (July–December 2005): 464–68.

Carruthers, Bruce G., and Sarah L. Babb. *Economy/Society: Markets, Meanings, and Social Structure*. Thousand Oaks, Calif.: Pine Forge Press, 2000.

Carson, P., S. Ziesche, G. Johnson, J. N. Cohn, and Vasodilator-Heart Failure Trial Study Group. "Racial Differences in Response to Therapy for Heart Failure: Analysis of the Vasodilator-Heart Failure Trials." *Journal of Cardiac Failure* 5 (1999): 178–87.

CDER [Department of Health and Human Services, Food and Drug Administration Center for Drug Evaluation and Research]. "Cardiovascular and Renal Drugs Advisory Committee, Volume II." Gaithersburg, Md., June 16, 2005. At http://circ.ahajournals.org/.

Chambers, Jason. "Equal in Every Way: African Americans, Consumption and Materialism from Reconstruction to the Civil Rights Movement." *Advertising and Society Review* 7, no. 1 (2006): DOI: 10.1353/asr.2006.0017.

Chepesiuk, Ron, and Joyce Jones. "Are Race-Specific Drugs Unethical?" *Black Enterprise* (November 2005): 37.

Chun, Wendy Hui Kyong. *Control and Freedom: Power and Paranoia in the Age of Fiber Optics*. Cambridge: MIT Press, 2006.

Clarke, Adele, Janet K. Shim, Laura Mamo, Jennifer Ruth Fosket, and Jennifer R.

Fishman. "Biomedicalization: Technoscientific Transformations of Health, Illness, and U.S. Biomedicine." *American Sociological Review* 68, no. 2 (April 2003): 161–94.

Clough, Patricia Ticineto, and Jean Halley, eds. *The Affective Turn: Theorizing the Social.* Durham: Duke University Press, 2007.

Cohen, Lizabeth. *A Consumers' Republic: The Politics of Mass Consumption in Postwar America.* New York: Vintage, 2003.

Cohn, J. N., et al. "Effect of Vasodilator Therapy on Mortality in Chronic Congestive Heart Failure: Results of a Veterans Administration Cooperative Study." *New England Journal of Medicine* 314 (1986): 1547–52.

——. "A Comparison of Enalapril with Hydralazine-Isosorbide Dinitrate in the Treatment of Chronic Congestive Heart Failure." *New England Journal of Medicine* 325 (1991): 303–10.

Cohn, Jay. "The Use of Race and Ethnicity in Medicine: Lessons from the African American Heart Failure Trial." *Journal of Law, Medicine and Ethics* 34 (Fall 2006): 552–54.

Conrad, Peter. "Medicalization and Social Control." *Annual Review of Sociology* 18 (1992): 209–32.

——. "The Shifting Engines of Medicalization." *Journal of Health and Social Behavior* 46 (2005): 3–14.

Conroy, R. M. "From Epidemiological Risk to Clinical Practice by Way of Statistics—A Personal View." In *Therapeutic Strategies in Cardiovascular Risk,* edited by I. M. Graham and R. B. D'Agostino. Oxford: Clinical Publishing, 2008.

Cooper, R., and C. Rotimi. "Hypertension in Populations of West African Origin: Is There a Genetic Predisposition?" *Journal of Hypertension* 12 (1994): 215–27.

——. "Hypertension in Blacks," *American Journal of Hypertension* 10 (July 1997): 804–12.

Cooper, R., et al. "The Prevalence of Hypertension in Seven Populations of West African Origin." *American Journal of Public Health* 87, no. 2 (1997): 160–68.

Cooper, Richard, and Richard David. "The Biological Concept of Race and Its Application to Public Health and Epidemiology." *Journal of Health Politics, Policy and Law* 11 (Spring 1986): 97–116.

Crawley, LaVera. "The Paradox of Race in the BiDil® Debate." *Journal of the National Medical Association* 99, no. 7 (July 2007): 821–22.

Crenshaw, Kimberlé Williams. "Race, Reform, and Retrenchment: Transformation and Legitimation in Anti-discrimination Law." *Harvard Law Review* 101, no. 7 (May 1988): 1331–87.

Curtin, Philip D. "The Slavery Hypothesis for Hypertension among African Americans: The Historical Evidence." *American Journal of Public Health* 82, no. 12 (1992): 1681–86.

Das, Veena, and Ranendra K. Das. "Pharmaceuticals in Urban Ecologies: The Register of the Local." In *Global Pharmaceuticals: Ethics, Markets, Practices,* edited by Adriana

Petryna, Andrew Lakoff, and Arthur Kleinman, 171–205. Durham: Duke University Press, 2006.

Davis, B. R., J. A. Cutler, D. J. Gordon, C. D. Furberg, J. T. Wright Jr., W. C. Cushman, R. H. Grimm, J. LaRosa, P. K. Whelton, H. M. Perry, M. H. Alderman, C. E. Ford, S. Oparil, C. Francis, M. Proschan, S. Pressel, H. R. Black, and C. M. Hawkins, for the ALLHAT Research Group. "Rationale and Design for the Antihypertensive and Lipid Lowering Treatment to Prevent Heart Attack Trial (ALLHAT)." *American Journal of Hypertension* 9 (1996): 342–60.

Davis, Sharon K., Rakale Collins Quarells, and Gary H. Gibbons. "Hypertension in African American Communities." In *Health Issues in the Black Community*, edited by Ronald L. Braithwaite and Sandra E. Taylor, 233–58. San Francisco: Wiley, 2009.

Dawber, Thomas Royle. *The Framingham Study: The Epidemiology of Atherosclerotic Disease*. Cambridge: Harvard University Press, 1980.

Dawber, T. R., W. B. Kannel, and G. D. Friedman. "The Use of Computers in Cardiovascular Epidemiology." *Progress in Cardiovascular Diseases* 5 (1963): 406–17.

Dawber, Thomas, William B. Kannel, Nicholas Revotskie, Joseph Stokes III, Abraham Kagan, and Tavia Gordon. "Some Factors Associated with the Development of Coronary Heart Disease—Six Years' Follow-Up Experience in the Framingham Study." *American Journal of Public Health* 49 (October 1959): 1349–56.

Dawber, Thomas R., Gilcin F. Meadors, and Felix Moore Jr. "Epidemiological Approaches to Heart Disease: The Framingham Study." *American Journal of Public Health* 41, no. 3 (March 1951): 279–86.

Dawber, Thomas R., and Felix E. Moore. "Longitudinal Study of Heart Disease in Framingham, Massachusetts: An Interim Report." *Research in Public Health: 1951 Annual Conference of the Milbank Memorial Fund*. New York: Milbank Memorial Fund, 1952.

Dawber, Thomas R., Felix E. Moore, and George V. Mann. "Coronary Heart Disease in the Framingham Study." *American Journal of Public Health* 47 (April 1957): 4–24.

Dawber, Thomas R., Georgiana Pearson, Patricia Anderson, George V. Mann, William Kannel, Dewey Shurtleff, and Patricia McNamara. "Dietary Assessment in the Epidemiologic Study of Coronary Heart Disease: The Framingham Study." *American Journal of Clinical Nutrition* 11 (September 1962): 226–34.

Dawber, Thomas R., et al. 1967. "Environmental Factors in Hypertension." In *The Epidemiology of Hypertension: Proceedings of an International Symposium*, a meeting sponsored by the Chicago Heart Association and the American Heart Association, Chicago, February 3–7, 1964. Edited by J. Stamler, R. Stamler, and T. N. Pullman. New York: Grune and Stratton, 1967.

Denton, Derek. 1982. *The Hunger for Salt: An Anthropological, Physiological, and Medical Analysis*. New York: Springer Verlag.

Derrida, Jacques. "Plato's Pharmacy." In *Dissemination*, translated by Barbara Johnson, 61–171. Chicago: University of Chicago Press, 1981.

——. *The Gift of Death*. Translated by David Wills. Chicago: University of Chicago Press, 1996.

——. "Remarks on Deconstruction and Pragmatism." In *Deconstruction and Pragmatism*, edited by Chantal Mouffe, 77–88. New York: Routledge, 1997.

DHEW (U.S. Department of Health, Education, and Welfare, Public Health Service). *National High Blood Pressure Education Program: Report to the Hypertension Information and Education Advisory Committee: Task Force III Community Education*, September 1, 1973. National Library of Medicine, Bethesda, Md.

——. *Diagnosis and Management of Hypertension: A Nationwide Survey of Physicians' Knowledge, Attitudes, and Reported Behavior: Conducted for the Food and Drug Administration and the National High Blood Pressure Education Program, National Heart, Lung, and Blood Institute*. DHEW Publication No. (NIH) 79-1056, 1979. National Library of Medicine, Bethesda, Md.

Diamond, Jared, and Jerome I. Rotter. "Evolution of Human Genetic Diseases." In *The Genetic Basis of Common Diseases*, edited by Richard Allen King, Jerome I. Rotter, and Arno G. Motulsky. New York: Oxford University Press, 2002.

Dimsdale, Joel E. "Stalked by the Past: The Influence of Ethnicity on Health." *Psychosomatic Medicine* 62 (2000): 161–70.

Din-Dzietham, R., W. N. Nembhard, R. Collins, and S. K. Davis. "Perceived Stress Following Race-Based Discrimination at Work Is Associated with Hypertension in African-Americans: The Metro Atlanta Heart Disease Study, 1999–2001." *Social Science and Medicine* 58, no. 3 (February 2004): 449–61.

Douglas, Janice G., George L. Bakris, Murray Epstein, Keith C. Ferdinand, Carlos Ferrario, John M. Flack, Kenneth A. Jamerson, et al. "Management of High Blood Pressure in African Americans: Consensus Statement of the Hypertension in African Americans Working Group of the International Society on Hypertension in Blacks." *Archives of Internal Medicine* 163 (March 10, 2003): 525–41.

Dublin, Louis I. "Factors in American Mortality: A Study of Death Rates in the Race Stocks of New York State, 1910." *American Economic Review* 6, no. 3 (September 1916): 523–48.

——. "The Health of the Negro." *Annals of the American Academy of Political and Social Science* 140 (1928): 77–85.

——. "The Problem of Negro Health as Revealed by Vital Statistics." *Journal of Negro Education* 6 (1937): 268–75.

Du Bois, W. E. B. *The Philadelphia Negro*. New York: Lippincott, 1899.

——. *The Health and Physique of the Negro American: Report of a Social Study Made under the Direction of Atlanta University; Together with the Proceedings of the Eleventh Conference for the Study of the Negro Problems* (Atlanta: Atlanta University Press, 1906). Excerpts reprinted as W. E. Burghardt Du Bois, "Voices from the Past: The Health and Physique of the Negro American," *American Journal of Public Health* 93, no. 2 (February 2003): 272–76.

Duhart, Olympia. "Killing Us Softly: The Hypertension Threat," *Healthquest: Total Wellness for Mind, Body, and Spirit* 12 (February 28, 1996): 6–9.

Dumit, Joseph. "Drugs for Life." *Molecular Interventions* 2, no. 3 (2002): 124–27.

——. "Is It Me or My Brain? Depression and Neuroscientific Facts." *Journal of Medical Humanities* 24, nos. 1–2 (Summer 2003): 35–47.

——. *Picturing Personhood: Brain Scans and Biomedical Identity.* Princeton: Princeton University Press, 2003.

——. "Pharmaceutical Witnessing: Drugs for Life in an Era of Direct-to-Consumer Advertising." In *Technologized Images, Technologized Bodies,* edited by Jeanette Edwards, Penelope Harvey, and Peter Wade, 37–60. Oxford: Berghahn Books, 2010.

——. *Drugs for Life: How Pharmaceutical Companies Define Our Health.* Durham: Duke University Press, forthcoming.

Dunklee, Brady, Jenny Reardon, and Kara Wentworth. 2006. "Race and Crisis." *Social Science Research Council Forum: Is Race Real?* At http://raceandgenomics.ssrc.org/Reardon/.

Duster, Troy. "Buried Alive: The Concept of Race in Science." In *Genetic Nature/Culture: Anthropology and Science Beyond the Two-Culture Divide,* edited by Alan H. Goodman, Deborah Health, and M. Susan Lindee, 258–77. Berkeley: University of California Press, 2003.

——. "Comparative Perspectives and Competing Explanations: Taking on the Newly Reconfigured Reductionist Challenge to Sociology." *American Sociological Review* 71, no. 1 (February 2006): 1–15.

Dyer, George S. M., and Leonard S. Lilly. "Heart Failure." In *Pathophysiology of Heart Disease: A Collaborative Project of Medical Students and Faculty,* 3rd ed., edited by Leonard S. Lilly, 211–36. Philadelphia: Lippincott Williams and Wilkins, 2003.

Eagan, Catherine M. "The Invention of the White Race[s]." Review of *Whiteness of a Different Color: European Immigrants and the Alchemy of Race,* by Matthew Frye Jacobson, *American Quarterly* 51 (1999): 921–30.

Ecks, Stefan. "Pharmaceutical Citizenship: Antidepressant Marketing and the Promise of Demarginalization in India." *Anthropology and Medicine* 12, no. 3 (December 2005): 239–54.

——. "Global Pharmaceutical Markets and Corporate Citizenship: The Case of Novartis' Anti-cancer Drug Glivec," *BioSocieties* 3, no. 2 (2008): 165–81.

Ecks, Stefan, and Soumita Basu. "The Unlicensed Lives of Antidepressants in India: Generic Drugs, Unqualified Practitioners, and Floating Prescriptions." *Transcultural Psychiatry* 46, no. 1(2009): 86–106.

Embree, Edwin R. "Negro Illness and Its Effect upon the Nation's Health." *Modern Hospital* 30 (1928): 49–54.

Emslie, Carol, Kate Hunt, and Graham Watt. "Invisible Women? The Importance of Gender in Lay Beliefs about Heart Problems." *Sociology of Health and Illness* 23, no. 2 (2001): 203–33.

Epstein, Steven. *Impure Science: AIDS, Activism, and the Politics of Knowledge*. Berkeley: University of California Press, 1998.

——. "Bodily Differences and Collective Identities: The Politics of Gender and Race in Biomedical Research in the United States." *Body and Society* 10 (2004): 183–203.

——. *Inclusion: The Politics of Difference in Medical Research*. Chicago: University of Chicago Press, 2007.

——. "The Rise of 'Recruitmentology': Clinical Research, Racial Knowledge, and the Politics of Inclusion and Difference." *Social Studies of Science* 38, no. 5 (2008): 801–32.

Ernst, Waltraud, and Bernard Harris. *Race, Science and Medicine, 1700–1960*. New York: Routledge, 1999.

Farmer, Harold E. "The Incidence of Heart Disease among Negroes." *Journal of the National Medical Association* 32, no. 5 (1940): 198–203.

Farmer, Paul. *Pathologies of Power: Health, Human Rights, and the New War on the Poor*. Berkeley: University of California Press, 2003.

Fausto-Sterling, Anne. "Refashioning Race: DNA and the Politics of Health Care." *differences: A Journal of Feminist Cultural Studies* 15, no. 3 (2004): 1–37.

Ferdinand, Keith. "Lessons Learned from the Healthy Heart Community Prevention Project in Reaching the African American Population." *Journal of Health Care for the Poor and Underserved* 8, no. 3 (August 1997): 366–71.

Fields, Barbara J. "Ideology and Race in American History." In *Region, Race and Reconstruction*, edited by J. Morgan Kousser and James McPherson, 143–77. New York: Oxford University Press, 1982.

Fisher, Jill. *Medical Research for Hire: The Political Economy of Pharmaceutical Clinical Trials*. Piscataway, N.J.: Rutgers University Press, 2009.

Fishman, Jennifer. "Manufacturing Desire: The Commodification of Female Sexual Dysfunction." *Social Studies of Science* 34 (2004): 187–218.

Flack, John M., Domenic A. Sica, George Bakris, Angela L. Brown, Keith C. Ferdinand, Richard H. Grimm Jr., W. Dallas Hall, Wendell E. Jones, David S. Kountz, Janice P. Lea, Samar Nasser, Shawna D. Nesbitt, Elijah Saunders, Margaret Scisney-Matlock, Kenneth A. Jamerson, on behalf of the International Society on Hypertension in Blacks. "Management of High Blood Pressure in Blacks: An Update of the International Society on Hypertension in Blacks Consensus Statement." *Hypertension* 56 (2010): 780–800.

Fleck, Ludwik. "Some Specific Features of the Medical Way of Thinking." In *Cognition and Fact: Materials on Ludwik Fleck*, edited by Robert S. Cohen and Thomas Schnelle, 39–46. 1927; Dordrecht, Holland: Reidel, 1986.

Fleming, Peter. *A Short History of Cardiology*. Amsterdam: Rodopi, 1997.

Flexner, Abraham. "The Medical Education of the Negro." In *The Flexner Report on Medical Education in the United States and Canada*. New York: Carnegie Foundation, 1910. Reprinted in *Journal of the National Medical Association* 85 (1993): 152.

Fortun, Mike. "Race in the Meantime: The 'Care for the Data' for Complex Conditions." Paper presented at the conference "The Business of Race," MIT Center for the Study of Diversity in Science, Technology and Medicine, March 30 2007. At http://web.mit.edu/csd/BRS/Program.html.

Foucault, Michel. *The Birth of the Clinic: An Archeology of Medical Perception.* Translated by A. M. Sheridan Smith. London: Tavistock Publications, 1973.

——. *Archeology of Knowledge.* 1972; Oxford: Routledge, 2002.

Fox, Nick J., and Katie J. Ward. "Pharma in the Bedroom . . . and the Kitchen . . . : The Pharmaceuticalisation of Daily Life." *Sociology of Health and Illness* 30, no. 6 (September 2008): 856–68.

France, J. J. "Cardio-Vascular Syphilis." *Journal of the National Medical Association* 14, no. 3 (1922): 151–53.

Fujimura, Joan. "Constructing 'Do-Able' Problems in Cancer Research: Articulating Alignment." *Social Studies of Science* 17 (May 1987): 257–93.

——. "Postgenomic Futures: Translations across the Machine-Nature Border in Systems Biology." *New Genetics and Society* 24, no. 2 (2005): 195–225.

Fullwiley, Duana. "The Molecularization of Race: Institutionalizing Human Difference in Pharmacogenetics Practice." *Science as Culture* 16, no. 1 (March 2007): 1–30.

——. "The Biologistical Construction of Race: 'Admixture' Technology and the New Genetic Medicine." *Social Studies of Science* 38 (2008): 695–735.

Fye, W. Bruce. "A History of the Origin, Evolution, and Impact of Electrocardiography." *American Journal of Cardiology* 73, no. 13 (1994): 937–49.

——. *American Cardiology: A History of a Specialty and Its College.* Baltimore: Johns Hopkins University Press, 1996.

Gager, Leslie. "Changing Conditions in Medical Practice." *Journal of the National Medical Association* 25, no. 2 (1933): 72–76.

Gamble, Vanessa Northington, ed. *Germs Have No Color Line: Blacks and American Medicine 1900–1940.* New York: Garland Publishing, 1989.

——. *Making a Place for Ourselves: The Black Hospital Movement, 1920–1945.* New York: Oxford University Press, 1995.

Garrety, Karin. "Social Worlds, Actor-Networks and Controversy: The Case of Cholesterol, Dietary Fat, and Heart Disease." *Social Studies of Science* 27 (1997): 727–73.

Gates, Henry Louis, Jr., ed. *"Race," Writing, and Difference.* Chicago: University of Chicago Press, 1986.

——. *Figures in Black: Words, Signs, and the "Racial" Self.* New York: Oxford University Press, 1987.

——. *The Signifying Monkey: A Theory of Afro-American Literary Criticism.* New York: Oxford University Press, 1988.

Geest, Sjaak van der, Susan Reynolds Whyte, and Anita Hardon. "The Anthropology of Pharmaceuticals: A Biographical Approach." *Annual Review of Anthropology* 25 (1996): 153–78.

Ghali, J. K., S. W. Tam, M. L. Sabolinski, A. L. Taylor, J. Lindenfeld, J. N. Cohn, and M. Worcel. "Exploring the Potential Synergistic Action of Spironolactone on Nitric

Oxide-Enhancing Therapy: Insights from the African-American Heart Failure Trial." *Journal of Cardiac Failure* 14 (2008): 718–23.

Gieryn, Thomas. "Boundary-Work and the Demarcation of Science from Non-science: Strains and Interests in Professional Ideologies of Scientists." *American Sociological Review* 48 (December 1983): 781–95.

Gillum, Richard F. "Pathophysiology of Hypertension in Blacks and Whites: A Review of the Basis of Racial Blood Pressure Differences." *Hypertension* 1 (1979): 468–75.

Gilroy, Paul. *Against Race: Imagining Political Culture beyond the Color Line*. Cambridge: Harvard University Press, 2000.

Glieberman, Lillian. "Sodium, Blood Pressure, and Ethnicity: What Have We Learned?" *American Journal of Human Biology* 21 (2009): 679–86.

Gravlee, Clarence C. "How Race Becomes Biology: Embodiment of Social Inequality." *American Journal of Physical Anthropology* 139 (2009): 47–57.

Gravlee, Clarence C., Amy L. Non, and Connie J. Mulligan. "Genetic Ancestry, Social Classification, and Racial Inequalities in Blood Pressure in Southeastern Puerto Rico." *PLoS ONE* 4, no. 9 (September 2009): e6821. At http://www.plosone.org/article/info:doi/10.1371/journal.pone.0006821.

Greene, Jeremy. "Releasing the Flood Waters: Diuril and the Reshaping of Hypertension." *Bulletin of the History of Medicine* 79 (2005): 749–94.

——. *Prescribing by Numbers: Drugs and the Definition of Disease*. Baltimore: Johns Hopkins University Press, 2007.

——. "What's in a Name? Generics and the Persistence of the Pharmaceutical Brand in American Medicine." *Journal of the History of Medicine and Allied Sciences* 66, no. 4 (2011): 468–506.

Greene, Jeremy, and Scott Podolsky. "Keeping Modern in Medicine: Pharmaceutical Promotion and Physician Education in Postwar America." *Bulletin of the History of Medicine* 83, no. 2 (Summer 2009): 331–77.

Greenlee, Edwin J. "Biomedicine and Ideology: A Social History of the Conceptualization and Treatment of Essential Hypertension in the United States." Ph.D. dissertation, Temple University, 1989.

——. "Discourse, Foucault, and Critical Medical Anthropology." *Central Issues in Anthropology* 9, no. 1 (1991): 79–87.

Greenslit, Nathan. "Dep®ession and Consum♀tion: Psychopharmaceuticals, Branding, and New Identity Practices." *Culture, Medicine and Psychiatry* 29 (2005): 477–502

——. "Pharmaceutical Relationships: Intersections of Illness, Fantasy and Capital in the Age of Direct-to-Consumer Marketing." Ph.D. dissertation, Massachusetts Institute of Technology, 2007.

Greenslit, Nathan, and Joseph Dumit. *Medi(c)ating Illness: An Ethnographic Exploration of Women's Health in the Age of Direct to Consumer Advertising*. National Science Foundation Dissertation Improvement Grant (NSF Award 0426130), 2004.

Griggers, Cathy. "Lesbian Bodies in the Age of (Post)Mechanical Reproduction." In *The Lesbian Postmodern*, edited by Laura L. Doan, 118–33. New York: Columbia University Press, 1994.

Grim, C. E., et al. "Racial Differences in Blood Pressure Evans Co., Georgia: Relationship to Sodium Intake and Plasma Renin Activity." *Journal of Chronic Diseases* 33 (1980): 87–94.

Grim, C. E., T. W. Wilson, G. D. Nicholson, et al. "Blood Pressure in Blacks: Twin Studies in Barbados." *Hypertension* 15 (1990): 803–9.

Grim, Clarence, and Miguel Robinson. "Salt, Slavery and Survival: Hypertension in the African Diaspora." *Epidemiology* 14, no. 1 (January 2003): 120–22.

Grimm, R. H., K. L. Margolis, V. Papademetriou, W. C. Cushman, C. E. Ford, J. Bettencourt, M. H. Alderman, J. N. Baslie, H. R. Black, V. DeQuattro, J. Echfeldt, C. M. Hawkins, and M. Proschan, for the ALLHAT Collaborative Research Group. "Baseline Characteristics of the 42,448 High Risk Hypertensives Enrolled in the Antihypertensive and Lipid Lowering Treatment to Prevent Heart Attack Trial (ALLHAT)." *Hypertension* 37 (2001): 19–27.

Hacking, Ian. *Representing and Intervening: Introductory Topics in the Philosophy of Natural Science*. Cambridge: Cambridge University Press, 1983.

——. "The Self-Vindication of the Laboratory Sciences." In *Science as Practice and Culture*, edited by Andrew Pickering, 29–64. Chicago: University of Chicago Press, 1992.

Hadden, David R. "Holidays in Framingham?" *British Medical Journal* 325 (2002): 544.

Haga, Susanne B., and Geoffrey S. Ginsburg. "Prescribing BiDil: Is It Black and White?" *Journal of the American College of Cardiology* 48, no. 1 (2006): 12–14.

Hall, W. Dallas, Elijah Saunders, and Neil Shulman. *Hypertension in Blacks: Epidemiology, Pathophysiology, and Treatment*. Chicago: Year Book Medical Publishers, 1985.

Hamilton, Jennifer. "The Case of the Genetic Ancestor." In *Genetics and the Unsettled Past: The Collision of DNA, Race, and History*, edited by Keith Wailoo, Alondra Nelson, and Catherine Lee, 266–78. Piscataway, N.J.: Rutgers University Press, 2012.

Hammonds, Evelynn. "Missing Persons: Black Women and AIDS." *Radical America* 24 (1990): 7–24.

——. "New Technologies of Race." In *The Gendered Cyborg: A Reader*, edited by Gill Kirkup, Linda Janes, and Kath Woodward, and Fiona Hovenden, 305–18. New York: Routledge, 2000.

——. "Straw Men and Their Followers: The Return of Biological Race." *Social Science Research Council Forum: Is Race "Real"?* June 7, 2006. At http://raceandgenomics.ssrc.org/Hammonds/.

Hammonds, Evelynn, and Rebecca Herzig, eds. *The Nature of Difference: Sciences of Race in the United States from Jefferson to Genomics*. Cambridge: MIT Press, 2009.

Haraway, Donna. "Manifesto for Cyborgs: Science, Technology, and Socialist Feminism in the 1980's." *Socialist Review* 80 (1985): 65–108.

——. "Situated Knowledges: The Science Question in Feminism and the Privilege of Partial Perspective." *Feminist Studies* 14 (1988): 575–99.

——. *Modest_Witness@Second_Millenium.FemaleMan©_Meets_OncoMouse™: Feminism and Technoscience.* New York: Routledge, 1997.

Harding, Sandra G. *The Feminist Standpoint Theory Reader: Intellectual and Political Controversies.* New York: Routledge, 2004.

Harlan, Louis R. *Booker T. Washington: The Wizard of Tuskegee, 1901–1915.* New York: Oxford University Press, 1983.

Harlan, Louis R., and Raymond W. Smock. "Introduction." In *The Booker T. Washington Papers*, vol. 13, 1913–1914, edited by Louis R. Harlan and Raymond W. Smock. Urbana: University of Illinois Press, 1984.

Hartigan, John, Jr. "Establishing the Fact of Whiteness." In *Race, Identity, and Citizenship: A Reader*, edited by Rodolfo D. Torres, Louis F. Miron, and Jonathan Xavier India, 183–99. Malden, Mass.: Blackwell, 1999.

Hartman, Stephanie. "Reading the Scar in Breast Cancer Poetry." *Feminist Studies* 30 (2004): 155–77.

Harvard Business School. "Merck-Medco: Vertical Integration in the Pharmaceutical Industry." Case Study, HBS 9–598–091. Cambridge: Harvard Business School, 1998.

Hatch, Anthony. "The Politics of Metabolism: The Metabolic Syndrome and the Reproduction of Race and Racism." Ph.D. dissertation, University of Maryland, 2009.

Hayden, Cori. "A Generic Solution? Pharmaceuticals and the Politics of the Similar in Mexico." *Current Anthropology* 48, no. 4 (August 2007): 475–95.

Hazen, H. H. *Syphilis.* 2nd ed. St. Louis: Mosby, 1928.

——. "A Leading Cause of Death among the Negroes: Syphilis." *Journal of Negro Education* 6, no. 3 (1937): 310–21.

Healy, David. "Shaping the Intimate: Influences on the Experience of Everyday Nerves." *Social Studies of Science* 34, no. 2 (April 2004): 219–45.

Hertz, Robin P., Alan N. Unger, Jeffrey A. Cornell, and Elijah Saunders. "Racial Disparities in Hypertension Prevalence, Awareness, and Management." *Archives of Internal Medicine* 165, no. 18 (2005): 2098–104.

Herzberg, David L. *Happy Pills in America: From Miltown to Prozac.* Baltimore: Johns Hopkins University Press, 2009.

Hester, Jennifer. "Bricolage and Bodies of Knowledge: Exploring Consumer Responses to Controversy about the Third Generation Oral Contraceptive Pill." *Body and Society* 11, no. 3 (September 2005): 77–95.

Hindman, S. S. "Syphilis among Insane Negroes." *American Journal of Public Health* 5, no. 3 (1915): 218–24.

Hoberman, John. "Medical Racism and the Rhetoric of Exculpation: How Do Physicians Think about Race?" *New Literary History* 38 (2007): 505–25.

Hoffman, Frederick. *Race Traits and Tendencies of the Negro.* 1896; Reprint, New York: AMS Press, 1973.

Hoffman, Sharona. " 'Racially-Tailored' Medicine Unravelled." *American University Law Review* 55 (2005): 396–452.

Holloway, Edward E. "Approach to Cardiac Diagnosis." *Journal of the National Medical Association* 35, no. 2 (1943): 58–60.

Holmes, S. J. "The Principal Causes of Death among Negroes: A General Comparative Statement." *Journal of Negro Education* 6 (1937): 289–302.

Hoover, Eddie L. "There Is No Scientific Rationale for Race-Based Research." *Journal of the National Medical Association* 99, no. 6 (June 2007): 690–92.

Howell, Joel D. "The Changing Face of Twentieth-Century American Cardiology." *Annals of Internal Medicine* 105 (1986): 772–82.

Huggett, Brady. "BiDil Flops." *Nature Biotechnology* 26, no. 3 (March 2008): 252.

Hunt, Susan. "The Flexner Report and Black Academic Medicine: An Assignment of Place." *Journal of the National Medical Association* 85 (1993): 151–55.

Illich, Ivan. *Medical Nemesis.* New York: Pantheon, 1976.

Inda, Jonathan Xavier. "Materializing Hope: Racial Pharmaceuticals, Suffering Bodies, and Biological Citizenship." In *Corpus: An Interdisciplinary Reader on Bodies and Knowledge*, edited by Monica Casper and Paisley Currah, 61–80. New York: Palgrave-Macmillan, 2011.

Jackson, Algernon Brashear. "Public Health and the Negro." *Journal of the National Medical Association* 15 (1923): 256–59.

Jackson, Fatimah L. C. "A Response to George Armelagos' Commentary." *Transforming Anthropology* 13, no. 2 (October 2005): 125–35.

——. "Anthropological Science and the Salt-Hypertension Hypothesis." *Transforming Anthropology* 14, no. 2 (October 2006): 173–75.

Jacobson, Matthew Frye. *Whiteness of a Different Color: European Immigrants and the Alchemy of Race.* Cambridge: Harvard University Press, 1998.

Jasanoff, Sheila, ed. *States of Knowledge: The Co-production of Science and the Social Order.* New York: Routledge, 2004.

Jasanoff, Sheila, and Sang-Hyun Kim. "Containing the Atom: Sociotechnical Imaginaries and Nuclear Power in the United States and South Korea." *Minerva* 47 (2009): 119–46.

Jenks, Angela. "What's the Use of Culture? Heath Disparities and the Development of Culturally Competent Care." In *What's the Use of Race? Modern Governance and the Biology of Difference*, edited by Ian Whitmarsh and David S. Jones, 207–24. Cambridge: MIT Press, 2010.

JNMA. "On Dr. Taylor of Philadelphia." Editorial. *Journal of the National Medical Association* 7 (1915): 206–8.

Johnmar, Fard. "Conversations about Race-Based Medicine: NitroMed's Michael L. Sabolinksi." July 27, 2006. At http://fardj.prblogs.org/2006/06/27/conversations-about-race-based-medicine-nitromeds-michael-l-sabolinski-md/.

Jones, Camara. "Levels of Racism: A Theoretic Framework and a Gardener's Tale." *American Journal of Public Health* 90, no. 8 (2000): 1212–15.

Jones, David S. "Visions of a Cure: Visualization, Clinical Trials, and Controversies in Cardiac Therapeutics, 1968–1998." *Isis* 91, no. 3 (2000): 504–41.

——. "Virgin Soils Revisited." *William and Mary Quarterly* 60, no. 4 (October 2003): 703–42.

——. *Rationalizing Epidemics: Meanings and Uses of American Indian Mortality since 1600.* Cambridge: Harvard University Press, 2004.

Kahn, H. A. "Use of Computers in Analyzing Framingham Data." *Circulation Research* 11 (1962): 585–86.

Kahn, Jonathan. "How a Drug Becomes 'Ethnic': Law, Commerce, and the Production of Racial Categories in Medicine." *Yale Journal of Health Policy, Law, and Ethics* 4 (2004): 1–46.

——. "From Disparity to Difference: How Race-Specific Medicines May Undermine Policies to Address Inequalities in Health Care," *Southern California Interdisciplinary Law Journal* 15 (2005): 105–29.

——. "Misreading Race and Genomics after BiDil." Letter to the editor. *Nature Genetics* 37 (July 2005): 655–56.

——. "Exploiting Race in Drug Development: BiDil's Interim Model of Pharmaco-genomics." *Social Studies of Science* 38, no. 5 (October 2008): 737–58.

Kaiser, Robert M. "The Introduction of the Thiazides: A Case Study in Twentieth-Century Therapeutics." In *The Inside Story of Medicines: A Symposium*, edited by Gregory J. Higby and Elaine C. Stroud, 121–38. Madison, Wisc.: American Institute of the History of Pharmacy, 1997.

Kannel, William B. Letter to the editor. "The Framingham Study." *British Medical Journal* 2, no. 6046 (November 20, 1976): 1255.

Kannel, William B., Thomas R. Dawber, Abraham Kagan, Nicholas Revotskie, and Joseph Stokes III. "Factors of Risk in the Development of Coronary Heart Disease —Six-Year Follow-Up Experience." *Annals of Internal Medicine* 55 (July 1961): 33–50.

Kaufman, Jay S. "No More 'Slavery Hypothesis' Yarns." Letter to the editor. *Psychosomatic Medicine* 63 (2001): 324.

Kaufman, Jay S., and Susan A. Hall. "The Slavery Hypertension Hypothesis: Dissemination and Appeal of a Modern Race Theory." *Epidemiology* 14 (January 2003): 111–18.

Kawachi, Ichiro, and Peter Conrad. "Medicalization and the Pharmacological Treatment of Blood Pressure." In *Contested Ground: Public Purpose and Private Interest in the Regulation of Prescription Drugs*, edited by Peter Davis. New York: Oxford University Press, 1996.

Kenney, John A. "The Negro Hospital Renaissance." *Journal of the National Medical Association* 22 (July–September 1930): 109–12.

Keller, Evelyn Fox. *The Century of the Gene*. Cambridge: Harvard University Press, 2000.

Kelly, Ann, and P. Wenzel Geissler. "The Value of Transnational Medical Research." *Journal of Cultural Economy* 4 (2011): 3–10.

Kempner, Walter. "Treatment of Heart and Kidney Disease and of Hypertensive and Arteriosclerotic Vascular Disease with the Rice Diet." *Annals of Internal Medicine* 31 (1949): 821–56.

Kimberley, Margaret. "Rx for Black Hearts." *Black Commentator*, no. 143 (June 23, 2005). At http://www.blackcommentator.com/143/143_freedom_rider_rx.html; also at Alternet as "A Bitter Pill for Black Hearts," http://www.alternet.org/story/23185/.

Kirk, Dudley. "Demographic Transition Theory." *Population Studies* 50, no. 3 (1996): 361–87.

Klag, M. J., P. K. Whelton, and J. Coresh, et al. "The Association of Skin Color with Blood Pressure in US Blacks with Low Socioeconomic Status." *JAMA* 265 (February 6, 1991): 599–602.

Klawiter, Maren. *The Biopolitics of Breast Cancer: Changing Cultures of Disease and Activism*. Minneapolis: University of Minnesota Press, 2008.

Klein, Naomi. *No Logo: Taking Aim at the Brand Bullies*. New York: Picador, 2000.

Kleinman, Arthur. *What Really Matters: Living a Moral Life amidst Uncertainty and Danger*. New York: Oxford University Press, 2006.

Krieger, Nancy. "Embodying Inequality: A Review of the Concepts, Measures, and Methods for Studying Health Consequences of Discrimination." *International Journal of Health Services* 29, no. 2 (1999): 295–352.

——. "Does Racism Harm Health? Did Child Abuse Exist before 1962? On Explicit Questions, Critical Science, and Current Controversies: An Ecosocial Perspective." *American Journal of Public Health* 93 (2003): 194–99.

——. "Stormy Weather: Race, Gene Expression, and the Science of Health Disparities." *American Journal of Public Health* 95 (2005): 2155–60.

Lakoff, Andrew. "The Anxieties of Globalization: Antidepressant Sales and Economic Crisis in Argentina." *Social Studies of Science* 34 (2004): 247–69.

Landecker, Hannah. "Immortality, in Vitro: A History of the HeLa Cell Line," In *Biotechnology and Culture: Bodies, Anxieties, Ethics*, edited by Paul Brodwin, 53–72. Bloomington: University of Indiana Press, 2000.

Latour, Bruno. *Science in Action: How to Follow Scientists and Engineers through Society*. Cambridge: Harvard University Press, 1987.

——. "Technology Is Society Made Durable." In *Sociology of Monsters: Essays on Power, Technology and Domination*, edited by John Law, 103–31. London: Routledge, 1991.

——. *We Have Never Been Modern*. Translated by Catherine Porter. Cambridge: Harvard University Press, 1993.

Latour, Bruno, and Michel Callon. "Unscrewing the Big Leviathan: How Actors Macro-Structure Reality and How Sociologists Help Them to Do So." In *Advances in Social Theory and Methodology: Toward an Integration of Micro- and Macro-Sociologies*, edited by K. Knorr-Cetina and A. V. Cicourel, 277–303. London: Routledge and Kegan Paul.

Lauretis, Teresa de. *Technologies of Gender*. Bloomington: Indiana University Press, 1987.

Lawrence, Christopher. "'Definite and Material': Coronary Thrombosis and Cardiologists in the 1920s." In *Framing Disease: Studies in Cultural History*, edited by Charles E. Rosenberg and Janet Lynne Golden, 50–82. New Brunswick: Rutgers University Press, 1992.

Lee, Sandra Soo-Jin. "Racializing Drug Design: Implications of Pharmacogenomics for Health Disparities." *American Journal of Public Health* 95, no. 12 (2005): 2133–38.

Leibowitz, J. O. *The History of Coronary Heart Disease*. Berkeley: University of California Press, 1970.

Lerner, Barron H. *The Breast Cancer Wars: Hope, Fear, and the Pursuit of a Cure in 20th-Century America*. New York: Oxford University Press, 2001.

Lévi-Strauss, Claude. *Totemism*. Translated by Rodney Needham. Boston: Beacon Press, 1963.

Levitt, Steven D., and Stephen J. Dubner. *Freakonomics: A Rogue Economist Explores the Hidden Side of Everything*. New York: William Morrow, 2005.

Levy, Daniel, and Susan Brink. *A Change of Heart: How the Framingham Heart Study Helped Unravel the Mysteries of Cardiovascular Disease*. New York: Random House, 2005.

Lewontin, Richard. "The Apportionment of Human Diversity." *Evolutionary Biology* 6 (1972): 391–98.

Lilienfeld, David E. "Louis I. Dublin and the Development of the Observational Study: The Metropolitan Life Insurance Company Natural History (Cohort) Studies of Typhoid Fever and Scarlet Fever." *Annals of Epidemiology* 19, no. 6 (2009): 410–15.

Littlefield, Melissa. "Constructing the Organ of Deceit: The Rhetoric of fMRI and Brain Fingerprinting in Post-9/11 America." *Science, Technology and Human Values* 34, no. 3 (2009): 365–92.

Lock, Margaret. "Eclipse of the Gene and the Return of Divination." *Current Anthropology* 46 (December 2005): S47–S70.

Lorde, Audre. *The Cancer Journals*. San Francisco: Aunt Lute Books, 1980.

Löwy, Ilana. *Between Bench and Bedside: Science, Healing, and Interleukin-2 in a Cancer Ward*. Cambridge: Harvard University Press, 1997.

Lynch, James J. *The Broken Heart: The Medical Consequences of Loneliness*. New York: Basic Books, 1977.

Lynch, Michael, Simon A. Cole, and Ruth McNally, eds. *The Truth Machine: The Contentious History of DNA Fingerprinting*. Chicago: University of Chicago Press, 2008.

MacKinnon, Catharine. "Difference and Dominance: On Sex Discrimination." In *Feminism Unmodified*, 32–45. Cambridge: Harvard University Press, 1987.

Mackowiak, Philip A., ed. "Racial Characteristics." In *Post-mortem: Solving History's Great Medical Mysteries*, 305–38. Philadelphia: American College of Physicians, 2007.

Malik, Kenan. "A Colour Coded Prescription." BBC Radio 4, November 17, 2005. At http://www.kenanmalik.com/tv/analysis_race+medicine.html.

Mamo, Laura, and Jennifer R. Fishman. "Potency in All the Right Places: Viagra as a Technology of the Gendered Body." *Body and Society* 7 (2001): 13–35.

Mann, G. V., G. Pearson, T. Gordon, and T. R. Dawber. "Diet and Cardiovascular Disease in the Framingham Study." *American Journal of Clinical Nutrition* 11, no. 3 (September 1962): 200–225.

Maren, Thomas. "Diuretics and Renal Drug Development." In *Renal Physiology: People and Ideas*, edited by Carl W. Gottschalk, Robert W. Berliner, and Gerhard H. Giebisch, 407–36. Bethesda, Md.: American Physiological Society, 1987.

Marks, Harry M. *The Progress of Experiment: Science and Therapeutic Reform in the United States, 1900–1990.* Cambridge: Cambridge University Press, 1997.

Martin, Emily. "The Pharmaceutical Person." *BioSocieties* 1 (2006): 273–87.

——. *Bipolar Expeditions: Mania and Depression in American Culture.* Princeton: Princeton University Press, 2007.

Marx, Karl. *Capital.* Volume 1. Translated by Ben Fowkes. London: Penguin, 1990.

Massumi, Brian. *Parables for the Virtual: Movement, Affect, Sensation.* Durham: Duke University Press, 2002.

Materson, Barry J. "Variability in Response to Anti-hypertensive Drug Treatment." Comment. *Hypertension* 43 (2004): 1166–67.

Mauss, Marcel. *The Gift: Forms and Functions of Exchange in Primitive Societies.* Glencoe, Ill.: Free Press, 1954.

May, Elaine Tyler. *America and the Pill: A History of Promise, Peril, and Liberation.* New York: Basic Books, 2010.

McBride, David. *From TB to AIDS: Epidemics among Urban Blacks since 1900.* Albany: SUNY Press, 1991.

McDermott, Monica, and Frank L. Samson. "White Racial and Ethnic Identity in the United States." *Annual Review of Sociology* 31 (2005): 245–61.

McDonough, John R., Curtis G. Hames, Sarah C. Stulb, and Glen E. Garrison. "Cardiovascular Disease Field Study in Evans County, Ga." *Public Health Reports* 78, no. 12 (December 1963): 1051–60.

McGoey, Linsey. "Pharmaceutical Controversies and the Performative Value of Uncertainty." *Science as Culture* 18, no. 2 (June 2009): 151–64.

Meltzer, Jay I. "A Specialist in Clinical Hypertension Critiques ALLHAT." *American Journal of Hypertension* 16 (May 2003): 416–20.

Menard, J. "Oil and Water? Economic Advantage and Biomedical Progress Do Not Mix Well in a Government Guidelines Committee." *American Journal of Hypertension* 7 (1994): 877–85.

Metzl, Jonathan. *Prozac on the Couch: Prescribing Gender in the Era of Wonder Drugs.* Durham: Duke University Press, 2003.

——. *The Protest Psychosis: How Schizophrenia Became a Black Disease.* Boston: Beacon Press, 2010.

Michaels, Leon. *The Eighteenth-Century Origins of Angina Pectoris: Predisposing Causes, Recognition, and Aftermath*. London: Wellcome Trust, 2001.

Michener, James. *Hawaii*. New York: Random House, 1959.

Mihaly, John P., and Neville C. Whiteman. "Myocardial Infarction in the Negro: Historical Survey as It Relates to Negroes." *American Journal of Cardiology* 2, no. 4 (October 1958): 464–74.

Millman, Joel, "Going Nativist: How the Press Paints a False Picture of the Effects of Immigration." *Columbia Journalism Review* (January/February 1999). At http://archives.cjr.org/year/99/1/nativist.asp.

Mitchell, Robert, and Catherine Waldby. "National Biobanks: Clinical Labor, Risk Protection, and the Creation of Biovalue." *Science, Technology and Human Values* 35, no. 3 (2010): 330–55.

Mokwe, Evan, Suzanne E. Ohmit, Samar A. Nasser, Tariq Shafi, Elijah Saunders, Errol Crook, Amanda Dudley, and John M. Flack. "Determinants of Blood Pressure Response to Quinapril in Black and White Hypertensive Patients." *Hypertension* 43 (2004): 1202–7.

Mol, Annemarie. *The Body Multiple: Ontology in Medical Practice*. Durham: Duke University Press, 2002.

Moloney, Kevin. *Rethinking Public Relations: PR, Propaganda, and Democracy*. New York: Routledge, 2000.

Montoya, Michael. *Making the Mexican Diabetic: Race, Science, and the Genetics of Inequality*. Berkeley: University of California Press, 2011.

Moore, Felix E. "Committee on Design and Analysis of Studies." *American Journal of Public Health* 50 (1960): S10–S19.

Moore, William W. *Fighting for Life: The Story of the American Heart Association, 1911–1975*. Dallas: American Heart Association, 1983.

Moser, Marvin. "Epidemiology of Hypertension with Particular Reference to Racial Susceptibility." *Annals of the New York Academy of Sciences* 84 (1960): 989–99.

Mouffe, Chantal. "Deconstruction, Pragmatism, and the Politics of Democracy." In *Deconstruction and Pragmatism*, ed. Chantal Mouffe, 1–12. New York: Routledge, 1997.

Munly, William C. "Problems in the Prevention and Relief of Heart Disease." *American Journal of Public Health and the Nation's Health* 18 (September 1928): 1098–104.

National High Blood Pressure Education Program. *The Seventh Report of the Joint National Committee on Prevention, Detection, Evaluation, and Treatment of High Blood Pressure (JNC 7)*, December 2003. At http://www.nhlbi.nih.gov/.

Nelkin, Dorothy, and Laurence Tancredi. *Dangerous Diagnostics: The Social Power of Biological Information*. New York: Basic Books, 1989.

Nelson, Alondra. "Bio Science: Genetic Genealogy Testing and the Pursuit of African Ancestry." *Social Studies of Science* 38 (2008): 759–83.

———. "The Factness of Diaspora: The Social Sources of Genetic Genealogy Testing."

In *Revisiting Race in a Genomic Age*, edited by Barbara Koenig, Sandra Soo-Jin Lee, and Sarah S. Richardson, 253–70. Piscataway, N.J.: Rutgers University Press, 2008.

——. "The Inclusion-and-Difference Paradox: Review of *Inclusion: The Politics of Difference in Medical Research*, by Steven Epstein. *Social Identities* 15, no. 5 (September 2009): 741–43.

——. *Body and Soul: The Black Panther Party and the Fight against Medical Discrimination.* Minneapolis: University of Minnesota Press, 2011.

Nguyen, Vinh-Kim. "Antiretroviral Globalism, Biopolitics, and Therapeutic Citizenship." In *Global Assemblages: Technology, Politics, and Ethics as Anthropological Problems*, edited by Aihwa Ong and Stephen Collier, 124–44. Malden, Mass.: Blackwell, 2005.

NHLBI [National Heart, Lung, and Blood Institute]. Congestive Heart Failure Fact Sheet. At http://library.thinkquest.org/27533/facts.html.

——. "Data Fact Sheet: Congestive Heart Failure in the United States: A New Epidemic." September 1996. At http://www.vidyya.com/2pdfs/dfschf.pdf.

——. "Framingham Heart Study: Design, Rationale, and Objectives." At http://www.nhlbi.nih.gov/about/framingham/design.htm.

——. "Jackson Heart Study: Design, Rationale, and Objectives." At http://www.nhlbi.nih.gov/about/jackson/2ndpg.htm.

NHLBI and Boston University. *You Changed America's Heart: A 50th Anniversary Tribute to the Participants in the Framingham Heart Study.* Pamphlet. 1998.

Nissen, Steven E. "Report from the Cardiovascular and Renal Drugs Advisory Committee: U.S. Food and Drug Administration; June 15–16, 2005; Gaithersburg, Md." *Circulation* 112 (2005): 2043–46.

Omi, Michael, and Howard Winant. *Racial Formation in the United States: From the 1960s to the 1990s.* 2nd ed. New York: Routledge, 1994.

Omran, A. R. "The Epidemiologic Transition: A Theory of the Epidemiology of Population Change." *Milbank Quarterly* 49, no. 4 (1971): 509–38.

Oppenheimer, Gerald. "Becoming the Framingham Study, 1947–1950." *American Journal of Public Health* 95 (2005): 602–10.

——. "Profiling Risk: The Emergence of Coronary Heart Disease Epidemiology in the United States (1940–1970)." *International Journal of Epidemiology* 35 (2006): 720–30.

Osborne, Newton G., and Marvin D. Feit. "The Use of Race in Medical Research." *JAMA* 267 (1992): 275–79.

Page, Irvine H. *Hypertension Research: A Memoir, 1920–1960.* New York: Pergamon Press, 1988.

Parthasarathy, Shobita. *Building Genetic Medicine: Breast Cancer, Technology, and the Comparative Politics of Health Care.* Cambridge: MIT Press, 2007.

Patton, Cindy. "Migratory Vices." In *Queer Diasporas*, edited by Cindy Patton and Benigno Sanchez-Eppler, 15–36. Durham: Duke University Press, 2000.

Payne, Thomas J., et al. "Sociocultural Methods in the Jackson Heart Study: Conceptual and Descriptive Overview, Ethnicity and Disease." *Ethnicity and Disease* 15 (Autumn 2005): S6-38–48.

Peniston, Reginald L., and Otelio S. Randall. "Coronary Artery Disease in Black Americans, 1920–1960: The Shaping of Medical Opinion." *Journal of the National Medical Association* 81, no. 5 (1989): 591–600.

Penner, D'Ann R., and Keith C. Ferdinand, eds. *Overcoming Katrina: African American Voices from the Crescent City and Beyond.* New York: Palgrave Macmillan, 2009.

Persson, Asha. "Incorporating *Pharmakon*: HIV, Medicine, and Body Shape Change." *Body and Society* 10 (2004): 45–67.

Peters, Rosalind M. "Racism and Hypertension among African Americans." *Western Journal of Nursing* 26, no. 6 (2004): 612–31.

Petryna, Adriana. *Life Exposed: Biological Citizens after Chernobyl.* Princeton: Princeton University Press, 2002.

Pollock, Anne. "Cultural Economy of Racialized Pharmaceuticals in the U.S.," in *Value of Transnational Medical Research: Labour, Participation and Care,* edited by Ann Kelly and P. Wenzel Geissler. London: Routledge, 2012.

——. "Pharmaceutical Meaning-Making beyond Marketing: Racialized Subjects of Generic Thiazide." *Journal of Law, Medicine, and Ethics* 36, no. 3 (September 2008): 530–36.

——. "Reading Friedan toward a Feminist Articulation of Heart Disease." *Body and Society* 16, no. 4 (2010): 77–97.

——. "Transforming the Critique of Big Pharma." *BioSocieties* 6, no. 1 (March 2011): 106–18.

Porter, Theodore M. *Trust in Numbers: The Pursuit of Objectivity in Science and Public Life.* Princeton: Princeton University Press, 1995.

Postel-Vinay, Nicolas, ed. *A Century of Arterial Hypertension: 1896–1996.* Chichester, England: Wiley, 1996.

Postel-Vinay, Nicolas, and Pierre Corvol. *Le retour du Dr Knock: Essai sur le risque cardiovasculaire.* Paris: Editions Odile Jacob, 2000.

Puckrein, Gary A. "The Acquisitive Impulse: Plantation Society, Factions, and the Origins of the Barbadian Civil War (1627–1652)." Ph.D. dissertation, Brown University, 1978.

——. *Little England: Plantation Society and Anglo-Barbadian Politics, 1627–1700.* New York: New York University Press, 1984.

Rabinow, Paul. "Artificiality and Enlightenment: From Sociobiology to Biosociality." *Essays on the Anthropology of Reason,* 91–111. Princeton: Princeton University Press, 1996.

Race, Kane. *Pleasure Consuming Medicine: The Queer Politics of Drugs.* Durham: Duke University Press, 2009.

Rajan, Kaushik Sunder. *Biocapital: The Constitution of Postgenomic Life.* Durham: Duke University Press, 2006.

Rankins, J., J. Wortham, and L. L. Brown. "Modifying Soul Food for the Dietary

Approaches to Stop Hypertension Diet (DASH) Plan: Implications for Metabolic Syndrome (DASH of Soul)." *Ethnicity and Disease* 17 (Suppl 4) (Summer 2007): S4–7-12.

Rapp, Rayna. "Cell Life and Death, Child Life and Death: Genomic Horizons, Genetic Diseases, Family Stories." In *Remaking Life and Death: Toward an Anthropology of the Biosciences*, edited by Sarah Franklin and Margaret Lock, 129–64. Santa Fe: School of American Research Press, 2003.

Rasmussen, Nicolas. "The Moral Economy of the Drug Company—Medical Scientist Collaboration in Interwar America." *Social Studies of Science* 34, no. 2 (2004): 161–85.

Reardon, Jenny. *Race to the Finish: Identity and Governance in an Age of Genomics*. Princeton: Princeton University Press, 2004.

——. "Race and Biology: Beyond the Perpetual Return of Crisis." In "Race and Genomics: Old Wine in New Bottles? Documents from a Transdisciplinary Discussion," *NTM International Journal of the History of Science, Technology and Medicine* 16 (2008): 373–77.

——. "The Democratic, Anti-racist Genome? Technoscience at the Limits of Liberalism." *Science as Culture* 21, no. 1 (2012): 25–47.

——. "The Postgenomic Condition: Technoscience at the Limits of Liberal Democratic Imaginaries." Unpublished manuscript.

Reiser, Stanley Joel. *Medicine and the Reign of Technology*. Cambridge: Cambridge University Press, 1978.

"Report of the Committee on Medical Education on Colored Hospitals." *Journal of the National Medical Association* 2 (1910): 283–91.

"Report of the Joint National Committee on Detection, Evaluation, and Treatment of High Blood Pressure." *JAMA* 237, no. 3 (January 17, 1977): 255–61.

Reverby, Susan, ed. *Tuskegee's Truths: Rethinking the Tuskegee Syphilis Study*. Chapel Hill: University of North Carolina Press, 2000.

Riska, Elianne. "The Rise and Fall of Type A Man." *Social Science and Medicine* 51 (2000): 1665–74.

——. "From Type A Man to the Hardy Man: Masculinity and Health." *Sociology of Health and Illness* 24, no. 3 (2002): 347–58.

Roberts, Charles Stewart. *Life and Writings of Stewart R. Roberts, M.D.: Georgia's First Heart Specialist*. Spartanburg, S.C.: Reprint Company Publishers, 1993.

Roberts, Dorothy. *Killing the Black Body: Race, Reproduction, and the Meaning of Liberty*. New York: Pantheon Books, 1997.

——. "Is Race-Based Medicine Good for Us? African American Approaches to Race, Biomedicine, and Equality." *Journal of Law, Medicine and Ethics* 36, no. 3 (September 2008): 537–45.

——. "Race and the New Biocitizen." In *What's the Use of Race? Modern Governance and the Biology of Difference*, edited by Ian Whitmarsh and David S. Jones, 259–76. Cambridge: MIT Press, 2010.

——. *Fatal Invention: How Science, Politics, and Big Business Re-create Race in the Twenty-First Century*. New York: New Press Books, 2011.

Roberts, Stewart R. "The Larger View of Heart Disease." *Southern Medical Journal* 18 (1925): 391–95.

——. "Nervous and Mental Influences in Angina Pectoris." *American Heart Journal* 7 (1931): 21–35

Rodwin, Marc A. "Drug Advertising, Continuing Medical Education, and Physician Prescribing: A Historical Review and Reform Proposal." *Journal of Law, Medicine and Ethics* 38, no. 4 (Winter 2010): 807–15.

Roman, C. V. "Vitality of the Negroes: Comparison of Death Rate with That of the Whites." *Journal of the National Medical Association* 2, no. 3 (July–September 1910): 180–81.

Rose, Nikolas. *The Politics of Life Itself: Biomedicine, Power, and Subjectivity in the Twenty-First Century*. Princeton: Princeton University Press, 2006.

——. "Race, Risk and Medicine in the Age of 'Your Own Personal Genome.'" *BioSocieties* 3, no. 4 (December 2008): 423–39.

Rose, Nikolas, and Carlos Novas. "Biological Citizenship." In *Global Assemblages: Technology, Politics, and Ethics as Anthropological Problems*, edited by Aihwa Ong and Stephen Collier, 439–63. Oxford: Blackwell, 2005.

Rosenberg, Charles E. "What Is Disease? In Memory of Owsei Temkin." *Bulletin of the History of Medicine* 77, no. 3 (Fall 2003): 491–505.

Rosengarten, Marsha. *HIV Interventions: Biomedicine and the Traffic between Information and Flesh*. Seattle: University of Washington Press, 2009.

Rothstein, William G. *Public Health and the Risk Factor: A History of an Uneven Medical Revolution*. Rochester: University of Rochester Press, 2003.

Sade, Robert M. "What's Right (and Wrong) with Racially Stratified Research and Therapies." *Journal of the National Medical Association* 99, no. 6 (June 2007): 693–96.

Sailer, Steve. "Race Flat-Earthers Dangerous to Everyone's Health." May 11, 2003. At http://www.vdare.com/.

Samsky, Ari. "Since We Are Taking the Drugs: Labor and Value in Two International Drug Donation Programs." *Journal of Cultural Economy* 4, no. 1 (2011): 27–43.

Sankar, Pamela, and Jonathan Kahn. "BiDil: Race Medicine or Race Marketing?" *Health Affairs* 24 (July–December 2005): W5-455–63.

Savitt, Todd L. "Abraham Flexner and the Black Medical Schools." In *Race and Medicine in Nineteenth- and Early-Twentieth-Century America*, 252–66. Kent, Ohio: Kent State University Press, 2007.

Schwab, Edward H., and Victor E. Schulze. "Heart Disease in the American Negro of the South." *American Heart Journal* 7 (1932): 710–17.

Scott, James. *Seeing Like a State: How Certain Schemes to Improve the Human Condition Have Failed*. New Haven: Yale University Press, 1999.

Sehgal, Ashwini R. "Overlap between Whites and Blacks in Response to Antihypertensive Drugs." *Hypertension* 43 (2004): 566–72.

Sempos, Christopher T., Diane E. Bild, and Teri Manolio. "Overview of the Jackson Heart Study: A Study of Cardiovascular Diseases in African American Men and Women." *American Journal of the Medical Sciences* 317, no. 3 (March 1999): 142–46.

Shah, Nayan. *Contagious Divides: Epidemics and Race in San Francisco's Chinatown.* Berkeley: University of California Press, 2001.

Shamsham, Fadi, and Judith Mitchell. "Essentials of the Diagnosis of Heart Failure." *American Family Physician* 61, no. 5 (2000): 1319–28.

Shim, Janet K. "Bio-power and Racial, Class, and Gender Formation in Biomedical Knowledge Production." *Research in the Sociology of Health Care* 17 (2000): 173–95.

——. "Understanding the Routinised Inclusion of Race, Socioeconomic Status and Sex in Epidemiology: The Utility of Concepts from Technoscience Studies." *Sociology of Health and Illness* 24, no. 2 (2002): 129–50.

——. "Constructing 'Race' across the Science-Lay Divide: Racial Formation in the Epidemiology and Experience of Cardiovascular Disease." *Social Studies of Science* 35, no. 3 (2005): 405–36.

Skinner, David. "Racialised Futures: Biologism and the Changing Politics of Identity." *Social Studies of Science* 36, no. 3 (2006): 459–88.

——. "Groundhog Day? The Strange Case of Sociology, Race and 'Science.'" *Sociology* 41, no. 5 (2007): 931–43.

Sloane, David Charles, and Beverlie Conant Sloane. *Medicine Moves to the Mall.* Baltimore: Johns Hopkins University Press, 2003.

Smedley, B. D., A. Y. Stith, and A. R. Nelson, eds. *Unequal Treatment: Confronting Racial and Ethnic Disparities in Health Care.* Washington: National Academies Press, 2002.

Smith, David Barton. *Health Care Divided: Race and Healing a Nation.* Ann Arbor: University of Michigan Press, 1999.

Smith, Lindsay. *Subversive Genes: Re(con)stituting Identity, Family, and Human Rights in Argentina.* Ph.D. dissertation, Harvard University, 2008.

Smith, Susan. *Sick of Being Sick and Tired: Black Women's Health Activism in America, 1890–1950.* Philadelphia: University of Pennsylvania Press, 1995.

Smith, T. Manuel. "Coronary Atherosclerosis in the Negro." *Journal of the National Medical Association* 38, no. 6 (1946): 193–202.

Sontag, Susan. *Illness as Metaphor.* New York: Farrar, Straus and Giroux, 1978.

Stark, David. *The Sense of Dissonance: Accounts of Worth in Economic Life.* Princeton: Princeton University Press, 2009.

Steenburgh, Jason van. "Diuretics for Hypertension Get a Big Boost, But Will Data Change Prescribing Patterns?" *American College of Physicians Observer,* April 2003, at http://www.acpinternist.org/.

Stevens, Rosemary. *In Sickness and in Wealth: American Hospitals in the Twentieth Century.* New York: Basic Books, 1989.

Stocking, George, Jr. "The Turn-of-the-Century Concept of Race." *Modernism/Modernity* 1, no. 1 (1994): 4–16.

Stoler, Ann Laura. *Race and the Education of Desire: Foucault's History of Sexuality and the Colonial Order of Things*. Durham: Duke University Press, 1995.

——. "Racial Histories and Their Regimes of Truth." *Political Power and Social Theory* 11 (1997): 183–206.

——. *Along the Archival Grain: Epistemic Anxieties and Colonial Common Sense*. Princeton: Princeton University Press, 2009.

Susser, Mervyn. "Epidemiology in the United States after World War II: The Evolution of Technique." *Epidemiologic Reviews* 7 (1985): 147–77.

Tallbear, Kimberly. "Narratives of Race and Indigeneity in the National Genographic Project." *Journal of Law, Medicine and Ethics* 35, no. 3 (Fall 2007): 412–24.

Tapper, Melbourne. *In the Blood: Sickle Cell Anemia and the Politics of Race*. Philadelphia: University of Pennsylvania Press, 1999.

Taylor, A. L., S. Ziesche, C. Yancy, P. Carson, R. D'Agostino Jr., K. Ferdinand, M. Taylor, K. Adams, M. Sabolinski, M. Worcel, and J. N. Cohn; the African-American Heart Failure Trial Investigators. "Combination of Isosorbide Dinitrate and Hydralazine in Blacks with Heart Failure." *New England Journal of Medicine* 351 (2004): 2049–57.

Taylor, Herman A. "The Jackson Heart Study: An Overview." *Ethnicity and Disease* 15 (Autumn 2005): S6-1–3.

Taylor, Herman A., et al. "Toward Resolution of Cardiovascular Health Disparities in African Americans: Design and Methods of the Jackson Heart Study." *Ethnicity and Disease* 15 (Autumn 2005) (Suppl 6): S6 4–17.

Taylor, J. Madison. "Remarks on the Health of the Colored People." Address to the Colored Convention, Varrick Memorial Temple, February. *Journal of the National Medical Association* 7 (1915): 160–63.

Taylor, Verta. *Rock-a-By Baby: Feminism, Self-Help, and Post-partum Depression*. New York: Routledge, 1996.

Temple, Robert, and Norman L. Stockbridge. "BiDil for Heart Failure in Black Patients: The U.S. Food and Drug Administration Perspective." *Annals of Internal Medicine* 146 (January 2, 2007): 57–62.

Terry, C. E. "The Negro: His Relation to Public Health in the South." *American Journal of Public Health* 3 (1913): 300–306.

Thomas, Patricia. "In the Trenches of Framingham." *Medical World News*, October 12, 1987, 68–70.

Thompson, Warren S. "Population." *American Journal of Sociology* 34, no. 6 (May 1929): 959–75.

Timmermans, Stefan. "Making the Case for Heart Disease." In *Postmortem: How Medical Examiners Explain Suspicious Deaths*, 35–73. Chicago: University of Chicago Press, 2006.

Timmermans, Stefan, and Marc Berg. *The Gold Standard: The Challenge of Evidence-Based Medicine and Standardization in Health Care*. Philadelphia: Temple University Press,

2003.

Tobbell, Dominique. "Allied against Reform: Pharmaceutical Industry–Academic Physician Relations in the United States, 1945–1970." *Bulletin of the History of Medicine* 82, no. 4 (Winter 2008): 878–912.

Tomes, Nancy. "The Great American Medicine Show Revisited." *Bulletin of the History of Medicine* 79, no. 4 (Winter 2005): 627–63.

Tone, Andrea. *Devices and Desires: A History of Contraceptives in America*. New York: Hill and Wang, 1994.

Townes, Emilie M. *Breaking the Fine Rain of Death: African American Health Issues and a Womanist Ethic of Care*. New York: Continuum, 1998.

Trask, Larry. "Guide to Punctuation: Scare Quotes." University of Sussex, England. At http://www.cogs.susx.ac.uk/.

Turkle, Sherry. "Whither Psychoanalysis in Computer Culture?" *Psychoanalytic Psychology* 21 (2004): 16–30.

——, ed. *Evocative Objects: Things We Think With*. Cambridge: MIT Press, 2007.

——. *Alone Together: Why We Expect More from Technology and Less from Each Other*. New York: Basic Books, 2011.

Tutton, Richard. "Promising Pessimism: Reading the Futures to Be Avoided in Biotech." *Social Studies of Science* 41, no. 3 (June 2011): 411–29.

Vonderlehr, R. A. "Untreated Syphilis in the Male Negro." *Venereal Disease Information* 17 (1936): 260–65.

Vrecko, Scott. "Birth of a Brain Disease: Science, the State and Addiction Neuropolitics." *History of the Human Sciences* 23, no. 4 (2010): 52–67.

Wade, Peter. *Race, Nature and Culture: An Anthropological Perspective*. London: Pluto Press, 2002.

Wagner, Sarah. *To Know Where He Lies: DNA Technology and the Search for Srebrenica's Missing*. Berkeley: University of California Press, 2008.

Wailoo, Keith. *Dying in the City of the Blues: Sickle Cell Anemia and the Politics of Race and Health*. Chapel Hill: University of North Carolina Press, 2001.

——. "Stigma, Race, and Disease in 20th Century America." *Lancet* 367 (2006): 531–33.

——. *How Cancer Crossed the Color Line*. Oxford: Oxford University Press, 2011.

Wailoo, Keith, and Stephen Pemberton. *The Troubled Dream of Genetic Medicine: Ethnicity and Innovation in Tay-Sachs, Cystic Fibrosis, and Sickle Cell Disease*. Baltimore: Johns Hopkins University Press, 2006.

Wald, Priscilla. *Contagious: Cultures, Carriers, and the Outbreak Narrative*. Durham: Duke University Press, 2008.

Washington, Harriet A. *Medical Apartheid: The Dark History of Medical Experimentation on Black Americans from Colonial Times to the Present*. New York: Doubleday, 2006.

Watson, Karol E., and Greg Fonarow. "Adherence to Best Practices: How Do Patient

Race and Gender Affect Physician Performance?" *Cardiovascular Risk Reports* 1 (2007): 102–7.

Weatherford, W. D. *Negro Life in the South: Present Conditions and Needs*. Rev. ed. New York: New York Association Press, 1918.

Weiner, Kate. "Exploring Genetic Responsibility for the Self, Family and Kin in the Case of Hereditary Raised Cholesterol." *Social Science and Medicine* 72 (June 2011): 1760–67.

Weiner, Kate, and Paul Martin. "A Genetic Future for Coronary Heart Disease?" *Sociology of Health and Illness* 30, no. 3 (2008): 380–95.

Weisse, Allen B. *Heart to Heart: The Twentieth-Century Battle against Cardiac Disease: An Oral History*. New Brunswick: Rutgers University Press, 2002.

Welsing, Frances Cress. "Blacks, Hypertension, and the Active Skin Melanocyte." *Urban Health* 4 (1975): 64–72.

——. *The Isis Papers: The Keys to the Colors*. Chicago: Third World Press, 1990.

West, C. S'thembile. "Honoring the Body: Rituals of Breath and Breathing." In *Faith, Health, and Healing in African American Life*, edited by Stephanie Mitchem and Emilie M. Townes, 96–108. Westport, Conn.: Praeger, 2008.

West, Cornel. "On Prophetic Pragmatism." In *The Cornel West Reader*, 149–74. New York: Basic Books, 1999.

Wheelwright, Jeff. "Human, Study Thyself: Learning Series: Genes, Race, and Medicine." *Discover* 26, no. 3 (March 2005). At http://discovermagazine.com/.

White, Paul Dudley. *Heart Disease*. New York: Macmillan, 1931.

White, Paul Dudley, with Margaret Parton. *My Life and Medicine: An Autobiographical Memoir*. Boston: Gambit, 1971.

Whitmarsh, Ian. "Biomedical Ambivalence: Asthma Diagnosis, the Pharmaceutical, and Other Contradictions in Barbados." *American Ethnologist* 35, no. 1 (February 2008): 49–63.

Williams, Patricia. "Spare Parts, Family Values, Old Children, Cheap." In *Critical Race Feminism: A Reader*, edited by Adrien Katherine Wing, 159–66. New York: New York University Press, 1997.

Williams, Richard Allen. *Textbook of Black Related Diseases*. New York: McGraw-Hill, 1975.

——. *Eliminating Healthcare Disparities in America: Beyond the IOM Report*. Totowa, N.J.: Humana Press, 2007.

Williams, Simon J., Paul Martin, and Jonathan Gabe. "The Pharmaceuticalisation of Society? A Framework for Analysis." *Sociology of Health and Illness* 33, no. 5 (July 2011): 710–25.

Wilson, Elizabeth. *Psychosomatic: Feminism and the Neurological Body*. Durham: Duke University Press, 2004.

——. "The Work of Antidepressants: Preliminary Notes on How to Build an Alliance between Feminism and Psychopharmacology." *BioSocieties* 1 (2006): 125–31.

Wilson, T. W., and C. E. Grim. "Biohistory of Slavery and Blood Pressure Differences in Blacks Today: A Hypothesis." *Hypertension* 17 (1991) (Suppl I): 122–28.

Woodward, G. N. "Racial Health: Presidential Address." Presented at the annual meeting of the John A. Andrew Clinical Society, Tuskegee Institute, Ala., April 1924. *Journal of the National Medical Association* 16 (1924): 177–79.

Wright, Jackson T., Jr., W. Fitzhugh Brundage, and Philip A. Mackowiak. "A 59-Year-Old Man with 'Racial Characteristics.'" *Journal of Clinical Hypertension* 9 (2007): 128–33.

Wright, Jackson T., Jr., J. Kay Dunn, Jeffrey A. Cutler, Barry R. Davis, William C. Cushman, Charles E. Ford, L. Julian Haywood, Frans H. H. Leenen, Karen L. Margolis, Vasilios Papademetriou, Jeffrey L. Probstfield, Paul K. Whelton, and Gabriel B. Habib; for the ALLHAT Collaborative Research Group. "Outcomes in Hypertensive Black and Nonblack Patients Treated with Chlorthalidone, Amlodipine, and Lisinopril." *JAMA* 293 (April 6, 2005): 1595–608.

Wright, Louis T. "Health Problems of the Negro." *Interracial Review* 8 (January 1935): 6–8.

Wyatt, Sharon, Nancy Diekelmann, Frances Henderson, Michael E. Andrew, Gloria Billingsley, Sherry H. Felder, Sonja Fuqua, and Priscilla B. Jackson. "A Community-Driven Model of Research Participation: The Jackson Heart Study Participant Recruitment and Retention Study." *Ethnicity and Disease* 13 (2003): 438–55.

Wyatt, Sharon, et al. *Community-Driven Model of Recruitment: The Jackson Heart Study: A Final Report of the Jackson Heart Study Participant Recruitment and Retention Study.* Presented to the NHBLI, November 30, 1999. The Jackson Heart Study, Jackson, Miss.

Wyatt, S. B., D. R. Williams, R. Calvin, F. C. Henderson, E. R. Walker, and K. Winters. "Racism and Cardiovascular Disease in African Americans." *American Journal of the Medical Sciences* 325, no. 6 (June 2003): 315–31.

Yu, Joon-Ho, Sara Goering, and Stephanie Fullerton. "Race-Based Medicine and Justice as Recognition: Exploring the Phenomenon of BiDil," *Cambridge Quarterly of Healthcare Ethics* 18 (2009): 57–67.

Zane, Jeffrey, and Judson L. Jeffries. "A Panther Sighting in the Pacific Northwest: The Seattle Chapter of the Black Panther Party." In *On the Ground: The Black Panther Party in Communities across America*, edited by Judson L. Jeffries. Jackson: University of Mississippi Press, 2010.

Žižek, Slavoj. *The Sublime Object of Ideology.* London: Verso, 1989.

———. *The Puppet and the Dwarf: The Perverse Core of Christianity.* Cambridge: MIT Press, 2003.

Žižek, Slavoj, and John Milbank. "Dialectical Clarity versus the Misty Conceit of Paradox." In *The Monstrosity of Christ: Paradox or Dialectic?*, edited by Creston Davis. Cambridge: MIT Press, 2009.

Zola, Irving. "Medicine as an Institution of Social Control." *Sociological Review* 20 (1972): 487–504.

INDEX

access to pharmaceuticals, 144–48, 165–69, 185, 189–90, 229nn49–50

ACE inhibitors, 135–36, 161, 164–65, 216n18, 229n44

activism, 2, 5, 11, 26, 94, 167, 169. *See also* social justice projects

affiliative self-fashioning, 127

African Americans, 1–2; in cardiology and cardiac surgery, 40–43; death rates of, 36, 38, 44–46, 50; discourses on disease and constitution of, 37–40, 43; diseases of, 88–89; heart disease rates of, 5, 36–37; racial terminology for, 20–23

African American Heart Failure Trial (A-HeFT), 80, 161–65, 170, 176

African American hypertension, 83–106; as civil rights project, 84–85, 90–95, 103–4; controllable and uncontrollable factors in, 100–101; as disease category, 17, 20, 24, 85–95, 102, 115, 132; etiology debates on, 48, 85, 89, 95–100, 211n46; genetic theories of, 20, 48, 83, 100–101, 132–36, 211n46; multi-drug therapy for, 137, 139–40; racialized associations of, 30, 84–85, 87–88, 92–93, 210nn31–32; rates of, 87; recordability of race in, 101–6, 164, 185; risk factors for, 100–101, 210nn31–32, 212n65; salt sensitivity in, 110–12, 132–33; slavery hypothesis of, 17, 24–25, 107–30, 174, 212nn6–7;

socioeconomic contexts of, 96–98; treatment for, 87, 89–91, 96, 99–100, 103–4, 106. *See also* hypertension; Jackson Heart Study; thiazide diuretics

African hypertension, 109–10

Afrocentrism, 89

Against Race (Gilroy), 9

Agamben, Giorgio, 36

Agar, Jon, 63

age, 100–101

A-HeFT. *See* African American Heart Failure Trial

alcohol use, 100–101

ALLHAT. *See* Antihypertensive and Lipid Lowering Treatment to Prevent Heart Attack Trial

allostasis, 98–99

ALTACE, 229n44

Althusser, Louis, 102, 124–25

American College of Surgeons, 41

American Heart Association (AHA): Council for High Blood Pressure Research of, 93; formation of, 30–31, 200n9; on risk factors for hypertension, 100–101; Scientific Sessions of, 197n19

American Indians, 14, 92, 133

American Medical Association (AMA), 41

American Society of Hypertension (ASH), 21, 83–85, 93–94, 113–14, 197n19

American way of life, 2, 29, 79–82; as an unequal democracy, 14, 40, 146, 150,

Anne Pollock is an assistant professor of
science and technology studies at Georgia Tech.

Library of Congress Cataloging-in-Publication Data
Pollock, Anne, 1975–
Medicating race : heart disease and durable preoccupations
with difference / Anne Pollock.
p. cm. — (Experimental futures : technological lives,
scientific arts, anthropological voices)
Includes bibliographical references and index.
ISBN 978-0-8223-5329-4 (cloth : alk. paper)
ISBN 978-0-8223-5344-7 (pbk. : alk. paper)
1. African Americans—Medical care. 2. African Americans—
Health and hygiene. 3. Cardiology—United States.
4. Heart—Diseases—United States. I. Title.
II. Series: Experimental futures.
RA448.5.N4P65 2012
616.1′2008996073—dc23
2011053305